Biotech's

DICTIONARY *Of* Microbiology

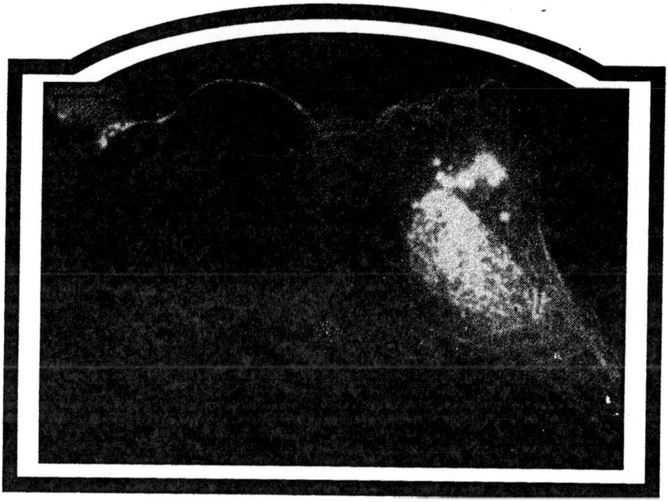

Compiled & Edited by
Dinesh Arora

BIOTECH
2023
BIOTECH BOOKS

Biotech's

DICTIONARY
Of
Microbiology

Compiled & Edited by
Dinesh Arora

First Indian Edition **2023**

ISBN 81-7622-125-2

Published by : **BIOTECH BOOKS**
4762-63/23, Ansari Road, Darya Ganj,
New Delhi - 110002
Phones : 011 4300 3222
Email : biotechbooks@yahoo.co.in

PRINTED IN INDIA

PREFACE

Microbes, organisms so tiny that they cannot be seen with naked eyes, have been around for billions of years. It is in the form of microorganisms that the story of life on this planet begins. But only in the last two hundred years has man understood their significance and only in the second half of 20th century, scientists learnt to manipulate genetic code of microorganisms (or microbes) and learned the biotechnological revolution.

Louis Pasteur came up with his theory of tiny organisms and full-proof method of preserving milk by boiling it and then packing it in evacuated (a process called pasteurisation). Thus was born the science of Microbiology. The field of Microbiology is the specialised field of biology and is defined as study of microorganisms that do not constitute a well-defined taxonomic group. Microorganisms are included in the two kingdoms of Archaebacteria and Eubacteria. Viruses are also an important constituent, albeit they are not quite 'organisms'.

This dictionary gives all the important and even unimportant terms useful for budding microbiologist. The definitions are lucid and explanatory. This provides the most accurate viewpoint regarding the terms pertaining to the field of Microbiology. With the recent advancement of technology in the previous decade, the field of Microbiology has taken a different shape. This dictionary of Microbiology covers all the recent advancements in the field of Microbiology. We hope students will find it a good reference book and dip into it from time to time.

alpha level
probability of a false positive result, or of rejecting the hypothesis of no treatment difference when there is no real difference or of a false positive. Also referred to as the probability of a type I error.

alpha spending function
function or rule that governs how the total level or probability of a type I error can be spread out over the interim analysis. Limits the chance of a false positive result when trial data is looked at multiple times. Can be used to set up guidelines for trial monitoring.

16s RRNA
large polynucleotide (about 1,500 bases) that functions as a part of the small subunit of the ribosome of prokaryotes and from whose sequence evolutionary information can be obtained, the eukaryotic counterpart is 18s RRNA.

3tc
also known as lamivudine, 3tc is composed of the enantiomer of the racemic mixture 2' deoxy 3' thiacytidine. Like other nucleoside analogs, 3tc inhibits HIV replication through viral DNA chain termination. It has been used in clinical trials in combination with AZT.

ABC transport systems
a type of active transport system that requires ATP as an energy source (ATP Binding Cassette).

abdomen
portion of body between thorax and pelvis. The abdomen contains the liver, the spleen and most of the digestive organs.

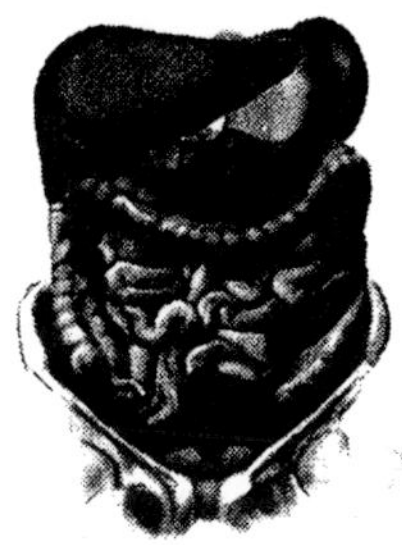

abscess
localised collection of pus within a tissue.

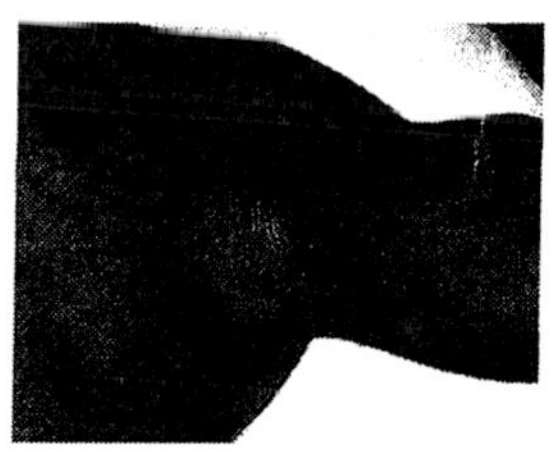

absorption
movement of ions and water into a organism as a result of

metabolic processes, frequently against an electrochemical potential gradient (active) or as a result of diffusion along an activity gradient (passive).

■ **acellular**
not composed of cells, therefore not living.

■ **acetaminophen (tylenol)**
analgesic and antipyretic.

■ **acetogenic bacterium**
prokaryotic organism that uses carbonate as a terminal electron acceptor and produces acetic acid as a waste product.

■ **acetyl COA**
product of the transition reaction, a precursor metabolite used in fatty acid synthesis.

■ **acetylene block assay**
estimates denitrification by determining release of nitrous oxide from acetylene treated soil.

■ **acetylene reduction assay**
estimates nitrogenase activity by measuring the rate of acetylene reduced to ethylene.

■ **acid fast bacillus**
bacteria capable of living in acidic environments, like inside macrophages. Tuberculosis and MAI/MAC are acid fast bacilli.

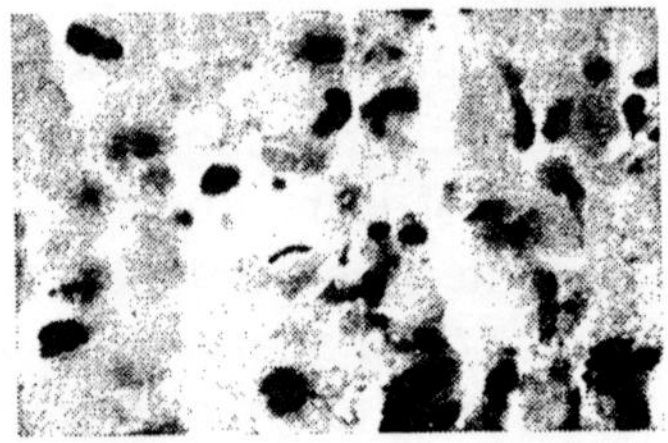

■ **acid soil**
soil with a ph value < 6.6.

■ **acid fast staining**
procedure used to stain organisms including members of the genus *mycobacterium* that do not readily take up stains. Once stained, mycobacterial cells resist decolourisation with an acidic solution of alcohol.

■ **acidic amino acids**
amino acids with more acid than amino groups.

■ **acidophile**
organism that grows best under acid conditions (down to a ph of 1).

■ **Acquired Immunodeficiency Syndrome (AIDS)**
most severe manifestation of infection with the Human Immunodeficiency Virus (HIV). The Centre For Disease Control And Prevention lists numerous opportunistic infections and neoplasm, which in the presence of HIV infection constitute

an Aids diagnosis. In addition, a cd4+ t cell count below 200/ mm3 in the presence of HIV infection constitutes an Aids diagnosis. The period between infection with HIV and the onset of Aids averages 10 years. People with Aids often suffer infections of the lungs, brain, eyes and other organs, and frequently suffer debilitating weight loss, diarrhoea and a type of cancer called Kaposi's Sarcoma. Even with treatment, most people with AIDS die within two years of developing infections or cancers that take advantage of their weakened immune systems.

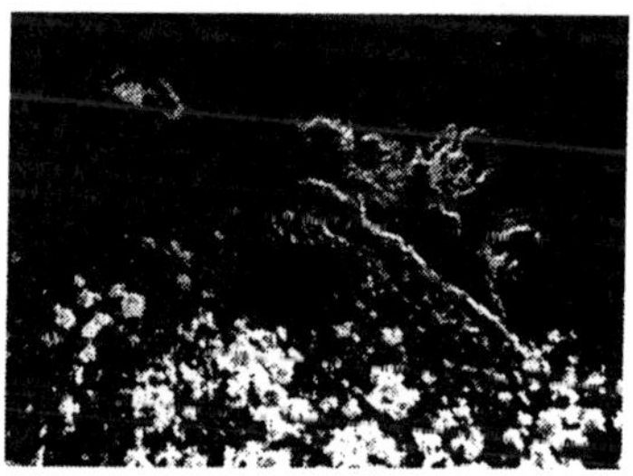

■ **acquired resistance**

development of antimicrobial resistance in a previously sensitive organism, occurs through spontaneous mutation or acquisition of new genetic information

■ **acremonium**

reported to be allergenic. Can produce a trichothecene toxin, which is toxic if ingested. It was the primary fungus identified in at least two houses where the occupant complaints of nausea, vomiting and diarrhoea. Asexual state of Emericellopsis sp., Chaetomium sp., and Nectripsis sp. It can produce mycetomas, infections of the cornea and nails.

■ **acridine orange**

fluorescent dye that binds DNA and can be used to determine the total number of micro-organisms in a sample.

■ **acromegaly**

chronic disease caused by hyper secretion of the pituitary growth hormones. It is characterised by enlargement of many parts of the skeleton, especially the nose, ears, jaws, fingers and toes.

■ **actin**

polymer that makes up microfilaments of eukaryotic cells, it can rapidly assemble and subsequently disassemble to cause motion.

■ **actinomycete**

nontaxonomic term applied to a group of high g + c base composition of gram positive bacteria that have a superficial resemblance to fungi. Includes many but not all organisms belonging to the order actinomycetales.

■ **actinomycetes**
filamentous bacteria, many are valuable in the production of antibiotics.

■ **activated (immune) T lymphocytes**
T cells activated by exposure to antigen.

■ **activated macrophages**
macrophages stimulated by cytokines to enlarge and become metabolically active, with greatly increased capability to kill and degrade intracellular organisms and materials.

■ **activated sludge method**
method of sewage treatment in which wastes are degraded by complex populations of aerobic micro-organisms.

■ **activation energy**
amount of energy required to bring all molecules in one mole of a substance to their reactive state at a given temperature.

■ **activator binding site**
site that precedes an ineffective promoter, binding of an activator to this site enhances the ability of RNA polymerase to initiate t.anscription at that promoter.

■ **active control treatment**
control treatment that involves use of a pharmacologically or medically active substance. Active controls are used when there is already an available treatment, so the use of a placebo or no treatment would be unethical.

■ **active immunity**
protective immunity produced by an individual in response to an antigenic stimulus.

■ **active site**
site on an enzyme molecule to which substrate binds, also known as the catalytic site.

■ **active transport**
energy requiring process by which molecules are carried across cell boundaries, can accumulate compounds against a concentration gradient.

■ **acute**
short term, intense symptomatology or pathology, as distinct from chronic. Many dis-

eases have an acute phase like HIV seroconversion disease and a chronic phase. This distinction is sometimes used in treatments, as in high dose ganciclovir for acute or induction treatment of CMV retinitis, followed by a lower dose for chronic or maintenance treatment

■ **acute infection**

infection causing disease with a sudden onset, severity and often short lasting. As related to HIV infection once the virus enters the body, HIV infects a large number of CD4+ t cells and replicates rapidly. During this acute or primary phase of infection, the blood contains man (viral particles that spread throughout the body, seeding themselves in various organs, particularly the lyophoid tissues.)

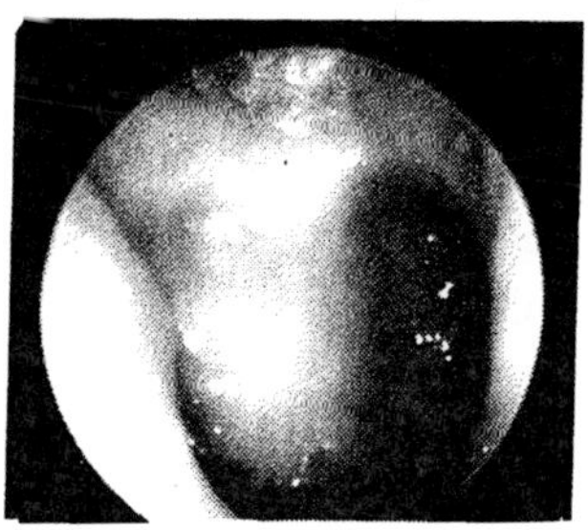

■ **acute infections**

infections in which the symptoms and signs have a rapid onset and are usually severe, often with fever, but short lived.

■ **acute phase response**

changes in the blood that occur early during an infection, with the production of acute phase proteins and cells that contribute to the inflammatory response.

■ **acute retroviral syndrome**

acute or primary HIV infection often passes unrecognised, but may be present as a mononucleosis like syndrome within three months of the infection. Demonstrating HIV antibody seroconversion makes the diagnosis.

■ **acyclovir (zovirax)**

acycloguanosine, a nucleoside analog. An antiviral drug used in the treatment of herpes simplex virus 1 (hsv 1, fever blisters, cold sores), herpes simplex virus 2 (hsv 2, genital herpes) and herpes zoster (shingles), and sometimes for acute varicella zoster virus (chickenpox).

■ **Acylated Homoserine Lactone (AHL)**

small molecules that can move freely in and out of a cell, provides cells with a mechanism of assessing cell density (quorum sensing).

■ **ad hoc review group**
review group that is created for the sole purpose of reviewing a specific application or set of applications. Also referred to as ad hoc study section, especially if the applications are for grant support.

■ **adcc (antibody dependent cellular cytotoxicity)**
non-specific killing of target cells by cells such as macrophages, granulocytes or natural killer cells, that contact the target via their FC receptors binding to FC of antibodies on the target.

■ **adenopathy**
any disease involving or causing enlargement of glandular tissues, especially the lymph nodes.

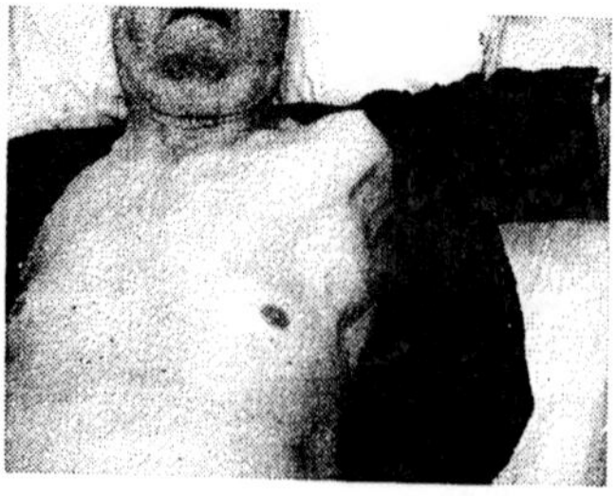

■ **adenosine diphosphate (ADP)**
acceptor of free energy in a cell; that energy is used to add a inorganic phosphate (P_i) to ADP, generating ATP.

■ **adenosine triphosphate (ATP)**
energy currency of a cell, serving as the ready and immediate donor of free energy.

■ **adherence**
degree to which patient care exactly follows study protocol.

■ **adjuvant**
ingredient, as in a prescription or solution that facilitates or modifies the action of the principal ingredient. May be used in HIV therapies or for HIV vaccines.

■ **administration**
term used to refer to how a drug or therapy is introduced into the body. Systemic administration means that the drug goes throughout the body usually carried in the bloodstream, and includes oral administration and intravenous administration i.e. injection into the vein. Local administration means that the drug is applied or introduced into the specific area affected by the disease, such as appli-

cation directly onto the affected skin surface i.e. topical administration. The effects of most therapies depend upon the ability of the drug to reach the affected area, thus the route of administration and consequent distribution of a drug in the body is an important determinant of its effectiveness.

■ **adsorption**
attachment of one substance to the surface of another.

■ **adverse event**
in a clinical trial, any unwanted effect detected in participants. The term is used whether or not the effect can be attributed to the intervention under study.

■ **adverse experience**
toxic reaction to a treatment under study. Typically, all grade 4, life threatening toxicities and deaths are adverse experiences, irrespective of whether or not they are believed to be due to study drug, as are any toxicities that require permanent discontinuation of study drug.

■ **adverse reactions**
any undesirable effect of a medication. All drugs may cause such reactions, so that periodic monitoring is necessary to detect any that do occur, even though their occurrence may be uncommon.

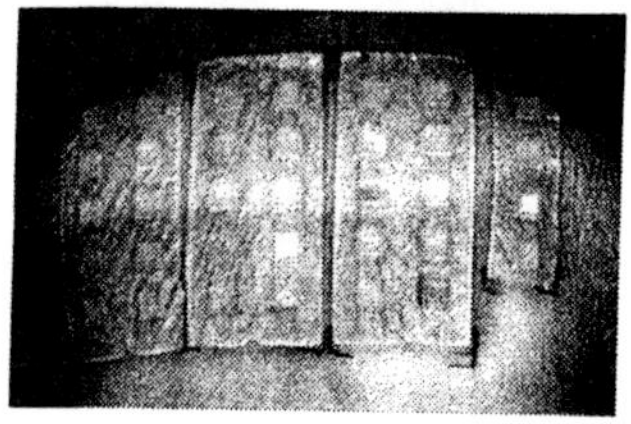

■ **AER**
adverse experience report, a document in a pre specified format used to collect information on all reportable adverse experiences

■ **aerobic**
having molecular oxygen as a part of the environment.

■ **aerobic respiration**
metabolic process in which electrons are transferred from the electron transport chain to molecular oxygen.

■ **aerosol**
material dispersed into the air as a fine mist.

■ **aerosolised**
form of administration of drug, in which a drug, such as pentamidine, is turned into a fine spray or mist by a nebuliser, and inhaled.

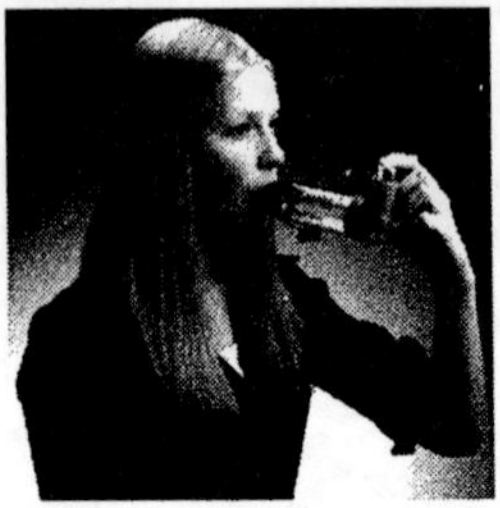

■ **aerotaxis**
movement towards, or away from molecular oxygen.

■ **aerotolerant anaerobes**
microbes that grow under both aerobic and anaerobic conditions, but do not shift from one mode of metabolism to another as conditions change. They obtain energy exclusively by fermentation.

■ **afb smear**
laboratory technique for visualising mycobacterium under the microscope. Smear results are usually available within a few days, and they correlate strongly with infectiousness, especially in untreated patients. However, a 'positive' result cannot distinguish between TB, MAI or other mycobacterial infections.

■ **afebrile**
without a fever.

■ **affected community**
includes HIV positive people, persons living with aids and other individuals, including their families, friends and advocates, directly impacted by HIV infection and its physical, psychological and sociological ramifications.

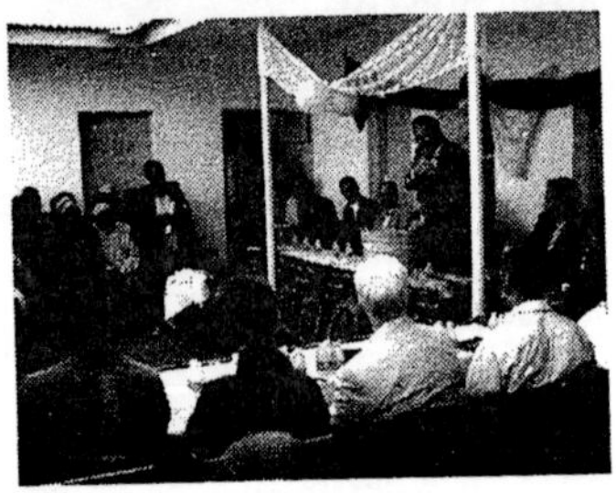

■ **aflatoxin**
potent toxin made by species of *aspergillus*, may contaminate peanuts and other grains.

■ **agammaglobulinemia**
near total absence of immunoglobulins.

■ **agar**
polysaccharide extracted from marine algae, used to solidify

microbiological media.

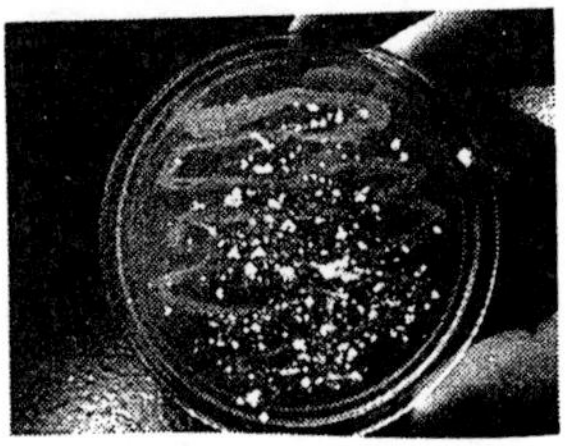

■ **agar slant**
microbiological medium that has been solidified with agar and stored in a tube that was held at a shallow angle as the medium solidified, creating a larger surface area.

■ **agarose**
highly purified form of agar used in gel electrophoresis.

■ **agglutination**
clumping together of cells or particles.

■ **AIDS dementia complex**
about half the people infected with HIV, the virus that causes aids, develop infections or other problems involving the brain or spinal cord. These neurological complications may include inflammation of the brain i.e. encephalitis, or of the membrane surrounding the brain i.e. meningitis, infections of the brain, brain or spinal cord tumours, nerve damage, difficulties in thinking and behavioural changes, loss of coordination, mood swings and loss of inhibitions, and finally wide spread cognitive deficit.

■ **AIDS knowledge base**
full text electronic database on AIDS, available in print as well as electronic form, produced and maintained by physicians and other health care professionals.

■ **aidsdrugs**
online database service, with references to drugs undergoing testing against AIDS, AIDS related complex and related opportunistic infections.

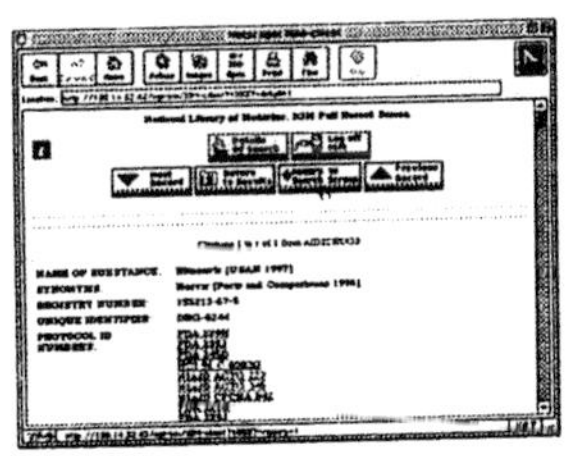

■ **aidsline**
online database service, with citations and abstracts covering the published scientific and medical literature on AIDS and related topics.

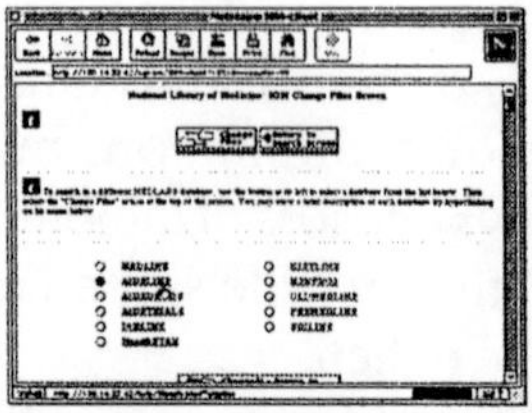

■ **AIDS related cancers**
several cancers are more common or more aggressive in people infected with HIV, the virus that causes aids. These malignancies include certain types of immune system cancers known as lymphomas, Kaposi's sarcoma and anogenital cancers primarily affecting the cervix and the anus. HIV, or the immune suppression it induces, appears to play a role in the development of these cancers.

■ **AIDS related complex (ARC)**
a group of symptoms, fever, fatigue, diarrhoea, and weight loss, that herald the onset of AIDS

■ **aidstrials**
an online database service, with information about clinical trials of agents under evaluation against HIV infection, aids and related opportunistic infections.

■ **akinete**
thick walled resting cell of cyanobacteria and algae.

■ **Alanine Aminotransferase (ALT)**
a liver enzyme, measured through a blood test that indicates the health of the liver. Lower counts are better. Levels may go up because of hepatitis and other infections, or because of drug toxicities

■ **alga (pl. Algae)**
primitive photosynthetic eukaryotic organism.

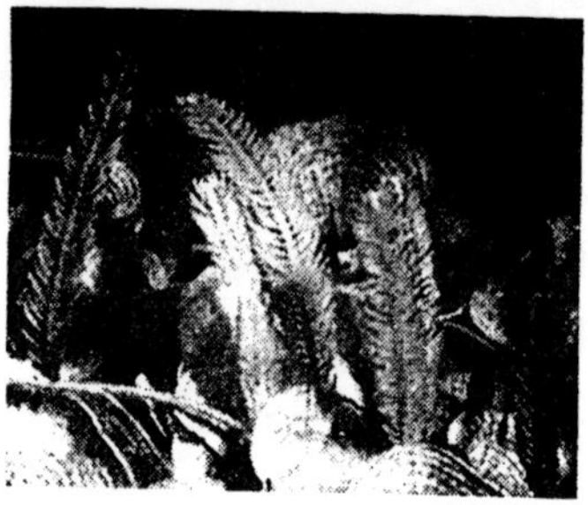

■ **aliphatic**
organic compound in which the main carbon structure is a straight chain.

■ **alkaline phosphatase**
enzyme that is normally present in certain cells within the liver, bone, kidney, intestine and placenta. When the cells are destroyed in those tissues, more of

the enzyme leaks into the blood, and levels rise in

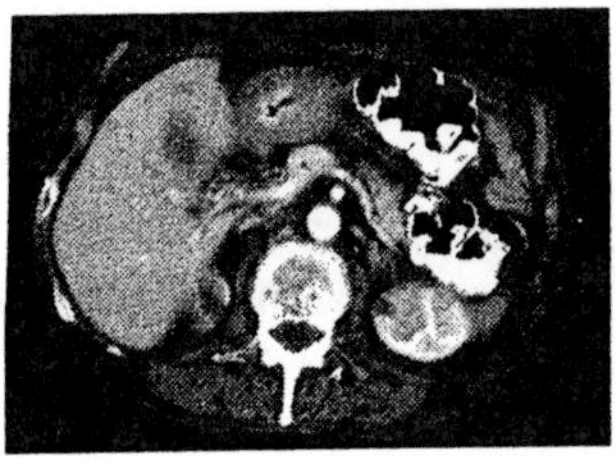

proportion to the severity of the condition. Measurement of this enz{me is used as an indication of the health of the liver.

■ **alkaline soil**
soil having a ph value >7.3.

■ **alkaliphiles**
organisms that grow optimally at a ph above 8.5.

■ **alkane**
straight chain or branched organic structure that lacks double bonds.

■ **alkene**
straight chain or branched organic structure that contains at least one double bond.

■ **alkyl group**
short chain or single carbon atom such as a methyl group.

■ **alkylating agent**
chemical that adds alkyl groups, short chains of carbon atoms to purines and pyrimidines, promotes mutations.

■ **allele**
form of a gene.

■ **allergen**
antigen that causes an allergy.

■ **allergic rhinitis**
hay fever, sneezing, runny nose, teary eyes resulting from exposure of a sensitised person to inhaled antigen, a mediated allergic reaction.

■ **allergy**
hypersensitivity, especially of the mediated type.

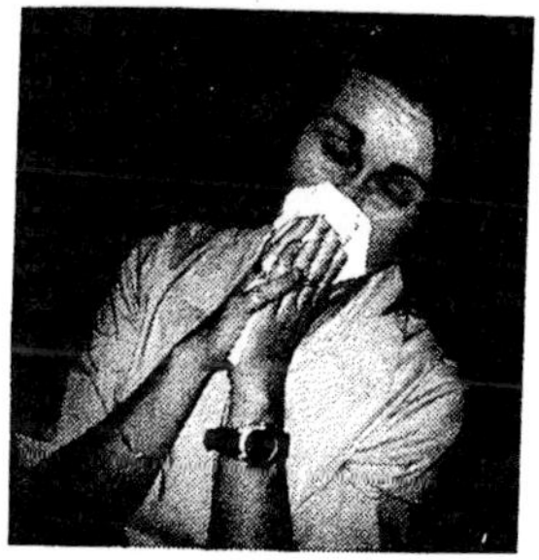

■ **allocation ratio**
treatment allocation ratio. For example, 1 1 is equal allocation, 3 1 is 75% in one group, and 25% in the other

■ **allocation strata**
treatment allocation strata. Allocations are generally balanced within strata.

■ **allochthonous flora**
organisms that are not indigenous to the soil but that enter soil by precipitation, diseased tissues, manure and sewage. They may persist for some time but do not contribute in a significant way to ecologically significant transformations or interactions.

■ **allograft**
organ or tissue graft transplanted between genetically non-identical members of the same species.

■ **allosteric site**
site on an allosteric enzyme that binds an effector molecule, binding alters the activity of the enzyme.

■ **alopecia**
loss of hair due to varied reasons, frequently occurs in patients undergoing chemotherapy for cancer or suffering from other diseases, such as aids, where cell killing, or cytotoxic, drugs are used.

■ **alpha (a) haemolysis**
type of haemolysis observed on blood agar characterised by zone of greenish clearing around the colonies.

■ **alternaria sp.**
very common allergen with an IgE mediated response. It is often found in carpets, textiles, and on horizontal surfaces in building interiors, often found on window frames. Outdoors it may be isolated from samples of soil, seeds and plants. It is commonly found in outdoor samples. The large spore sized 20 is 200 microns in length and 7 is 18 microns in sizes, suggests that the spores from this fungi get deposited in the nose, mouth and upper respiratory tract. It may be related to baker's asthma. It has been associated with hypersensitivity pneumonitis. The species *Alternaria alternata* is capable of producing tenuazonic acid and other toxic metabolites that may be associated with disease in humans or animals. Considered to be a common cause of extrinsic asthma i.e. immediate type hypersensitivity type I. Acute symptoms include oedema and bronchiospasms, chronic cases may develop pulmonary emphysema.

■ **alternative hypothesis**
in a trial, the alternative hypothesis might be that a treatment of

unknown efficacy has more benefit than the standard treatment. The alternative hypothesis is an alternative to the null hypothesis of no difference that specifies some true underlying difference of set of differences between two or more populations or groups with regard to some function, trait, characteristic, or effect. It may be stated in such a way so as to be concerned with a difference(s) in only one direction (one sided alternative hypothesis) or in either direction (two sided alternative hypothesis) relative to the null value.

■ **alternative pathway**

pathway of complement activation non-specifically initiated by bacterial substances such as endotoxin and polysaccharides.

■ **alternative therapy**

in western countries, alternative therapy refers to any type of medicine that supplements or is used in lieu of biomedicine i.e., conventional medicine or allopathic medicine. In other parts of the world, where traditional medicine predominates, the term may refer to biomedicine itself.

■ **alum**

potassium aluminium sulphate or ammonium aluminium sulphate, used especially as an emetic i.e., an agent that induces vomiting, an astringent i.e., a substance that contracts tissues and styptic i.e., a substance that tends to check bleeding by contracting the tissues or blood vessels.

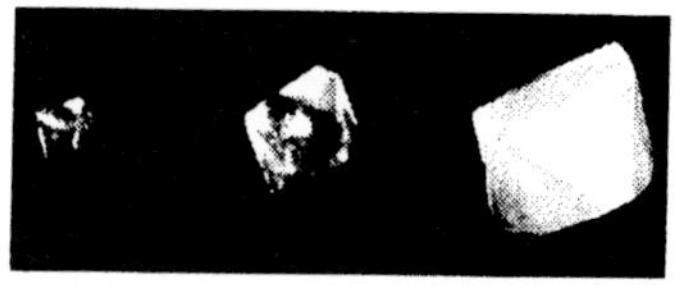

■ **alveolar**

pertaining to the alveoli sac, the site of gas exchange in the lungs.

■ **amalgam**

mixture of mercury with other metals to form a paste that hardens, used to fill cavities in teeth.

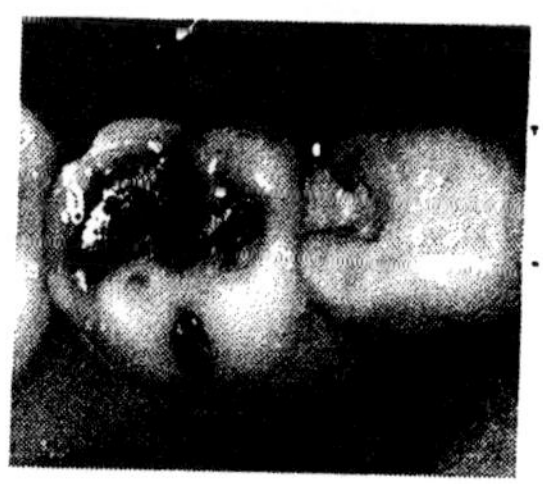

■ **amensalism (antagonism)**

production of a substance by one organism that is inhibitory to one or more other organisms.

The terms antibiosis and allelopathy also describe cases of chemical inhibition.

■ **amikacin**
antibiotic used as a component in combination therapy to treat tuberculosis or *mycobacterium avium* complex.

■ **amino (or n terminal)**
The end of the protein molecule that has an un-bonded – NH_2 group.

■ **amino acids**
any of a class of organic compounds having a carboxyl group (COOH) and an amino group (NH_2). Some 22 amino acids are commonly found in animals, and more than 100 less common forms are found in nature, chiefly in plants. When the carboxyl carbon atom of one amino acid binds to the nitrogen of another with the release of a water molecule, a linkage called a peptide bond is formed. Chains of amino acids, joined head to tail in this manner, are synthesised by living systems and are called polypeptides (up to about 50 amino acids) and proteins (over 50 amino acids).

■ **amino group**
an NH_2 group attached to a carbon skeleton as in the amines and amino acids.

■ **aminoglycosides**
group of antimicrobial medications that interferes with protein synthesis.

■ **ammonification**
the reactions that result in the release of ammonia from organic nitrogen containing molecules.

■ **amniocentesis**
the surgical insertion of a hollow needle through the abdominal wall and into the uterus of a pregnant female to obtain amniotic fluid i.e., the serous fluid in which the embryo is suspended especially to examine the foetal chromosomes for an abnormality or for the determination of the sex of the embryo..

■ **amoeba (pl. amoebae)**
protozoa that can alter their cell shape, usually by the extrusion of one or more pseudopodia.

■ **amoebiasis**
an inflammation of the intestines caused by infestation with *entamoeba histolytica* and

characterised by frequent, loose stools flecked with blood and mucus.

- **amphibolic pathways**
metabolic pathways that play roles in both catabolism and anabolism.

- **amphotericin b (fungizone)**
anti fungal drug that is used to treat fungal infections in persons with HIV, including candida, cryptococcus, histoplasmosis and others.

- **amylase**
pancreatic enzyme, high levels of which in the blood may indicate pancreatic damage.

- **amylases**
enzymes that digest starches.

- **anabolism**
cellular processes that use the energy stored in ATP to synthesise and assemble subunits such as amino acids, synonymous with biosynthesis.

- **anaemia**
condition in which there is a decreased volume of red cells in the blood. There are many causes for anaemia, including drug toxicities and chronic infections.

- **anaerobes**
organisms that grow in the absence of molecular oxygen.

- **anaerobic**
contains no molecular oxygen.

- **anaerobic respiration**
metabolic process in which electrons are transferred from the electron transport chain to an inorganic terminal electron acceptor other than O_2.

- **analgesic**
compound used to reduce or treat pain. Examples include aspirin, morphine, and acetaminophen.

- **analog (analogue)**
chemical compound with a structure similar to that of another but differing from it in respect to a certain component. It may have a similar or opposite action metabolically.

- **analysis by intention to treat**
method of data analysis in which the primary tabulations and companion summaries of outcome data are by assigned treatment, regardless of treatment adherence.

- **analysis by treatment administered**
  method of data analysis in which the primary tabulations and companion summaries of outcome data are by treatment administered, not by treatment assigned.

- **analytical study**
  an epidemiological study done to identify specific risk factors associated with developing a certain disease.

- **anamnestic response**
  heightened immunologic reaction elicited by a second or subsequent exposure to a particular pathogenic micro organism or antigen.

- **anamnestic response (memory response, secondary response)**
  enhanced immunological response to a second or subsequent dose of antigen.

- **anamorph**
  asexual stage of fungal reproduction in which cells are formed by the process of mitosis.

- **anaphylactic shock**
  life threatening allergic reaction characterised by a swelling of body tissues including the throat and a sudden decline in blood pressure, can be though rarely triggered by medication.

- **anaphylaxis**
  generalised hypersensitive reaction to an allergen that can cause a profound drop in blood pressure.

- **ancillary trial**
  investigation, stimulated by the trial and intended to generate information of interest to the trial, that is designed and carried out by investigators from one or more of the centres in the trial and that utilizes resources of the trials e.g., money, study patients, staff time, etc., but that is not a required part of the design or data collection procedures of the main trial.

- **androgen**
  masculinising hormone, e.g. testosterone.

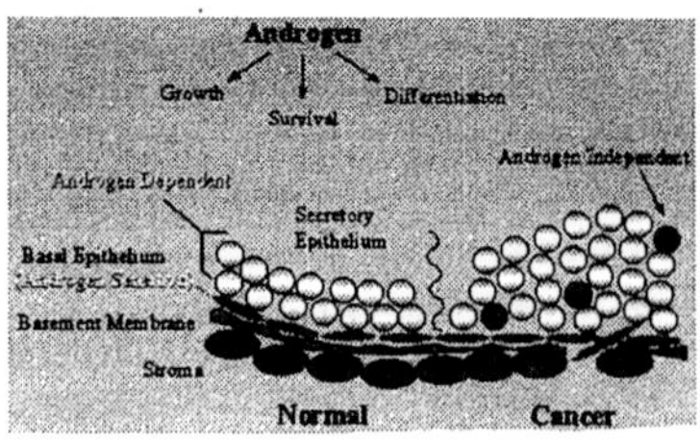

■ **anergic**
refers to the state of being so immunologically suppressed that one is unable to produce cutaneous delayed type hypersensitivity reaction (DTH). Such patients will usually not test positive for TB on a PPD (Mantoux) test.

■ **anergy**
loss or weakening of the body's immunity to an irritating agent, or antigen. The strength of the body's immune response is often quantitatively measured by means of a skin test where a solution containing an antigen known to cause a response, such as mumps or candida, is injected immediately under the skin. The lack of a reaction to these common antigens indicates anergy..

■ **angiogenesis**
process of forming new blood vessels. Angiogenesis is essential for the growth of tumours, especially Kaposi's sarcoma

■ **anion**
negatively charged ion.

■ **anion exchange capacity**
sum total of exchangeable anions that a soil can adsorb. Expressed as centimoles of negative charge per kilogram of soil.

■ **anorexia**
lack of or complete loss of appetite for food.

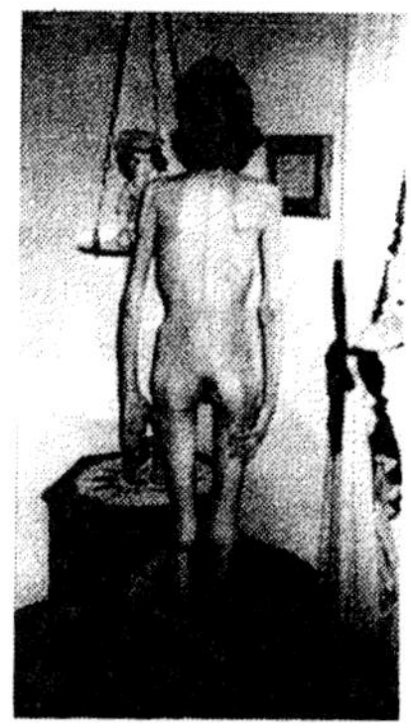

■ **anoxic**
literally 'without oxygen'. An adjective describing a microbial habitat devoid of oxygen.

■ **anoxygenic photosynthesis**
type of photosynthesis in green and purple bacteria in which oxygen is not produced.

■ **anoxygenic phototrophs**
photosynthetic bacteria that use hydrogen sulphide or organic compounds rather than water as a source of electrons for reducing power, they do not generate O_2.

■ **antagonism**
opposite of synergy. One factor (treatment) reduces or cancels the effect of another.

■ **antagonist**
biological agent that reduces the number or disease producing activities of a pathogen.

■ **antagonistic**
in antimicrobial therapy, a combination of antimicrobial medications in which the action of one interferes with the action of the other.

■ **antenatal**
before the time of birth.

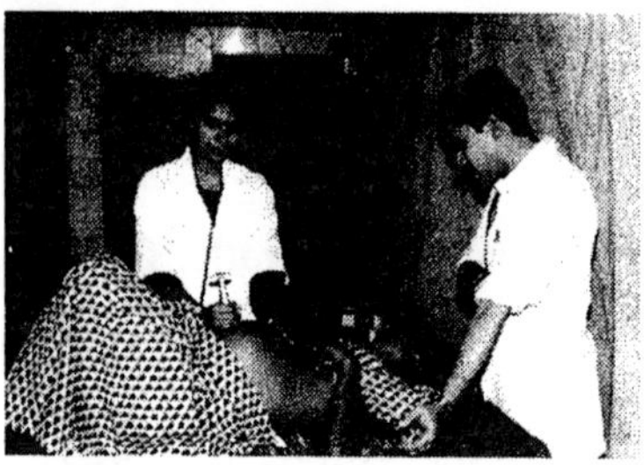

■ **antenna complex**
complex in photosynthetic organisms composed of hundreds of light gathering pigments, acts as a funnel, capturing light energy and transferring it to reaction centre chlorophyll.

■ **antheridium**
male gametangium found in the phylum oomycota (kingdom stramenopila) and phylum ascomycota (kingdom fungi).

■ **anthropogenic**
derived from human activities.

■ **antibacterial drug**
chemical used to treat bacterial infections.

■ **antibiogram**
antibiotic susceptibility pattern, used to distinguish different strains.

■ **antibiosis**
inhibition or lysis of an organism mediated by metabolic products of the antagonist, these products include lytic agents, enzymes, volatile compounds, and other toxic substances.

■ **antibiotic**
chemical substance that kills bacteria or inhibits their growth. An anti-microbial agent, derived from cultures of a micro organism or produced semi synthetically, used to treat infections.

■ **antibiotic associated colitis**
intestinal disease caused by overgrowth of toxin producing strains of *clostridium difficile*, typically, only occurs when a person is taking anti-microbial medications.

■ **antibodies**
molecules in the blood or secretory fluids that tag, destroy or neutralize bacteria, viruses or other harmful toxins. They are members of a class of proteins known as immunoglobulins, which are produced and secreted by b lymphocytes in response to stimulation by antigens. An antibody is specific to an antigen. The antigen/antibody reaction forms the basis of humoral (non cellular) immunity.

■ **antibody**
immunoglobulin protein produced by the body in response to a substance and that reacts specifically with that substance.

Production of Antibodies

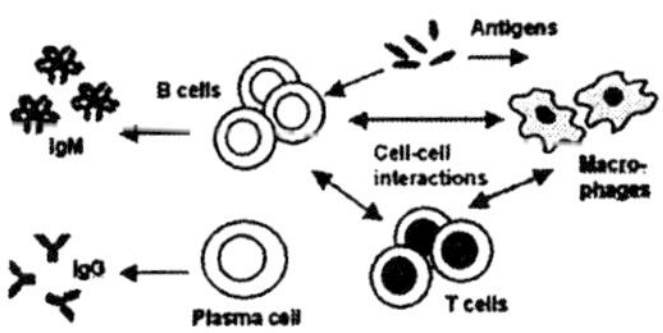

■ **Antibody Dependent Cell Mediated Cytotoxicity (ADCC)**
immune response in which antibodies bind to target cells, identifying them for attack by the immune system.

■ **anticodon**
sequence of three nucleotides of a TRNA molecule complementary to a particular codon in MRNA.

■ **anti-emetic**
an agent that prevents nausea and vomiting.

■ **antifolate**
agent that inhibits intracellular i.e., inside cells production of folinic acid.

■ **antigen**
any substance that antagonises or stimulates the immune system to produce antibodies. Antigens are often foreign substances such as bacteria or viruses that invade the body.

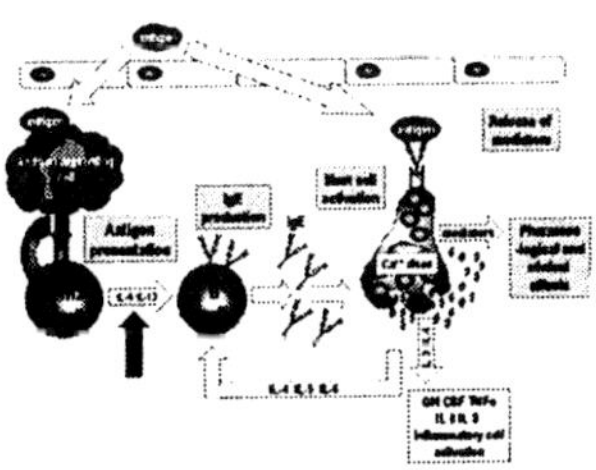

■ **antigen presentation**
process in which macrophages, dendritic cells or b cells ingest and partially degrade antigens which then appear on the cell surface in a form that can react with cd 4 t lymphocytes

■ **antigen binding sites**
hypervariable regions at the ends of the two arms of an antibody molecule that recognise specific antigen, there are two identical antigen binding sites on each monomer of antibody.

■ **antigenemia**
presence of detectable amounts of an antigen in the blood.

■ **antigenic determinant**
part of an antigen molecule that binds the specific antibody, an epitope.

■ **antigenic drift**
slight changes that occur in the antigens of a virus, specific antibodies made to the antigen before the change occurred are only partially effective.

■ **antigenic shift**
major changes that can occur in the antigen of a virus.

■ **antigenic variation**
routine alteration by an organism in the characteristics of certain of its surface proteins

■ **antigenicity**
ability of an antigen to combine with antibodies and t cell receptors to invoke a reaction from the immune system.

■ **anti idiotype**
antibody that recognises and binds to another antibody (idiotype).

■ **antimicrobial drug**
chemical used to treat microbial infections, also called an antimicrobial.

■ **anti neoplastic**
inhibiting or preventing the proliferation of tumour cells.

■ **antioxidant**
substance that inhibits oxidation or reactions promoted by oxygen or peroxides. Antioxidant nutrients protect human cells from damage caused by 'free radicals' highly reactive oxygen compounds.

■ **antiparallel**
term used to describe opposing orientations of the two strands of DNA in the double

helix, one strand is oriented in the 5' to 3' direction and its complement is oriented in the 3' to 5'direction.

■ **antiporter**
transport system that exchanges the location of one molecule or ion for another.

■ **antipyretic**
compound that reduces fever

■ **antiretroviral**
substance, drug, or process that destroys a retrovirus, or suppresses its replication. Often used to describe a drug active against HIV.

■ **antisense**
antisense compound is the mirror image of the genetic sequence that it is supposed to inactivate.

■ **antisense strand**
complement to the sense (or plus) strand of RNA. Also called the minus strand.

■ **antiseptic**
sterilised, or clean of any micro-organisms.

■ **antitoxins**
antibodies that recognise and inactivate toxins produced by certain bacteria, plants or animals..

■ **antiviral**
substance, drug or process that destroys a virus or suppresses its replication. Can apply to anti HIV activity, or other viruses, such as herpes or CMV.

■ **aphasia**
complete or partial loss of the ability to speak, or to understand speech.

■ **aplastic anemia**
potentially lethal condition in which the body is unable to make blood cells.

■ **apoptosis**
programmed cell death, with enzymatic degradation of DNA.

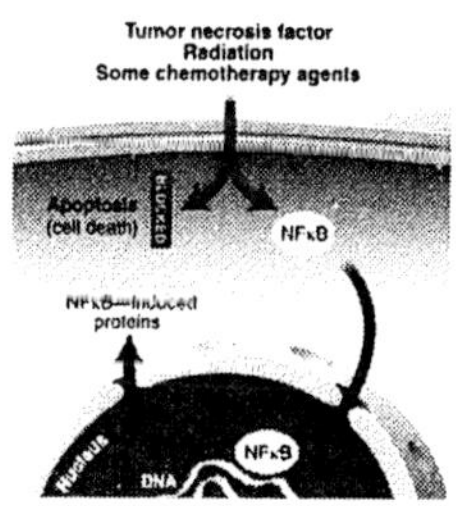

■ **apothecium**
open ascoma of fungi in the phylum ascomycota.

■ **apthous ulcer**
sore of indeterminate origin in the mouth or oesophagus. Some apthous ulcers have been linked to CMV or DDC use.

■ **arbovirus**
arthropod borne virus. One of a large group of RNA viruses carried by insects and mites that act as biological vectors.

■ **arbuscular mycorrhiza (AM)**
mycorrhizal type that forms highly branched arbuscules within root cortical cells.

■ **arbuscule**
special 'tree shaped' structure formed within root cortical cells by arbuscular mycorrhizal fungi.

■ **archaea**
domain name for single celled prokaryotes that usually grow in extreme environments.

■ **archaebacteria**
older term for the archaea.

■ **arm**
group of participants in a clinical trial, all of who receive the same treatment or placebo.

■ **aromatic**
organic compounds which contain a benzene ring, or a ring with similar chemical characteristics.

■ **arteriosclerosis**
condition characterised by thickening and loss of elasticity of the walls of arteries, 'hardening of the arteries'.

■ **arthralgia**
pain in a joint.

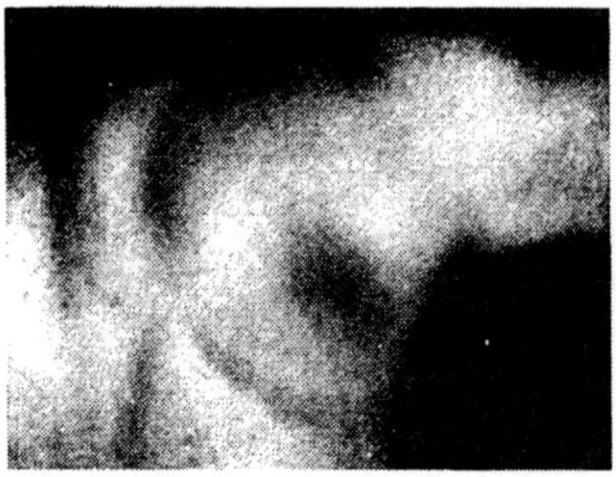

■ **arthropod**
invertebrate with jointed body and limbs (includes insects, arachnids and crustaceans).

Three Basic Characteristics of Arthropods
(Insects and their Relatives)

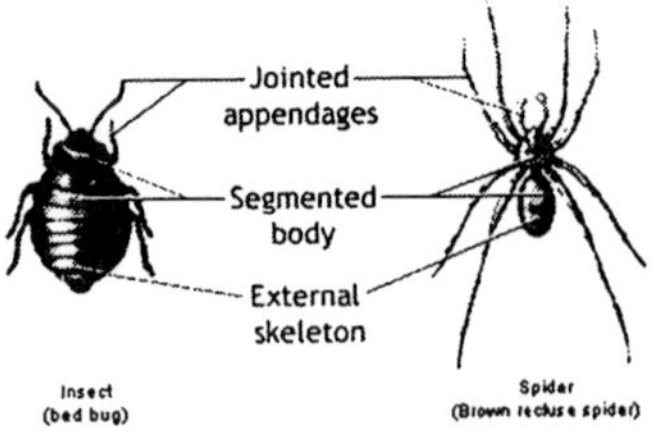

■ **arthus reaction**
hypersensitivity reaction caused by immune complexes and neutrophils

■ **artificial wetland method**
method of sewage treatment in which sewage is channelled into successive ponds where both aerobic and anaerobic stabilization occurs.

■ **ascoma (pl. ascomata)**
fungal fruiting body that contains ascospores, also termed an ascocarp.

■ **ascospore**
spores resulting from karyogamy and meiosis that are formed within an ascus. Sexual spore of the ascomycota.

■ **ascus (pl. asci)**
saclike cell of the sexual state formed by fungi in the phylum ascomycota containing ascospores.

■ **aseptic**
without the presence of disease causing micro-organisms.

■ **aseptic**
free of infectious agents, sterile.

■ **aseptic technique**
manipulating sterile instruments or culture media in such a way as to maintain sterility.

■ **asexual**
reproduction not preceded by the union of cells or genetic exchange.

■ **a site**
site on the ribosome to which TRNA's enter to donate their amino acid, acceptor site.

■ **aspartate aminotransferase**
liver enzyme, measured through a blood test that indicates the health of the liver. Lower counts are better. Levels may go up because of hepatitis and other infections, or because of drug toxicities

■ **aspergillosis**
fungal infection resulting from the fungus aspergillus of the lungs that can spread through the blood to other organs. Symptoms include fever, chills, difficulty in breathing and coughing up blood. If the infection reaches the brain, it may cause dementia.

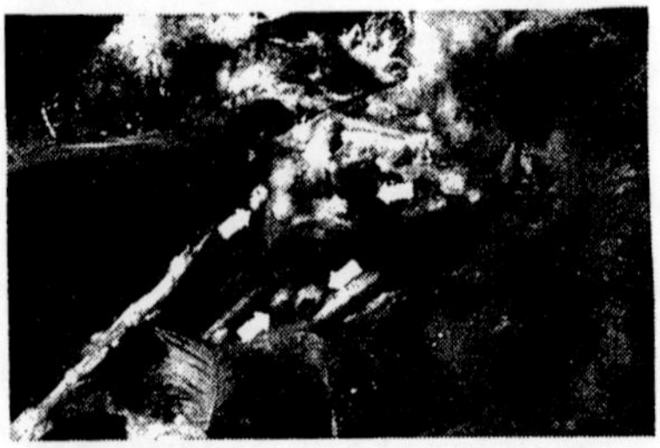

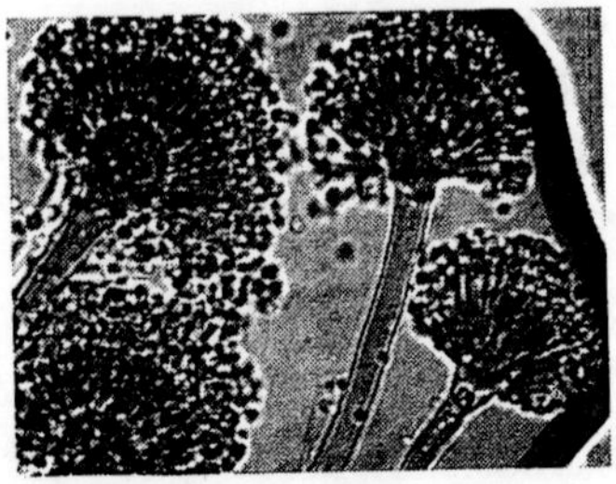

■ **aspergillus**
ubiquitous fungus, most commonly found in compost heaps. Aspergillus is a frequent cause of disease in transplant patients, and is increasingly seen in persons with HIV.

■ **aspergillus caesiellus**
this specie is only occasionally pathogenic.

■ **aspergillus candidus**
found in warm soils, grain and in the secondary decay of vegetation, associated with respiratory complaints. Can produce the toxin petulin that may be associated with disease in humans and other animals.

■ **aspergillus carneus**
this specie is only occasionally pathogenic.

■ **aspergillus clavatus**
conidia dimensions 3 4.5 x (2.5 - 4.5) microns. Found in soils and animal manure. Can produce the toxin petulin that may be associated with disease in humans and other animals. This species is only occasionally pathogenic.

■ **aspergillus deflectus**
this specie is only occasionally pathogenic.

■ **aspergillus flavus**
aw 0.78. Conidia dimensions 3 6 microns or 3 5 microns. It grows on mouldy corn and peanuts. It can be found in warm soil, foods and dairy products. Some strains are capable of producing a group of mycotoxins in the aflatoxin group. Aflatoxins are known animal carcinogen. There is limited evidence to suggest that this toxin is a human carcinogen. The toxin is poisonous to humans by inges-

tion. It may also result in occupational disease via inhalation. Experiments have indicated that it is teratogenic and mutagenic. It is toxic to the liver. It is reported to be allergenic. Its presence is associated with reports of asthma. It can be found in water damaged carpets. The production of the fungal toxin is dependent on the growth conditions and on the substrate used as a food source. This fungus is associated with aspergillosis of the lungs. This fungus is occasionally identified as the cause of corneal, otomycotic and nasoorbital infections.

■ **aspergillus fumigatus**

aw 0.8, optimum > 0.97. Conidia dimensions 2 3.5 microns. Major cause of aspergillosis. Both invasive and allergic aspergillosis are caused by this organism. Aspergillosis affects individuals who are immune compromised. It is considered a human pathogen. It grows well at 35 degrees C. It is commonly found outdoors in compost piles with temperatures higher than 40 degrees C, in mild to warm soils and on cereals.

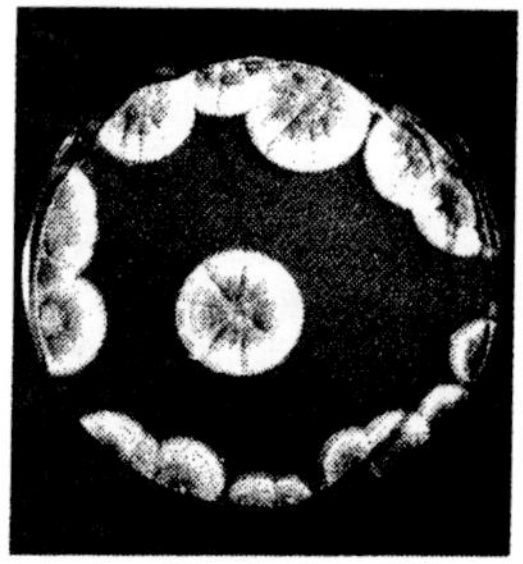

Aspergillus, the Green Mold, growing on malt agar media.

■ **aspergillus glaucus**

conidia dimensions 5 6.5 microns. Common outdoor fungus in the winter. It is reported to be allergenic. This species is only occasionally pathogenic. It can grow on leather. This fungus can grow at low moisture levels on grains, sugary food products, meat and wool. The ascomycetous state is Eurotium sp.

■ **aspergillus nidulans**

aw 0.78. conidia dimensions 2 4 microns. Found in mild to warm soils and on slowly decaying plants. Can produce the mycotoxin sterigmatocystin. This toxin has been shown to produce liver and kidney damage in lab animals. This fungus is associated with aspergillosis of the lungs and or disseminated aspergillosis. This species is only occasionally pathogenic.

aspergillus niger

aw 0.77, optimum > 0.97. Conidia dimensions 3.55 microns or 4 to 5 microns. Less common cause of aspergillosis. It has a musty odour. It is commonly found in the environment on textiles, in soils, grains, fruits and vegetables. It has been reported to cause skin and pulmonary infections. It is a common cause of fungal related ear infections otomycosis.

aspergillus ochraceus

aw 0.77. Conidia dimensions 2.5-3 microns. Found in grains, soil and salted food products. It is not usually associated with decaying vegetation. Can produce a kidney toxin ochratoxin A that may produce ochratoxicosis in humans. This is also known as Balkan nephropathy. The toxin is produced at optimum growth conditions at 25 degrees C and high moisture conditions. The ochratoxin may also be produced by other Aspergillus sp. & Penicillium sp. Other toxins that can be produced by this fungus include penicillic acid, xanthomegnin and viomellein. These are all reported to be kidney and liver toxins.

aspergillus oryzae

this specie is only occasionally pathogenic.

aspergillus parasiticus

some strains are capable of producing a group of mycotoxins in the aflatoxin group. Aflatoxins are known animal carcinogen. There is limited evidence to suggest that this toxin is a human carcinogen. The toxin is a poisonous to humans by ingestion. Experiments have indicated that it is teratogenic and mutagenic. It is toxic to the liver. The production of the fungal toxin is dependent on the growth conditions and on the substrate used as a food source.

aspergillus penicilloides

conidia dimensions 3 3.5 x 4 5 microns. Can grow in areas with low water activity. It is found in house dust and food.

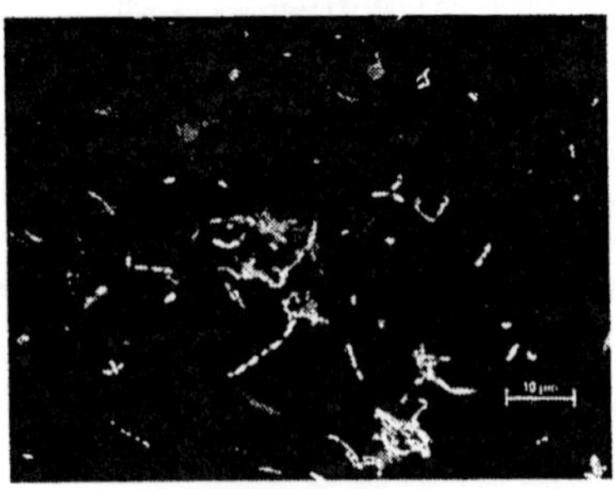

■ aspergillus restrictus
this species is only occasionally pathogenic.

■ aspergillus sp.
aw 0.75- 0.82. Reported to be allergenic. Members of this genus are reported to cause ear infections. Many species produce mycotoxins that may be associated with disease in humans and other animals. Toxin production is dependent on the species or a strain within a species and on the food source for the fungus. Some of these toxins have been found to be carcinogenic in animal species. Several toxins are considered potential human carcinogens. Considered to be a common cause of extrinsic asthma (immediate type hypersensitivity type I). Acute symptoms include edema and bronchiospasms, chronic cases may develop pulmonary emphysema

■ aspergillus sydowi
this specie is only occasionally pathogenic.

■ aspergillus terreus
aw 0.78. Conidia dimensions 1.8 -2.4 microns or 2- 2.5 microns. Aleurospores are 6-7 microns in diameter and are also produced. Found in warmer soil and in grains, straw. Cotton and decomposing vegetation. Can produce the toxin patulin and citrinin that may be associated with disease in humans and other animals. This fungus is associated with aspergillosis of the lungs and or disseminated aspergillosis. Found as an isolate from otomycosis ear infection and onychomycosis infection of finger or toenails.

■ aspergillus ustus
this specie is only occasionally pathogenic.

■ aspergillus versicolour
aw 0.78. Conidia dimensions 2 3.5 microns. It is commonly found in soil, hay, cotton and dairy products. It can produce a mycotoxin sterigmatocystin and cyclopiaxonic acid. These toxins can cause diarrhoea and upset stomach. It is reported to be a kidney and liver carcinogen. This species is only occasionally pathogenic.

■ assembly and budding
names for a portion of the process through which new HIV virus is formed in infected host cells. Viral core proteins, enzymes and RNA (ribonucleic acid) gather just in-

side the cell's membrane, while the viral envelope proteins aggregate within the membrane. An immature viral particle is formed and then pinches off from the cell, acquiring an envelope and the cellular and HIV proteins from the cell membrane. The immature viral particle then undergoes processing by an HIV enzyme called protease to become an infectious virus.

- **assembly of multiple ribosomes attached to a single MRN**
  molecule, also called a polysome.

- **assimilatory nitrate reduction**
  conversion of nitrate to reduced forms of nitrogen, generally ammonium, for the synthesis of amino acids and proteins.

- **association**
  synonyms for association include correlation and relationship. An association between two conditions or states means that if one is present, the other is likely to be so as well. Association does not necessarily imply a causal relationship. In addition, association does not necessarily imply a statistically significant relationship.

- **associative dinitrogen fixation**
  close interaction between a free living diazotrophic organism and a higher plant that results in an enhanced rate of dinitrogen fixation.

- **associative symbiosis**
  close but relatively casual interaction between two dissimilar organisms or biological systems. The association may be mutually beneficial but is not required for accomplishment of a particular function.

- **asthenia**
  weakness, debilitation.

- **asthma**
  immediate respiratory allergy resulting from mediator release from mast cells in the lower airways.

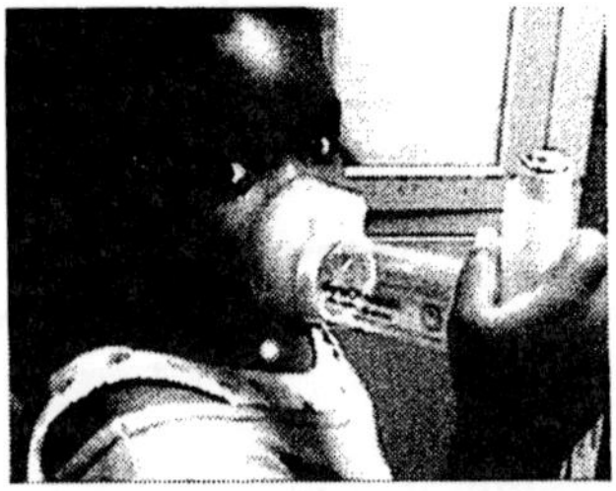

- **astrobiology**
  study of life in the universe.

- **asymptomatic**
  without signs or symptoms of disease.

- **asymptomatic infection**
  infection or phase of infection, without symptoms, usually used in aids literature to describe a person who has a positive reaction to one of several tests for HIV antibodies, but who shows no clinical symptoms of the disease.

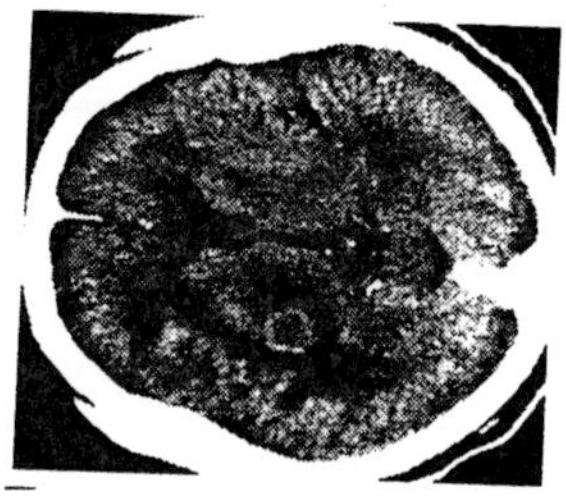

- **ataxia**
  problems with coordination or proper use of muscles.

- **atomic force microscope**
  type of scanning probe microscope that has a tip mounted so it can bend in response to the slightest force between the tip and the sample.

- **atovaquone (mepron)**
  antibiotic sometimes used in treatment of Pneumocystis carinii pneumonia (PCP), in trials for prophylaxis of PCP, and for treatment of toxoplasmosis.

- **ATP synthase**
  protein complex that harvests the energy of a proton motive force to synthesise ATP.

- **attack rate**
  proportional number of cases developing in a population exposed to an infectious agent.

- **attenuated virus**
  weakened virus with reduced ability to infect or produce disease. Some vaccines are based on attenuated viruses. An attenuated virus can no longer produce disease, but might be used to produce a vaccine.

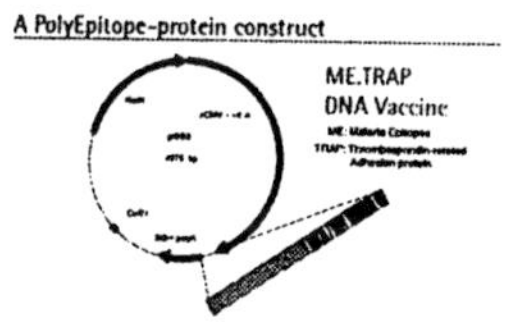

- **auramine**
  fluorescent dye that binds to a compound found only in the cell wall of members of the genus *mycobacterium*.

- **auto antibody**
  an antibody that is active against some of the tissues of the organism that produced it.

- **autoclave**
  device employing steam under pressure used for sterilising materials that are stable to heat and moisture.

■ **autoimmune disease**
disease produced as a result of an immune reaction against one's own tissues.

■ **auto immune diseases**
diseases caused when an organism's own immune system attacks its own cells.

■ **auto immunisation**
induction in an individual of an immune response to its own cells (tissue).

■ **auto inoculable**
susceptible of being inoculated with micro-organisms from one's own body.

■ **autologous**
pertaining to the same organism or one of its parts; originating within an organism itself.

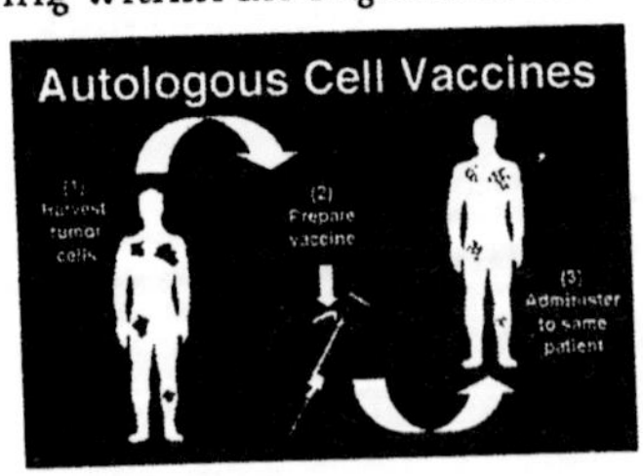

■ **autolysis**
spontaneous lysis.

■ **autolyse**
to spontaneously disintegrate as a result of enzymes within the cell

■ **autoradiography**
use of film to detect a radioactive molecule.

■ **autotroph**
organism which uses carbon dioxide as the sole carbon source.

■ **autotrophic nitrification**
oxidation of ammonium to nitrate through the combined action of two chemoautotrophic organisms, one forming nitrite from ammonium and the other oxidising nitrite to nitrate.

■ **auxotroph**
mutant of a micro-organism that requires an organic growth factor.

■ **avirulent**
lacking disease causing attributes, such as a capsule.

■ **aw**
abbreviation for water activity.

■ **axenic**
literally 'without strangers'. A system in which all biological populations are defined, such as a pure culture.

■ **axial filaments**
organ of motility found in spirochetes.

- **azithromycin (zithromax)**
  a macrolide antibiotic sometime used as a component in combination therapy for *mycobacterium avium* complex.

- **azoles**
  family of antifungal drugs e.g. fluconazole, itraconazole, etc., used to treat fungal infections in persons with HIV, including candida, cryptococcus, histoplasmosis and others.

- **azoles**
  large family of chemically synthesised medications, some of which have anti-fungal activity.

- **azt**
  also called zidovudine, retrovir, or azidothymidine, a thymidine (genetic building block) analog that suppresses replication of HIV. It is the only drug for the initial treatment of HIV infection. Adverse side effects may include anaemia, leukopenia, muscle fatigue, muscle wasting, nausea and headaches.

- **b cells**
  cells of the immune system that secrete antibody

- **B lymphocytes (B cells)**
  one among the two major classes of lymphocytes. During infections, these cells are transformed into plasma cells that produce large quantities of antibodies directed at specific pathogens. This transformation occurs through interactions with various types of t cells and other components of the immune system. In persons with aids, the functional ability of both the b and the t lymphocytes is damaged, with the t lymphocytes being the principal site of infection by the HIV virus.

- **bacillus**
  bacterium with an elongated, rod shape.

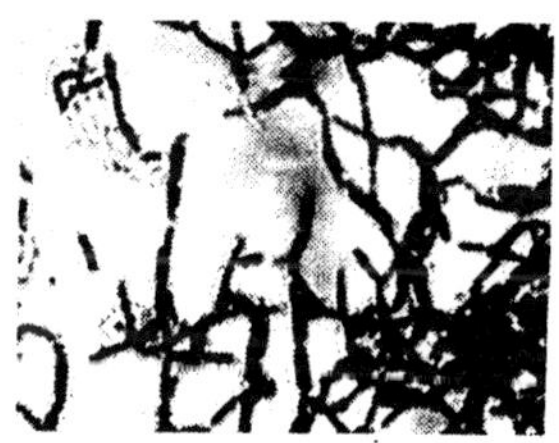

- **bacitracin**
  antimicrobial medication that inhibits cell wall biosynthesis by interfering with the transport of peptidoglycan precursors across the cytoplasmic membrane.

- **bacteremia**
  bacteria circulating in the bloodstream.

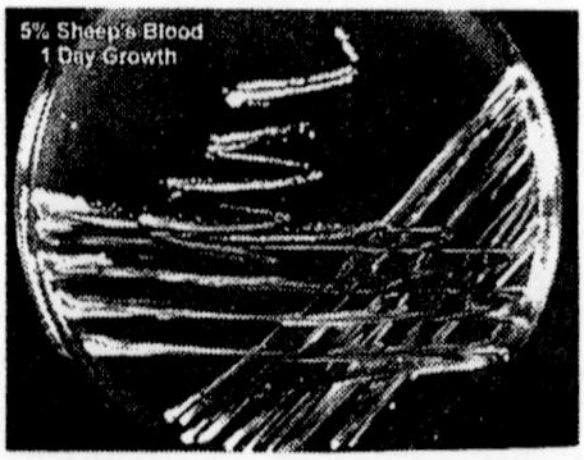

■ **bacteria**
all prokaryotes that are not members of the domain Archaea.

■ **bacterial artificial chromosome (BAC)**
derivative of the F plasmid used as vectors to clone DNA fragments as large as 3,00000 base pairs in length.

■ **bactericidal**
able to kill bacteria.

■ **bacteriochlorophyll**
light absorbing pigment found in green sulphur and purple sulphur bacteria.

■ **bacteriocin**
agent produced by certain bacteria that inhibits or kills closely related isolates and species.

■ **bacteriological specimen**
refers to any body fluid, secretion, or tissue sent to the laboratory where smears and cultures for bacteria will be performed. The specimen may consist of blood, sputum, urine, spinal fluid, material obtained at biopsy, etc.

■ **bacteriophages**
viruses that infect bacteria.

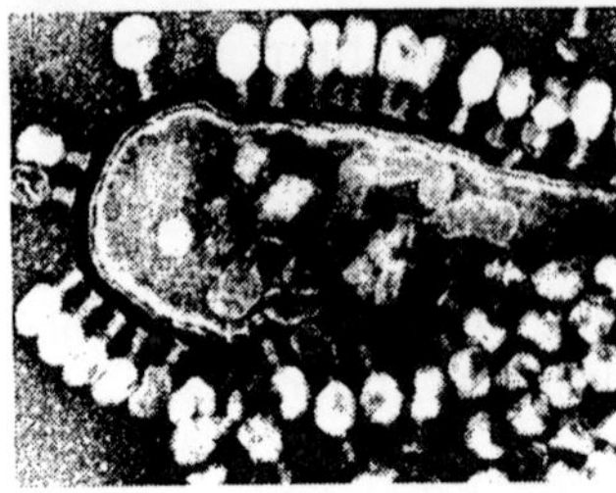

■ **bacteriorhodopsin**
pigment of some extreme halophiles that absorbs energy from sunlight and use it to expel protons from the cell, generating a proton gradient.

■ **bacteriostatic**
able to inhibit the growth of bacteria.

■ **bacterium**
microscopic organism composed of a single cell. Many bacteria can cause disease in humans.

■ **bacteroid**
altered form of cells of certain bacteria. Refers particularly to the swollen, irregular vacuolated cells of rhizobia in nodules of legumes.

■ **baculovirus**

virus of insects used in the production of some HIV vaccines.

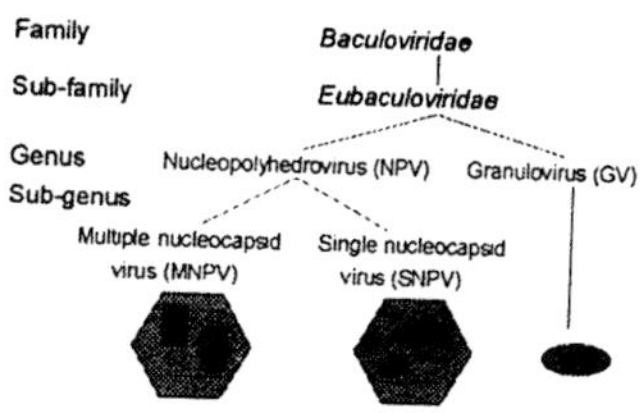

■ **balanced pathogenicity**

virus host relationship in which the virus persists in the host without causing obvious harm.

■ **barophiles**

bacteria that can grow under high pressure.

■ **basal body**

structure that anchors the flagella to the cell wall and plasma membrane.

■ **base**

refers to the purine or pyrimidine ring structure found in nucleic acids.

■ **base analog**

compound that resembles a purine or pyrimidine base closely enough to be incorporated into dna in place of a natural base.

■ **base composition**

proportion of the total bases consisting of guanine plus cytosine or thymine plus adenine base pairs. Usually expressed as a guanine + cytosine (g + c) value, e.g. 60% g+c.

■ **base pair**

pair of nucleotides contained in a double stranded nucleic acid, linked together by hydrogen bonds.

■ **base pairing**

hydrogen bonding of adenine (a) to thymine (t) and cytosine (c) to guanine (g), occurs between two complementary strands of DNA.

■ **baseline**

information gathered at the beginning of a study from which variations found in the study are measured.

■ **baseline characteristic**

variable that is measured, observed, or assessed on a patient at or shortly before treatment assignment and the initiation of treatment.

■ **baseline data**

set of data collected on a specific patient or set of patients prior to randomisation.

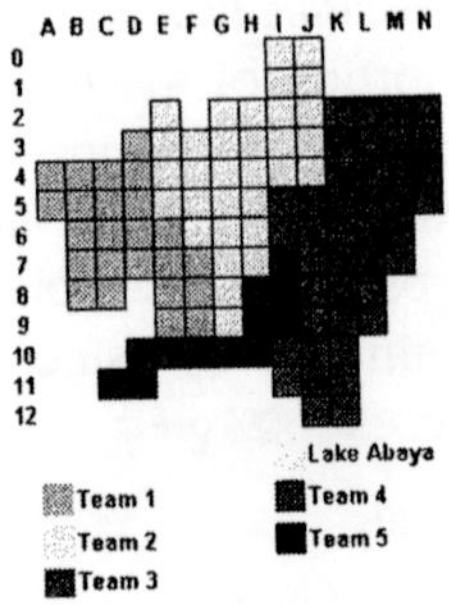

■ **baseline examination**
examination that is carried out as part of the baseline visit and that is designed to assess a patient's eligibility for enrolment into the trial and to produce required baseline data.

■ **basic amino acids**
amino acids with more basic groups than acid groups.

■ **basidioma (pl. basidiomata)**
fruiting body that produces basidia, also termed a basidiocarp.

■ **basidiomycetes**
fungal spores from mushrooms, the specific mushroom species cannot be identified on the culture plate. Many mushroom spores are reported to be allergenic.

■ **basidiospore**
spore resulting from karyogamy and meiosis that are formed on a basidium that usually is formed on a basidium. Sexual spore of the basidiomycota.

■ **basidium (pl. basidia)**
clublike cell of the sexual state formed by fungi in the phylum basidiomycota.

■ **basophil**
leukocyte with large dark staining granules that contain histamine and other mediators of inflammation, receptors on cell surfaces bind monomers of ige.

■ **BDNA (Branched DNA Assay)**
DNA test for detecting and measuring HIV in the blood plasma of people infected with HIV. The BDNA test is faster and probably more accurate than plasma culture, the test currently used. It is less sensitive than PCR, another new test. BDNA testing may eventually be useful to monitor the effectiveness of anti HIV drugs and to gauge HIV disease progression.

■ **beta (B) lactam drugs**
group of antimicrobial medications that inhibit peptidoglycan synthesis and have a shared chemical structure called a b lactam ring.

■ **beta (B) haemolysis**
type of haemolysis observed on blood agar that is characterised by a clear zone around a colony.

■ **beta carotene**
form of carotene, precursor to vitamin A, a red orange pigment found in plants and plant eating animals, is also found in dark green and dark yellow fruits and vegetables. Beta carotene may have beneficial effects on the immune system.

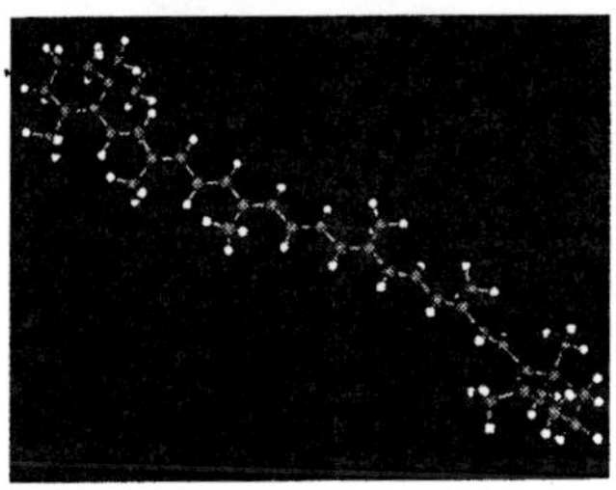

■ **bias**
deviation of results from the truth or mechanisms leading to such deviation, e.g., analysis bias, confounding factors, measurement bias, selection bias, withdrawal bias, and others.

■ **bias (analysis)**
deviation of results or inferences from the truth, resulting from flaws in the analysis or interpretation of results.

■ **bias (confounding factor)**
confounding factor is a variable, which is related to one or more of the variables defined in a study. A confounding factor may (1) mask an actual association or (2) falsely demonstrate an apparent association between the study variables where no real association between them exists. For example, alcohol intake may appear to be positively associated with laryngeal cancer but the actual association may be with the confounding factor of cigarette smoking, i.e., people who drink alcohol may be at increased risk for laryngeal cancer because they also smoke cigarettes. If confounding factors are not measured and considered, bias may result.

■ **bias (measurement bias)**
systematic measurement error. For example, a sphygmomanometer not correctly calibrated will produce biased blood pressure readings.

■ **bias (selection bias)**
error due to differences in characteristics of those participants who are selected for a study as compared to those not selected.

■ **bias (withdrawal)**
error due to specific characteristics of those participants who choose to withdraw from a study or become lost to follow up, as opposed to those who remain.

■ **bid**
common abbreviation for 'twice a day'.

■ **bilateral**
having, or being distributed on, two sides.

■ **bilayer (or unit) membrane**
double layer of phospholipid molecules that forms the major structure of the cytoplasmic (plasma) membrane

■ **bilirubin**
bile pigment whose measurement can be used as an indication of the health of the liver.

■ **binary fission**
asexual process of reproduction in which one cell divides into two independent daughter cells.

■ **binary outcome measure**
outcome measure that can assume only one of two values, such as in a trial with death as the outcome measure.

■ **binding antibody**
as related to HIV infection an antibody that attaches to some part of the HIV virus. Binding antibodies may or may not adversely affect the virus.

■ **binding protein**
protein that functions in the ABC transport system, resides immediately outside of the cytoplasmic membrane to deliver a given molecule to a specific transport complex within the membrane.

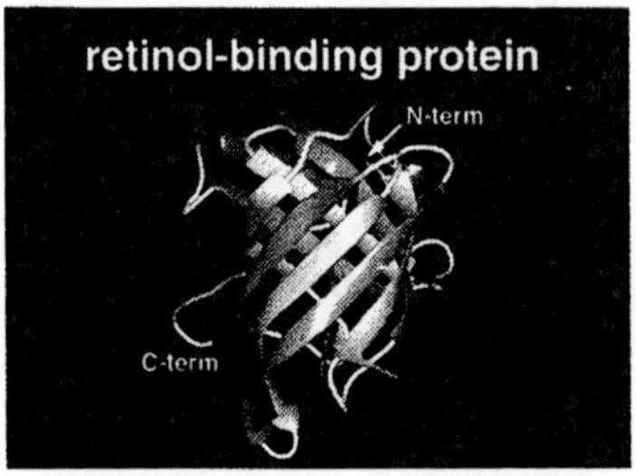

■ **binomial nomenclature**
system of having two names, genus and specific epithet, for each organism.

■ **bioaccumulation**
accumulation of a chemical substance in living tissue.

■ **bioavailability**
the rate and extent to which a substance is absorbed and circulated in the body.

■ **biochemical oxygen demand (BOD)**
measure of the amount of biologically degradable organic material in water.

■ **biocide**
compound such as a disinfectant that is toxic to many forms of life, including micro-organisms.

■ **biodegradable**
substance capable of being decomposed by biological processes.

■ **biodiversity**
diversity in the number of species of organisms inhabiting an ecosystem.

■ **biofilm**
polysaccharide encased community of micro-organisms attached to a surface.

■ **biofilm**
microbial cells encased in an adhesive, usually a polysaccharide material, and attached to a surface.

■ **biogeochemistry**
study of microbially mediated chemical transformations of geo-chemical interest, such as nitrogen or sulphur cycling.

■ **bioinformatics**
developing and using computer technology to store, retrieve and analyse nucleotide sequence data.

■ **bioleaching**
conversion of metals to a soluble form due to the metabolic oxidation of insoluble metal sulphides by micro-organisms such as *thiobacillus*species.

■ **Biological Response Modifiers (BRMS)**
substances, either natural or synthesised, that boost, direct, or restore normal immune defences. BRMS include interferons, interleukins, thymic hormones, and monoclonal antibodies.

■ **biological vector**
organism that acts as a host for a disease organism before it is transmitted to another organism; the pathogen can multiply to high numbers within it.

■ **bioluminescence**
biological production of light.

■ **biomagnification**
increase in the concentration of a chemical substance as it is progresses to higher tropic levels of a food chain.

■ **biomass**

total weight of all organisms in any particular environment.

■ **biopsy**

diagnostic technique involving the surgical removal of a small piece of tissue for microscopic examination conducted to make a diagnosis e.g. to determine whether abnormal cells such as cancer cells are present.

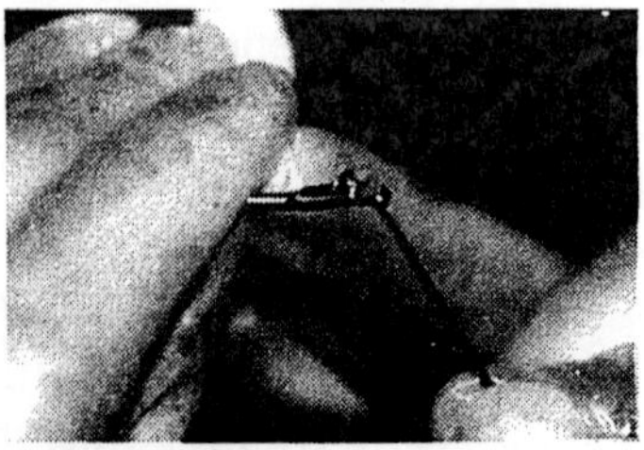

■ **bioremediation**

process that uses micro-organisms to degrade harmful chemicals.

■ **biosolid**

the resides of wastewater treatment. Formerly called sewage sludge.

■ **biosphere**

sum of all the regions of the earth where life exists.

■ **biosynthesis**

production of needed cellular constituents from other, usually simpler, molecules.

■ **biotechnology**

the use of living organisms or their products to make or modify a substance. These include recombinant DNA techniques (genetic engineering) and hybridoma technology.

■ **biotrophic**

nutritional relationship between two organisms in which one or both must associate with the other to obtain nutrients and grow.

■ **biotype**

strain that has a characteristic biochemical pattern, which differs from other strains, also called a biovar.

■ **bipolaris sp.**

fungus with large spores that is most likely to get deposited in the upper respiratory tract. This fungus can produce the mycotcxin sterigmatocystin that has been shown to produce liver and kidney damage when ingested by laboratory animals.

■ **blastomyces sp.**

human pathogen. The fungus is commonly found in soil. It is a dimorphic fungus having filamentous form when grown at 25 degrees C and a yeast form at 37 degrees C.

■ **blind**

a condition imposed on an individual or group of individuals for the purpose of keeping that individual or group of individuals from knowing or learning of some fact or observation, such as treatment assignment.

■ **blinded**

condition of having a blind in place, e.g., as in a single, double, or triple blinded trial.

■ **blinded study**

clinical trial in which participants are unaware as to whether or not they are in the experimental or control arm of the study.

■ **block**

group, quantity, section or segment that is considered as a unit for some purpose, procedure, process or action.

■ **block size**

the number of individual elements making up a block.

■ **blocking**

the process of establishing defined groups, as in a treatment allocation schedule designed to ensure a specific allocation ratio.

■ **blood agar**

type of agar medium that contains red blood cells, a rich medium that can be used to detect haemolysis.

■ **blood brain barrier**

property of the central nervous system blood vessels that restricts passage of infectious agents and certain molecules (such as medications) into the brain and spinal cord.

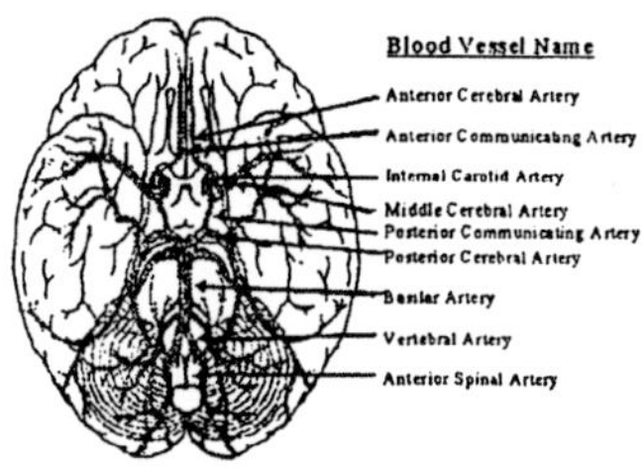

■ **blue green alga**

fungus that attacks cellulose and hemi cellulose in wood, leaving dark coloured lignin and phenolic materials behind.

■ **blunt end**

type of DNA ends generated by a restriction enzyme that cuts directly in the middle the recognition sequence.

■ **B lymphocytes**

B lymphocytes are blood cells of the immune system derived from the bone marrow and spleen involved in the production of antibodies. B lymphocytes float through all body fluids, are able to detect the presence of foreign invaders, and produce antibodies on their own and when primed by t lymphocytes. B lymphocytes can later differentiate into plasma and memory cells. B cells mediate the 'humeral' immune response.

■ **body fluids**
any fluid in the human body, such as blood, urine, saliva, sputum, tears, semen, mother's milk or vaginal secretions. Only blood, semen, mother's milk and vaginal secretions have been linked directly to the transmission of the HIV virus.

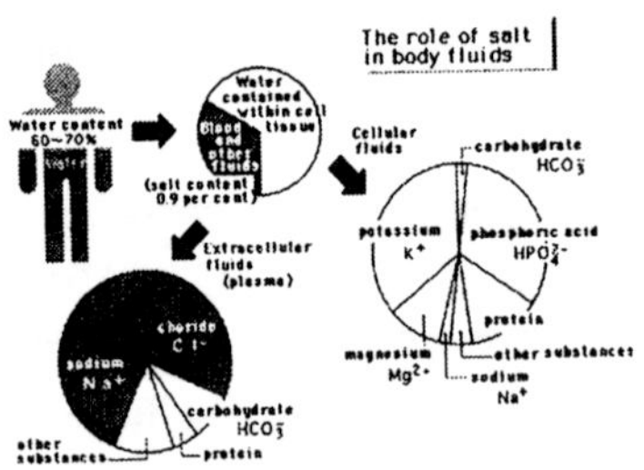

■ **boil**
painful localised collection of pus within the skin and subcutaneous tissue, a furuncle.

■ **bone marrow**
soft tissue located in the cavities of the bones where blood cells are formed, including erythrocytes, leukocytes and platelets.

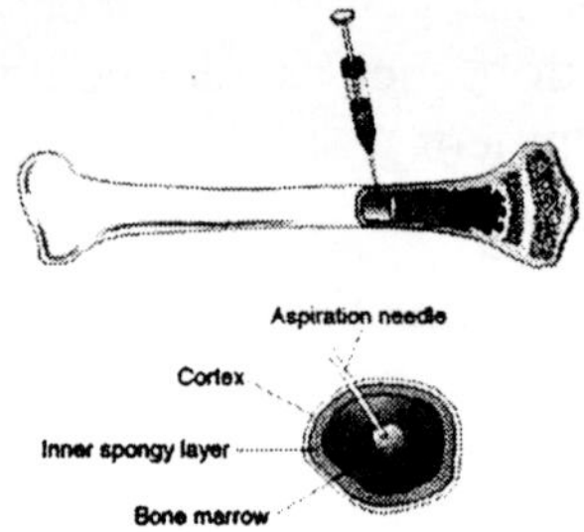

■ **booster**
second or later dose of a vaccine given to increase the immune response to the original dose.

■ **botrytis sp.**
aw 0.93. Conidia dimensions 7 14 x 5 9 microns. Reported to be allergenic. It is parasitic on plants and soft fruits. Found in soil and vegetables. Possibly associated with allergic symptoms (skin tests).

■ **botulinum toxin**
toxin produced by *clostridium botulinum* that can cause a fatal paralysis in people who consume it.

■ **breakthrough infection**
infection caused by the infectious agent the vaccine is de-

signed to protect against, that occurs during the course of a vaccine trial. These infections may be caused by exposure to the infectious agent before the vaccine has taken effect, or before all doses of the vaccine have been given. Breakthrough infections also occur in trial participants receiving placebos.

- **bright field microscope**

type of light microscope that illuminates the field of view evenly.

- **brine**

salty water, used to cure fish and meats.

- **broad spectrum antimicrobials**

antimicrobials that inhibit or kill a wide range of micro-organisms, often including both gram positive and gram negative bacteria.

- **bronchi**

hollow branches of the pulmonary tree which connects the trachea to the alveoli.

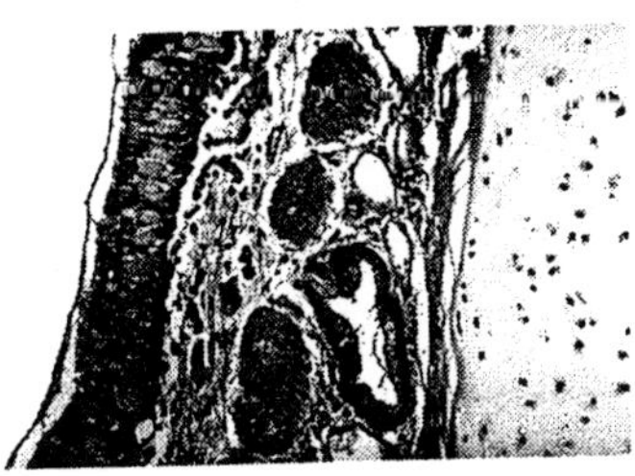

- **bronchitis**

inflammation of the bronchial tubes, generally accompanied by coughing, pain or shortness of breath.

- **bronchoscopy**

procedure for examining the respiratory tract by means of a fibre optic instrument i.e. bronchoscope, which is inserted through the mouth or nose into the trachea. Diagnostic specimens such as bronchial washings and transbronchial biopsies of lung tissue can be

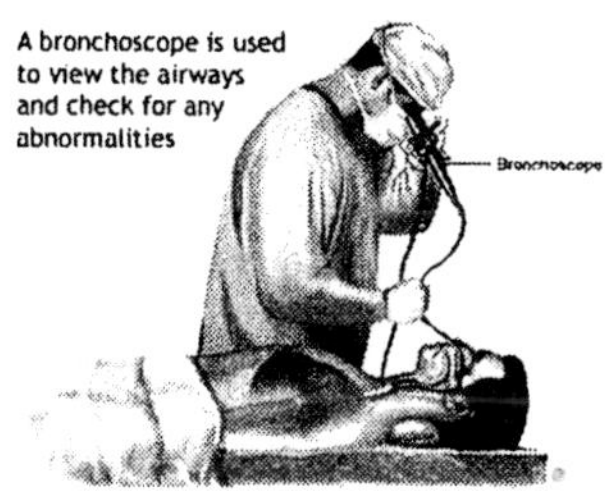

obtained during bronchoscopy.

- **bt toxin**

protein crystal naturally produced by the bacterium *Bacillus thuringiensis* as it forms endospores, toxic to insect larvae that consume it.

- **bubo**

enlarged, tender lymph node characteristic of plague and some venereal diseases.

■ **bubonic plague**
form of plague that typically develops when *yersinia pestis* is injected via the bite of an infected flea.

■ **budding**
step in the replication of some viruses in which the virus leaves the host cell encapsulated with a portion of the cell's membrane without killing the host cell in the process.

■ **budding**
asexual reproductive technique that involves a pushing out of a part of the parent cell that eventually gives rise to a new daughter cell.

■ **buffer**
substance in a solution that acts to prevent changes in ph.

■ **bulk density (soil)**
mass of dry soil per unit bulk volume (combined volume of soil solids and pore space).

■ **bulking**
Overgrowth of filamentous micro-organisms in sewage at treatment facilities, interferes with the separation of the solid sludge from the liquid effluent.

■ **burkitt's lymphoma**
lymphatic cancer that involves not only the lymphatic and the associated reticuloendothelial system, but also other body tissues. This disease, which is most common in Central Africa, is thought to be possibly caused by the epstein barr virus. Also called African lymphoma, burkitt's tumour.

■ **bursa**
tissue space lined by joint tissue, bursas are found in

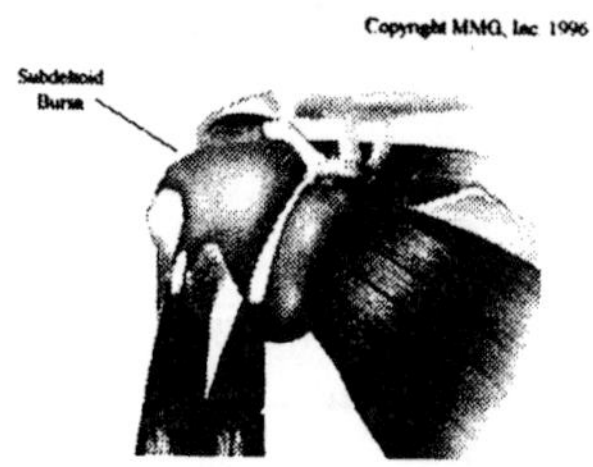

between tendon and bone, skin and bone and muscies.

■ **burst size**
number of newly formed virus particles released from a single cell.

■ **cachexia**
general ill health and malnutrition, marked by weakness and emaciation, usually associated with serious disease.

■ **calcofluor**
white fluorescent dye that binds to a component of fungal cells, causing them to fluoresce bright blue.

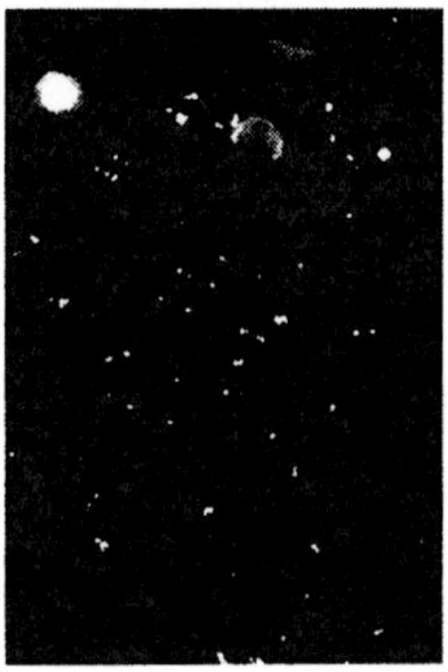

■ **calvin cycle**
biochemical route of carbon dioxide fixation in many autotrophic organisms.

■ **CAMP**
abbreviation for cyclic AMP.

■ **cancer**
abnormally growing cells that can spread from their site of origin, malignant tumours.

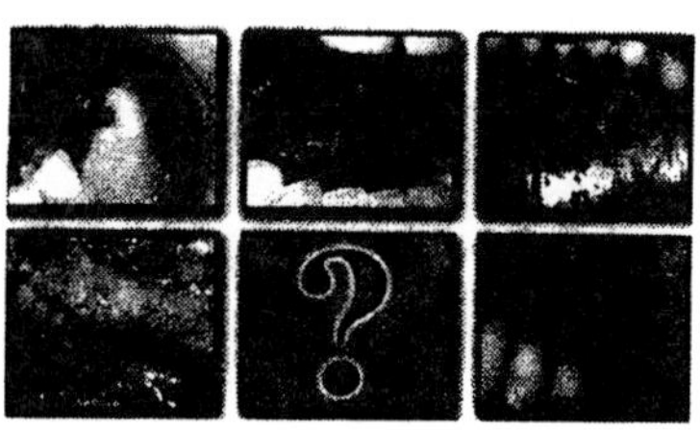

■ **candida albican**
yeast like fungi, commonly found in the normal flora of the mouth, skin, intestinal tract, and vagina. Generally, candida is harmless, but can become clinically infectious in immune compromised people.

■ **candida kruseii**
another candida species, similar to *candida albicans*, but often less susceptible to the common drugs used to treat *c albicans*

■ **candida sp.**
part of the normal flora of mouth and other mucous membranes in the body. Thrush and other diseases caused by Candida albicans usually occur after prolonged treatment with antibiotics or steroids. The environment is not a likely source of exposure for this fungus. Cells from the organism are usually not airborne. Reported to be allergenic.

■ **candidemia**
candida albicans in the blood.

■ **candidiasis**
fungal diseases caused by *candida albicans*.

■ **candle jar**
jar in which a lit candle converts some of the o_2 in air to co_2. used to cultivate capnophiles.

■ **CAP**
abbreviation for cyclic amp activating protein.

■ **capnophiles**
organisms that require increased concentrations of co_2 (5 to 10%) and approximately 15% oxygen.

■ **capsid**
protein coat that surrounds the nucleic acid of a virus.

■ **capsomer**
the ring shaped morphological unit of which icosahedral capsids are constructed.

■ **capsule**
compact layer of polysaccharide exterior to the cell wall in some bacteria.

■ **carbapenems**
group of antimicrobial medications that interferes with peptidoglycan synthesis; very resistant to b lactamases.

■ **carbohydrate**
compounds containing principally carbon, hydrogen and oxygen atoms in a ratio of 1:2:1.

■ **carbon cycle**
sequence where carbon dioxide is converted to organic forms by photosynthesis or chemosynthesis, recycled through the biosphere, with partial incorporation into sediments, and ultimately returned to its original state through respiration or combustion.

■ **carbon fixation**
conversion of carbon dioxide or other single carbon compounds to organic forms such as carbohydrates.

■ **carbon nitrogen (C/N) ratio**
ratio of the mass of organic carbon to the mass of nitrogen in soil or organic material.

■ **carboxy (or C terminal)**
the end of the protein molecule that has an unbonded –COOH group.

■ **carboxyl group**
a COOH group attached to a carbon skeleton as in the carboxylic acids and fatty acids.

■ **carbuncle**
painful infection of the skin and subcutaneous tissues, manifests as a cluster of boils.

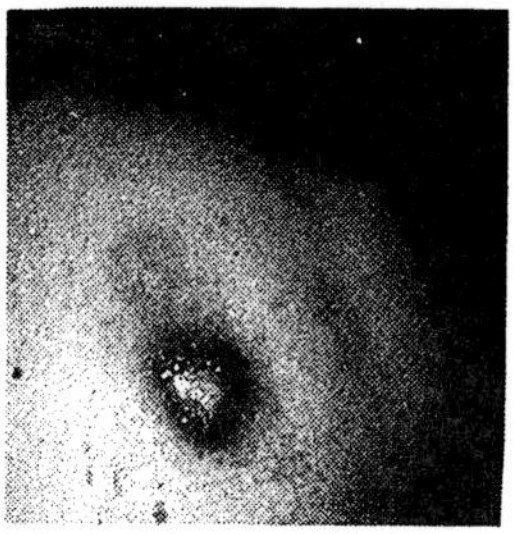

- **carcinogen**
  any cancer producing substance or agent.

- **cardiomyopathy**
  a degenerative condition of the heart muscle, cardiomyopathy may be caused by HIV, or by some drugs.

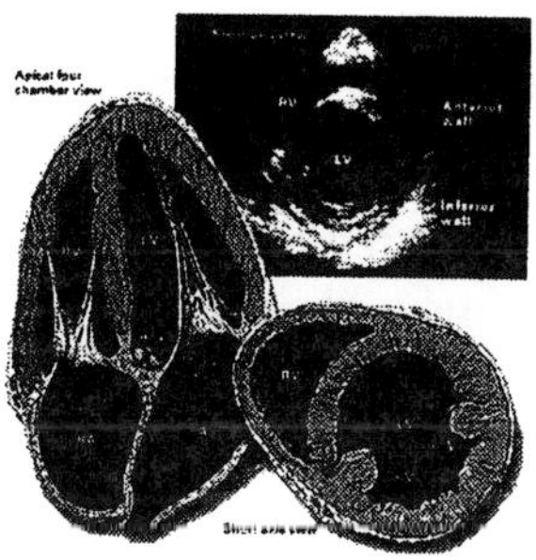

- **carrier**
  organism that carries a virus either in form of an infection or while it is in incubation.

- **carrier**
  1. type of protein found in cell membranes that transports certain compounds across the membrane; may also be called a permease or transporter protein.
  2. a human or other animal that harbours a pathogen without noticeable ill effects.

- **carrier state**
  state of infection in which the agent can be detected in body fluids without causing disease symptoms.

- **cascade**
  in biology, a series of reactions which, once started, continues to the final step by each step triggering the next in a special order, activation of complement is an example.

- **case report form**
  standardised data entry form used in a clinical trial. Generally, all information collected in trials appears on case report forms, or is referred to and explained by case report forms (as in the case of attached lab slips). Even in circumstances where there is other documentation in addition to CRF's (like the lab slips), generally all key values that will be analysed appear on the CRF.

- **case control study**
  a study that involves the identification of persons with the disease or condition of interest (cases) and a suitable group of persons

without the disease or condition of interest (controls). Cases and controls are compared with respect to some existing or past attribute or exposure believed to be causally related to the disease or condition. Also referred to as a retrospective study because the research approach proceeds from effect to cause. The term applies even if cases and controls are accumulated in a prospective manner.

■ **caseous necrosis**
type of localised tissue death having a cheese like consistency, characteristic of tuberculosis and certain other chronic infectious diseases.

■ **caspid**
the protein covering of some viruses made up of capsomeres, may stimulate the body's immune response.

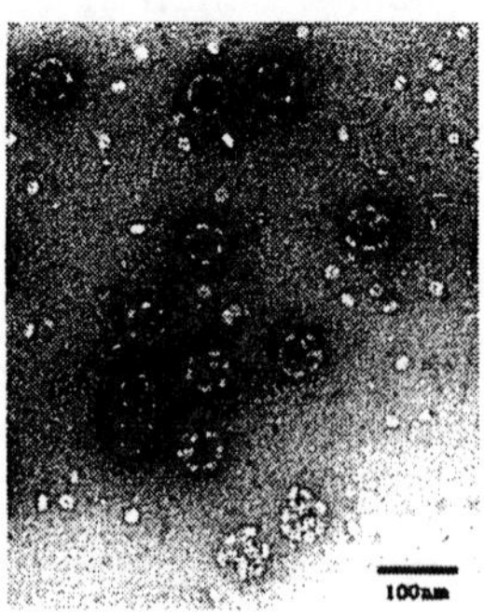

■ **catabolism**
cellular processes that harvest the energy released during the breakdown of compounds such as glucose and use that energy to synthesise ATP, the energy currency of all cells.

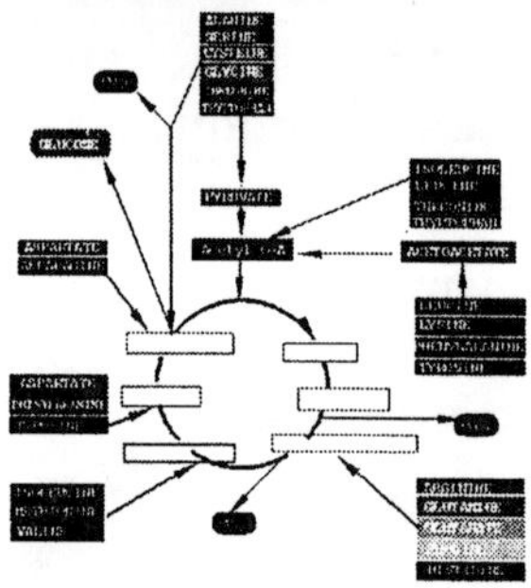

■ **catabolite**
of catabolism.

■ **catabolite repression**
inhibition of gene activity by an efficiently degraded catabolite.

■ **catalase**
enzyme that breaks down hydrogen peroxide (H_2O_2) to produce water (H_2O) and oxygen gas (O_2).

■ **catalyst**
substance that speeds up the rate of a chemical reaction without being altered or depleted in the process.

■ **catheter**

a semi permanently installed tubular medical device for insertion into canals, vessels, passageways or body cavities, usually to permit injection e.g., through an intravenous catheter into a vein or withdrawal of fluids, or to keep a passage open.

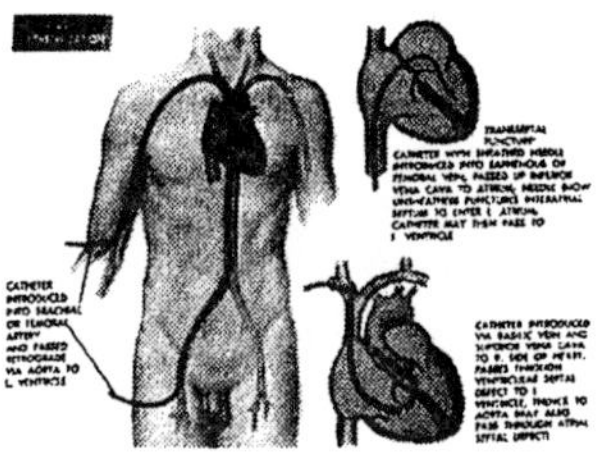

■ **Cation Exchange Capacity (CEC)**

sum of exchangeable cations that a soil can absorb at a specific ph. Expressed as centimoles of positive charge per kilogram of soil.

■ **cations**

positively charged ions.

■ **causation**

there is causation only when one factor necessarily alters the possibility of a second. Statistical methods alone cannot establish a causal relationship between factors. Examples of criteria to test causation include strength of the association, biologic credibility of the association, consistency of the findings with other investigations, temporal relationship of the association, presence of a dose response relationship.

Randomisation allows assessment of causation.

■ **cavitating**

eroding or creating holes. Often used to describe the characteristic destruction of lung tissue accompanying active tuberculosis.

■ **CD antigens**

abbreviation for cluster of differentiation antigens

■ **CD nomenclature**

this nomenclature was developed to standardise and compare monoclonal antibodies from different sources. Antibodies with similar reactivity patterns are assigned to cd groups representing 'clusters of differentiation'. T lymphocytes are cd3+ and can be separated into the cd4+ t helper cells and the cd8+ cytotoxic/suppressor cells. Although cd4+ cells are predominantly t lymphocytes, some monocytes are also cd4+.

■ **CD4 (T4)**

protein embedded in the cell surface of helper t lymphocytes, also found to a lesser degree on the surface of monocyte/macrophage, langerhans cells, astrocytes, keratinocytes and glial cells. One of the ways HIV invades cells is by first attaching to the cd4 molecule (cd4 receptor).

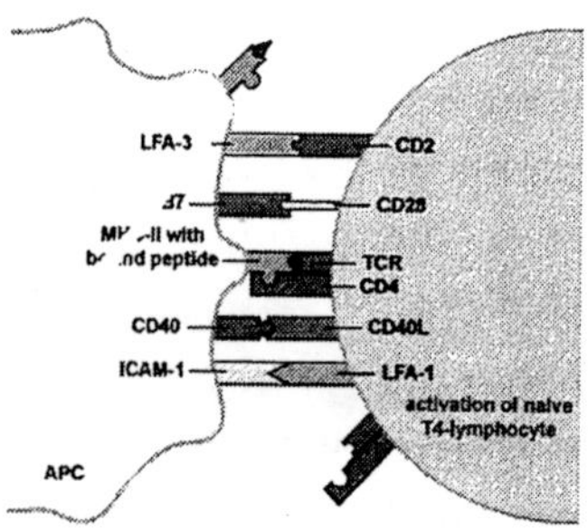

■ **CD4 (T4) or CD4+ cells**

white blood cells killed or disabled during HIV infection. These cells normally orchestrate the immune response, signalling other cells in the immune system to perform their special functions. Also known as T helper cells.

■ **CD4 cell**

'helper' T cell, responsible for coordinating much of the immune response. CD4 cells are one of the main targets damaged by HIV.

■ **CD4 count**

the number of t helper lymphocytes per cubic millimetre of blood. The CD4 count is a good predictor of immune health. A cd4 count less than 200 qualifies as a diagnosis of aids.

■ **CD 4 lymphocytes**

T lymphocytes bearing the CD 4 (cluster of differentiation) surface molecules, T helper cells are CD 4.

■ **CD8 (T8) cells**

protein embedded in the cell surface of suppressor T lymphocytes. Also called cytotoxic T cells.

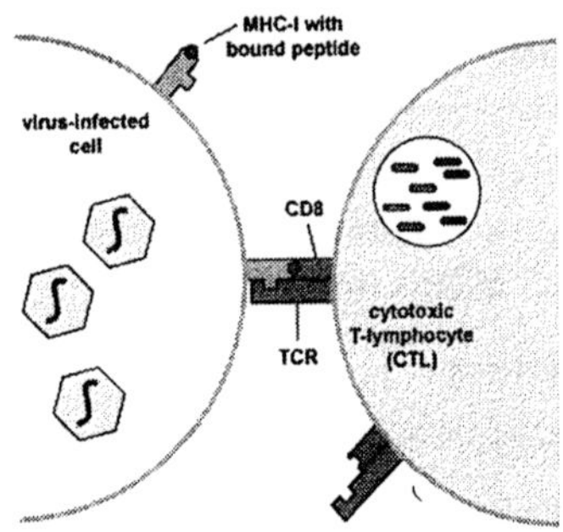

■ **CD 8 cells**

T lymphocytes bearing the CD 8 cluster of differentiation surface molecules, T cytotoxic cells and some T suppressor cells are CD 8 cells.

■ **CD8 count**
the number of killer/suppresser T lymphocytes in a cubic millimetre of blood.

■ **cdn a dn**
obtained by using reverse transcriptase to synthesise DNA from an RNA template *in vitro*. lacks introns that characterise eukaryotic DNA.

■ **cell**
fundamental unit of living matter.

■ **cell culture or tissue culture**
cultivation of animal or plant cells in the laboratory .

■ **cell lines**
specific cell types artificially maintained in the laboratory (in vitro) for scientific purposes.

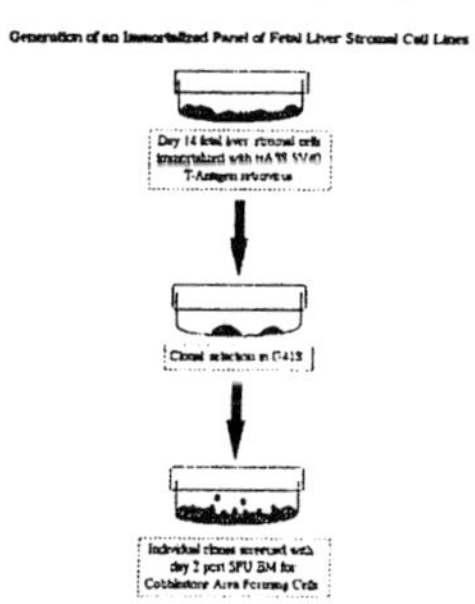

■ **cell wall**
rigid barrier that surrounds a cell, keeping the contents from bursting out. In prokaryotes, peptidoglycan provides rigidity to the cell wall.

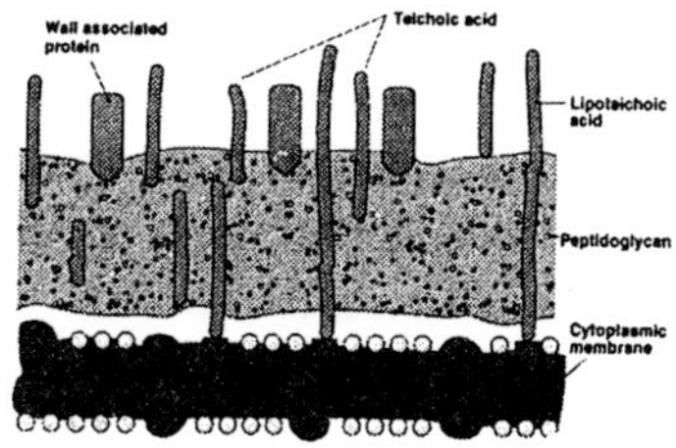

■ **cell mediated immunity (CMI)**
immune responses mediated by T lymphocytes.

■ **cellulose**
polymer of glucose subunits, principal structural component of plant cell walls.

■ **censoring**
term used in survival or time to event analyses to denote an individual who has not experienced the event of interest as of a specific point in follow up, e.g. Time of interim analysis, end of study, or time at lost to follow up. The process by which patient outcome data cannot be obtained beyond a specific point in time.

■ **centi**
prefix meaning one hundredth, as in a centimetre, which is a hundredth of a meter.

■ **cento**

prefix meaning a hundred times, as in centogram, a hundred grams.

■ **central metabolic pathways**

amphibolic pathways glycolysis, the tca cycle and the pentose phosphate pathway – that are used by most chemoheterotrophs.

■ **Central Nervous System (CNS)**

composed of the brain, spinal cord, and its coverings i.e. meninges.

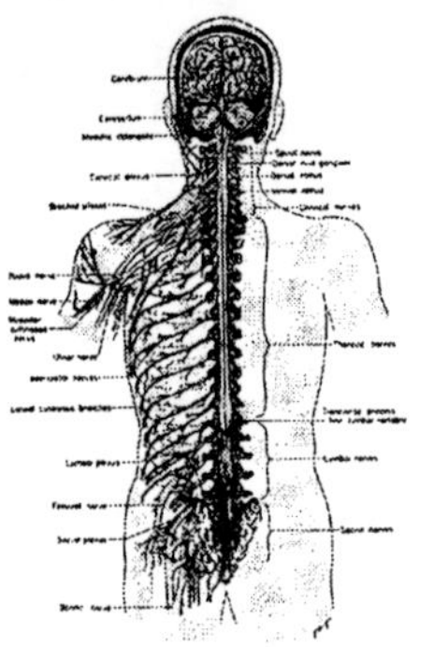

The human central nervous system, exposed by dissection from the dorsal aspect. Shows the brain, spinal cord and the proximal parts of the spinal nerves.

■ **Central Nervous System (CNS) damage**

although monocytes and macrophages can be infected by HIV, they appear to be relatively resistant to killing. However, these cells travel throughout the body and carry HIV to various organs, especially the lungs and the brain. People infected with HIV often experience abnormalities in the central nervous system. Investigators have hypothesised that an accumulation of HIV in brain and nerve cells or the inappropriate release of cytokines or toxic by products by these cells may be to blame for the neurological manifestations of HIV disease.

■ **cephalosporins**

group of antimicrobial medications that interfered with peptidoglycan synthesis.

■ **cerebral**

relating to the brain. Pertaining to the cerebrum, the main portion of the brain.

■ **Cerebrospinal Fluid (CSF)**

fluid that bathes the brain and spinal cord.

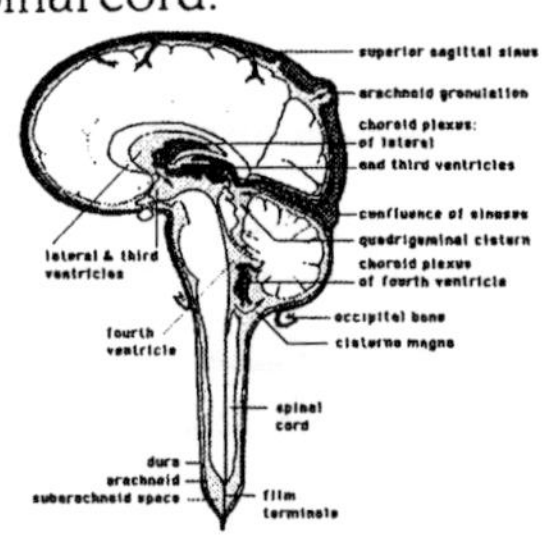

■ **cervical cancer**

neoplasm of the uterine cervix that can be detected in the early curable stage by the papanicolaou (PAP) test.

■ **cervical dysplasia**
development of abnormal tissue on the cervix, the lower part of the uterus. A precursor lesion for cervical cancer. Studies indicate an increase in prevalence of cervical dysplasia among HIV infected women. Additional studies have documented that a higher prevalence is associated with greater immuno suppression. HIV infection also may adversely affect the clinical course and treatment of cervical dysplasia and cancer.

■ **Cervical Intraepithelial Neoplasia (CIN1, CIN2, CIN3)**
dysplasia of the cervix epithelium, often pre malignant i.e., cancerous, characterised by various degrees of hyperplasia, abnormal keratinisation forming horny epidermal tissue and condylomata. Considerable evidence implicates Human Papilloma Virus (HPV) in the development of CIN. Immunosuppression may also play an important role in facilitating infection or persistence of HPV in the genital tract and progression of HPV induced neoplasia.

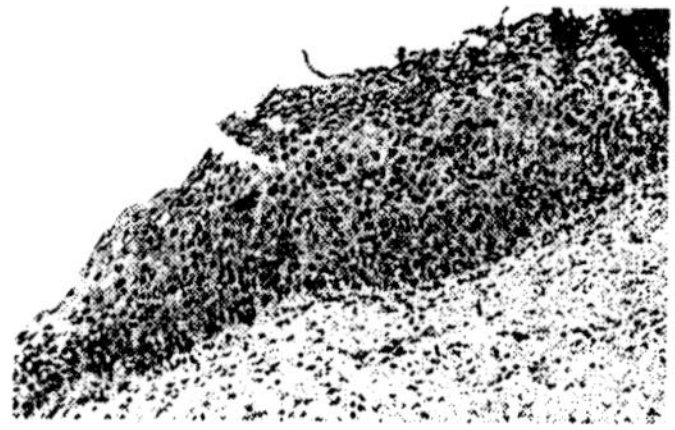

■ **cervix**
the cylindrical, lower part of the uterus that protrudes into the cavity of the vagina.

■ **cestode**
tapeworm.

■ **chaetomium sp.**
large ascomycetous fungus producing perithecia. It is found on a variety of substrates containing cellulose including paper and plant compost. It has been found on paper in sheetrock. It is reported to be allergenic. Can produce an Acremonium like state on fungal media.

■ **challenge**
in vaccine experiments, the exposure of an immunised animal to the infectious agent.

■ **chance**
random variation, i.e., the happening of events without an apparent cause.

■ **chancre**
sore resulting from an ulcerat-

ing infection. The 'hard chancre' of primary syphilis is typically firm and painless

■ **chaperones**
proteins that help other proteins fold properly.

■ **characteristics**
traits or attributes, those qualities that define or describe a thing or person

■ **chelate (chelator)**
organic chemical that forms ring compound in which a metal is held between two or more atoms strongly enough to diminish the rate at which it becomes fixed by soil, thereby making it more available for plant and microbial uptake.

■ **chemical bond**
force that holds atoms together to form molecules.

■ **chemically defined media**
bacteriological media composed of ingredients of known chemical composition, generally used for specific experiments when nutrients must be precisely controlled.

■ **chemiosmotic gradient**
accumulation of protons on one side of a membrane due to expulsion of protons by the electron transport chain, used to power the synthesis of ATP, fuel certain transport processes and drive the rotation of flagella. Also called the proton motive force.

■ **chemiosmotic theory**
theory that a proton gradient is formed by the electron transport chain and is then used to power the synthesis of ATP.

■ **chemoautotroph**
organism that obtains energy from the oxidation of chemical, generally inorganic, compounds and carbon from carbon dioxide.

■ **chemoautotrophs**
organisms that use inorganic chemicals as a source of energy and co_2 as the major source of carbon.

■ **chemoheterotroph**
organism that obtains energy and carbon from the oxidation of organic compounds.

■ **chemolithoautotrophs**
organisms that obtain energy by degrading reduced inorganic compounds such as hydrogen gas (H_2), and use CO_2 as a source of carbon.

■ **chemolithotroph**
organism that obtains energy from the oxidation of inorganic compounds and uses inorganic compounds as electron donors.

■ **chemoorganotroph**
organism that obtains energy and electrons (reducing power) from the oxidation of organic compounds.

■ **chemoprophylaxis**
prevention of disease by chemical means.

■ **chemostat**
device used to grow bacteria in the laboratory that allows nutrients to be added and waste products removed continuously.

■ **chemotaxis**
directed movement of an organism in response to a certain chemical in the environment.

■ **chemotherapeutic agent**
chemical used as a therapeutic medication to treat a disease.

■ **chemotherapy**
treatment of disease by chemical agents, usually, not always but mostly of cancer, by the use of a series of cytotoxic drugs that attack cancerous cells. This treatment commonly has adverse side effects that may include the temporary loss of the body's natural immunity to infections, loss of hair, digestive upset and a general feeling of illness. Although unpleasant, the adverse effects of treatment are tolerated considering the life threatening nature of the cancers usually treated by chemotherapy.

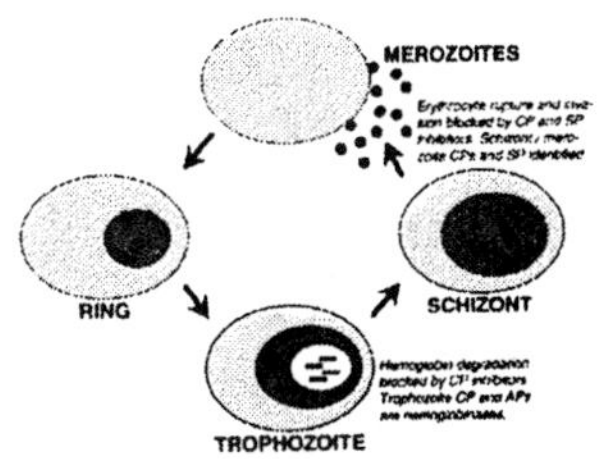

■ **chemotrophs**
organisms that obtain energy by degrading chemical compounds.

■ **chicken pox**
disease caused by the herpes virus, varicella.

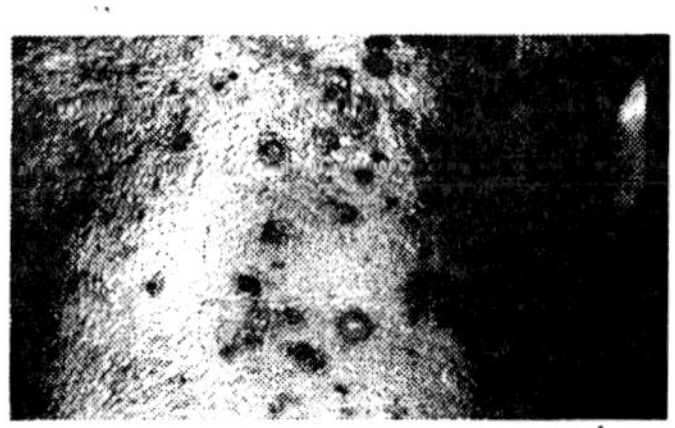

■ **chlamydospore**
thick walled resting structure that forms from the cell wall of

a fungal hypha, usually formed under conditions where the hypha is no longer able to function optimally.

■ **chloramphenicol**
antimicrobial medication that interferes with protein synthesis.

■ **chlorophyll**
green pigment required for photosynthesis.

■ **chloroplast**
chlorophyll containing organelle of photosynthetic eukaryotes.

■ **chocolate agar**
type of agar medium that contains red blood cells that have been heated under controlled conditions to lyse them, releasing their nutrients, used to culture fastidious bacteria.

■ **cholesterol**
sterol found in animal cell membranes, provides rigidity to eukaryotic membranes.

■ **chorea**
constant complex, rapid, jerky involuntary movements, an occasional sequel to untreated *streptococcus*

■ **chromatin**
complex of histones and DNA that make up the chromosomes of eukaryotic cells.

■ **chromatography**
any technique used to separate different species of molecules (or ions) by subjecting them to two different carrier phases mobile and stationary phases.

■ **chromosome**
array of genes responsible for the determination and transmission of hereditary characteristics.

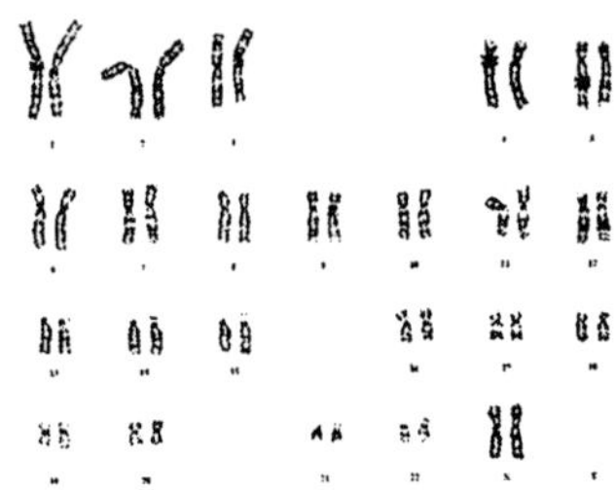

■ **chronic**
referring to a process, such as a disease process, that occurs slowly and persists over a long period of time, opposite of acute.

■ **Chronic Idiopathic Demyelinating Polyneuropathy (CIPD)**
chronic, spontaneous loss or destruction of myelin. Myelin is a

soft, white, somewhat fatty material that forms a thick sheath around the protoplasmic core of myelinated nerve fibre.

■ **chronic infections**
infections which develop slowly and persist for months or years.

■ **chytrid**
fungal organism in the phylum chytridiomycota that consists of a spherical cell from which short thin filamentous branches (rhizoids) grow that resemble fine roots.

■ **cidofovir**
experimental treatment for CMV

■ **ciliate**
protozoan that moves by means of cilia on the surface of the cell.

■ **cilium (pl. cilia)**
short, projecting hairline organelle of locomotion, similar to a flagellum.

Cilium/Flagellum Ultrastructure

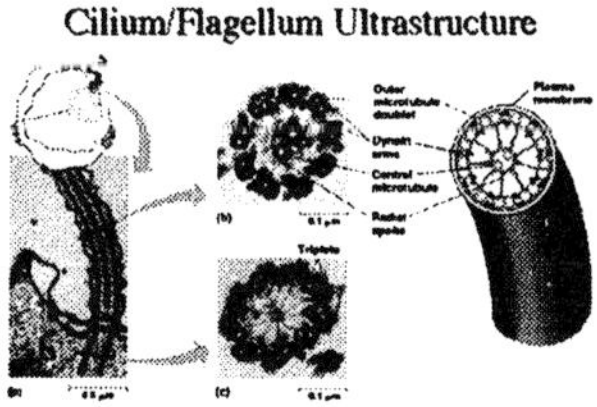

■ **ciprofloxacin (cipro)**
a flouroquinolone antibiotic, sometimes used in combination therapy for treatment of *mycobacterium avium* complex.

■ **circulative transmission**
transmission of viruses to plants by insects in which the virus circulates, but does not multiply in the body of the insect.

■ **citric acid cycle**
metabolic pathway that incorporates acetyl COA, ultimately generating co_2 and reducing power, also known as the tricarboxylic acid cycle (TCA cycle) and the krebs cycle.

■ **clade**
group of related HIV variants, classified according to degree of genetic similarity. HIV variants are currently grouped into clades A, B, C, D, E, F and O.

AN EXAMPLE OF A CLADE

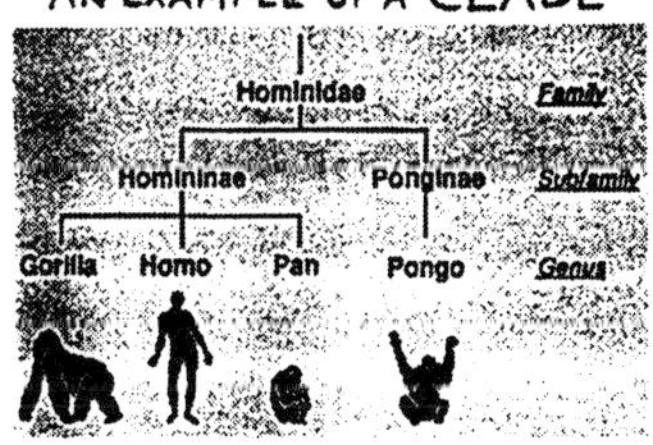

■ **cladosporium fulvum (fulvia fulva)**
conidia dimensions 12 47 x 4 10 microns. It is found on the leaves of tomatoes.

■ **cladosporium herbarum**
aw 0.88. Conidia dimensions 5 23 x 3 8 microns. It is found on dead plants, woody plants, food, straw, soil, paint and textiles.

■ **cladosporium macrocarpum**
conidia dimensions 9 29 x 5 13 microns. It is found on dead plants, woody plants, food, straw, soil, paint and textiles.

■ **cladosporium sp. (hormodendrum sp.)**
aw 0.88; Aw 0.84. Most commonly identified outdoor fungus. The outdoor numbers are reduced in the winter. The numbers are often high in the summer. Often found indoors in numbers less than outdoor numbers. It is a common allergen. Indoor Cladosporium sp. May be different than the species identified outdoors. It is commonly found on the surface of fibreglass duct liner in the interior of supply ducts. A wide variety of plants are food sources for this fungus. It is found on dead plants, woody plants, food, straw, soil, paint and textiles. It can cause mycosis. Produces greater than 10 antigens. Antigens in commercial extracts are of variable quality and may degrade within weeks of preparation. It is considered to be a common cause of extrinsic asthma (immediate type hypersensitivity type I). Acute symptoms include oedema and bronchiospasms, chronic cases may develop pulmonary emphysema.

■ **cladosporium sphaerospermum**
conidia dimensions 3 4.5 microns. It is found as a secondary invader of plants, food, soil, paint and textiles.

■ **clamp connection**
small branch of a fungal hypha that connects two compartments separated by a septum and helps to maintain a dikaryon in each hyphal compartment, characteristic of fungi in the phylum basidiomycota.

■ **clarithromycin (biaxin)**
macrolide antibiotic sometime used as a component in combination therapy for *mycobacterium avium* complex.

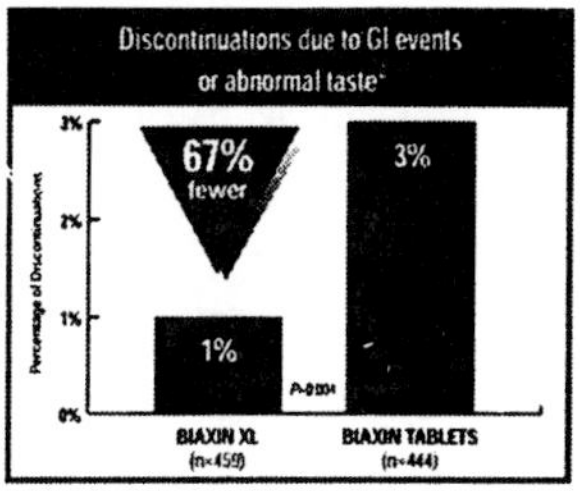

■ **class**

collection of similar orders, a collection of several classes makes up a phylum.

■ **classical pathway**

pathway of complement activation initiated by specific antigen antibody interaction.

■ **classification**

process of arranging organisms into similar or related groups, primarily to provide easy identification and study.

■ **clathrin**

proteins that line regions of eukaryotic cell membranes that are internalised during the process of endocytosis.

■ **clay**

soil particle < 0.002 mm in diameter.

■ **cleistothecium**

closed ascocarp of fungi in the phylum ascomycota.

■ **climax**

most advanced successional community of plants capable of development under, and in dynamic equilibrium with, the prevailing environment.

■ **clindamycin**

antibiotic sometimes used in the treatment of PCP and toxoplasmosis. Clindamycin usage has been associated with severe diarrhoea caused by the bacteria *c. Dificile.*

■ **clinic coordinator**

study nurse or other staff person who is the primary administrator and contact person for a research effort.

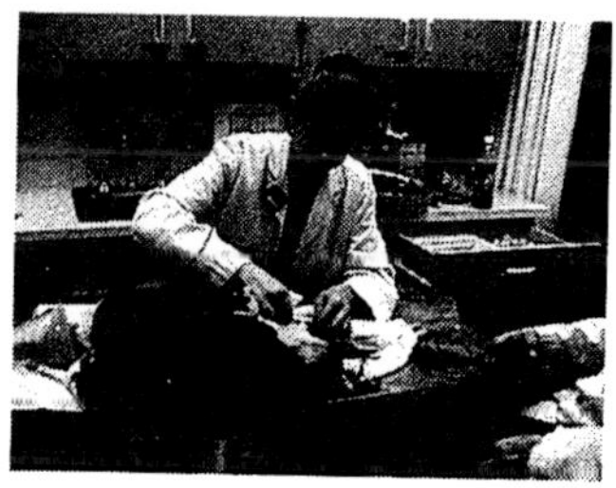

■ **clinical**

pertaining to or founded on actual observation and treatment of patients, as distinguished from theoretical or basic science.

■ **clinical alert**

mechanism for urgent cases in which timely and broad dissemination of results of clinical trials could prevent morbidity (sickness) and mortality (death). The clinical alert does not become a barrier to subsequent publication of the full research paper. Clinical alerts are widely distributed electronically through the national library of medicine and through standard mailings.

■ **clinical event committee**

group of physicians used to review endpoints in trials, and to evaluate their certainty.

■ **clinical latency**

state or period of an infectious agent, such as a virus or bacterium, living or developing in a host without producing clinical symptoms. As related to HIV infection although infected individuals usually exhibit a period of clinical latency with little evidence of disease, the virus is never truly latent. Even early in the disease, HIV is active within lymphoid organs where large amounts of virus become trapped in the FDC network. Surrounding germinal centres are areas rich in cd4+ t cells. These cells increasingly become infected and viral particles accumulate both in infected cells and as free virus.

HSV-1 Latency

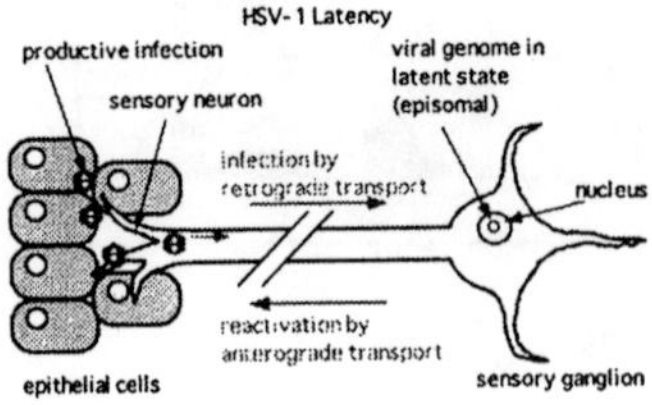

■ **clinical practice guidelines**

standards for physicians to adhere to, in prescribing care for a given condition or illness.

■ **Clinical Science Review Committee**

internal committee at the division of aids in charge of prioritising research, approving trial designs, coordinating intra and extramural efforts, and clearing specific protocols for implementation.

■ **clinical trial**

carefully designed and executed investigation of the effects of a drug or vaccine administered to human subjects. The goal is to define the clinical efficacy and pharmacological effects e.g. toxicity, side effects, incompatibilities or interactions of the drug.

■ **clofazimine**
anti leprosy drug that is used as a component in combination therapy of *mycobacterium avium* complex.

■ **clonal anergy**
inability of a clone of potentially responsive cells to respond immunologically.

■ **clonal deletion**
elimination of immature lymphocytes upon binding to self antigens to produce tolerance to self.

■ **clonal selection and expansion**
selection and activation of a lymphocyte by interaction of antigen and specific antigen receptor on the lymphocyte surface, causing the lymphocyte to proliferate to form an expanded clone.

■ **clone**
group of cells derived from a single cell.

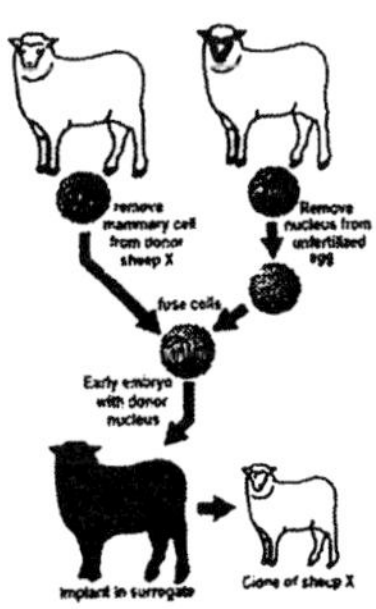

■ **cloning vector**
DNA molecule that is able to bring about the replication of foreign DNA fragments.

■ **cloning vehicle**
replicating piece of DNA into which genes of interest are introduced for the purpose of cloning the DNA.

■ **closed system**
batch system (such as a tube or flask of broth, or an agar plate) used for growing micro-organisms, nutrients are not replenished and wastes are not removed.

■ **clostridium dificile (c. dificile)**
normal gastrointestinal tract bacteria. Antibiotics can cause overgrowth of *c dificile*, and accompanying perforating enterocolitis

■ **clotrimazole**
topical antifungal drug that is used to treat fungal infections in persons with HIV, particularly candida.

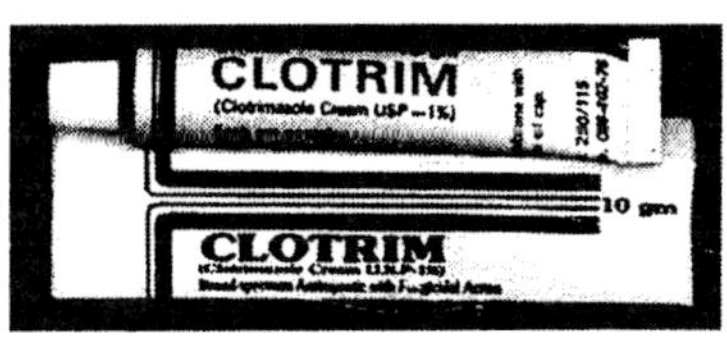

■ **clusters of differentiation (CD) antigens**
cell surface antigens identified by clusters or groups of monoclonal antibodies, used to distinguish subgroups of white blood cells

■ **CMI**
abbreviation for cell mediated immunity

■ **CO_2 fixation**
process of converting inorganic carbon (CO_2) to an organic form.

■ **coagulase**
non-enzymatic product of *staphylococcus aureus* that clots plasma.

■ **coccidioidomycosis**
infectious fungal disease caused by the inhalation of spores of coccidioides immitis, which is carried on windblown dust particles. The disease is endemic in hot dry regions of the South Western US and Central and South America, and is an opportunistic disease associated with aids. Also called desert fever, san joaquin fever, valley fever.

■ **coccus**
spherical bacterial cells.

■ **codon**
set of three nucleotides.

■ **coenocytic**
fungal hypha without crosswalls (septa), so that the nuclei present in the cytoplasm are free floating and mobile.

■ **coenzyme**
small organic molecule that transfers small molecules from one enzyme to another.

■ **coenzyme a**
coenzyme involved in decarboxylation.

■ **cofactors**
substances, micro-organisms or characteristics of individuals that may influence the progression of a disease or the likelihood of becoming ill.

■ **cognitive**
pertaining to thought, awareness, or the ability to rationally apprehend the world and abstract meaning.

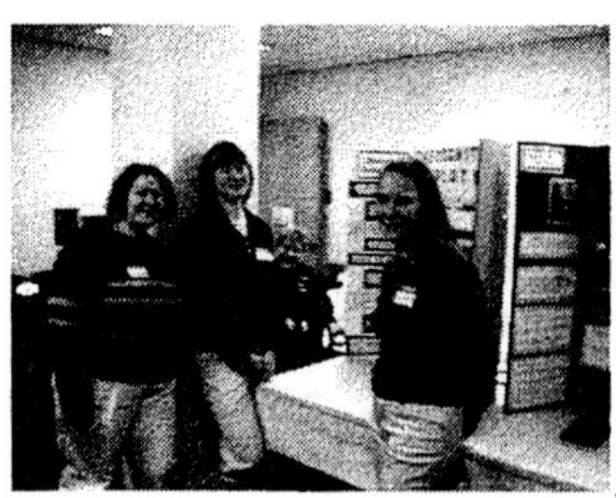

■ **cohesion**
force holding a solid or liquid together, owing to attraction between like molecules.

■ **cohesive ends**
single stranded overhangs generated when DNA is digested with a restriction enzyme that cuts asymmetrically within the recognition sequence, sticky ends.

■ **cohort**
in epidemiology, the term describes a group of individuals with some characteristics in common.

■ **cohort group**
population with a known exposure to a specific risk factor that is followed over time in a prospective study.

■ **coliform**
gram negative, nonspore forming facultative rod that ferments lactose with gas formation with 48 hours at 35°c. Often an indicator organism for faecal contamination of water supplies. *Escherichia coli* and *enterobacter* are important members.

■ **coliforms**
facultative, nonspore forming, gram negative rods that ferment lactose, producing acid and gas within 48 hours at 35°c, because most typically reside in the intestine they are used as indicators of faecal pollution.

■ **colitis**
inflammation of the colon

■ **colloid fraction**
organic and inorganic matter with very small particle size and a correspondingly large surface area per unit of mass.

■ **colon**
division of the lower intestine, extending from the caecum to the rectum; also called the large intestine.

■ **colonisation**
residence of bacteria in, or on, part of the body and causing neither disease nor a response from the individual's immune system.

■ **colony**
population of bacterial cells arising from a single cell.

■ **colony blot**
technique that uses a probe to detect a given DNA sequence in colony.

■ **colony forming unit**
unit that gives rise to a single colony, may be a single cell or

multiple cells attached to one another

■ **colourectal**
relating to the colon and rectum, or to the entire large bowel (large intestine).

■ **colposcopy**
type of examination of a living tissue surface, under magnification, to identify location and extent of lesions.

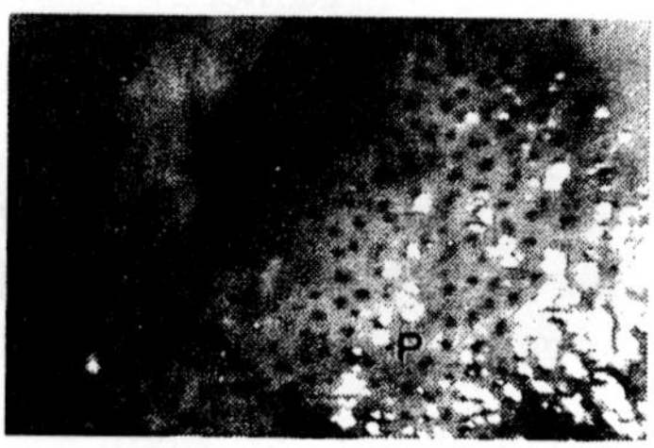

■ **combination therapy**
administration of two antibiotics simultaneously to prevent growth of mutants that might be resistant to one of the antibiotics

■ **cometabolism**
transformation of a substrate by a micro-organism without deriving energy, carbon, or nutrients from the substrate. The organism can transform the substrate into intermediate degradation products but fails to multiply at its expense.

■ **commensalism**
relationship between two organisms in which one partner benefits from the association and the other is unaffected.

■ **commercially sterile**
free of all micro-organisms capable of growing under normal storage conditions, the endospores of some thermophiles may remain.

■ **common source epidemic**
outbreak of disease due to contaminated food, water, or other single source of infectious agent.

■ **communicable diseases**
diseases that are spread from an infected animal or person to another animal or person.

■ **communities**
all of the living organisms in a given area.

■ **community**
all organisms that occupy a common habitat and interact with one another.

■ **compassionate use**
method of providing unapproved drugs to very sick patients who have no other treatment options.

■ **competent**
in a genetic sense, the ability to take up DNA.

■ **competition**
rivalry between two or more species for a limiting factor in the environment that usually results in reduced growth of participating organisms.

■ **competitive inhibition**
type of enzyme inhibition that occurs when the inhibitor competes with the normal substrate for binding to the active site.

■ **complement**
group of proteins in normal blood serum and plasma who combine with antibodies, causing the destruction of antigens (particularly bacteria and foreign blood corpuscles).

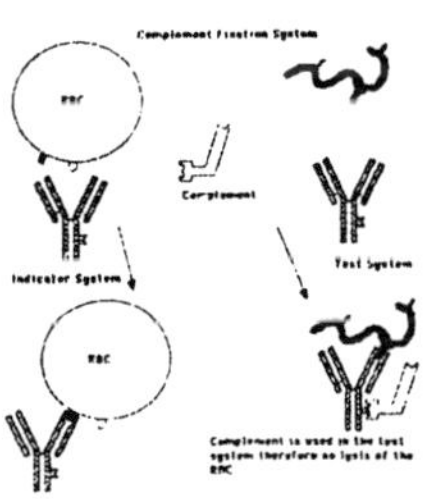

■ **complement cascade**
precise sequence of events, triggered by an antigen antibody complex where each component of the complement system is activated in turn, inactivating and occasionally destroying the pathogens.

■ **complement fixation test**
serological method in which antibody antigen reactions are detected by the consumption (fixation) of complement.

■ **complementary**
bases in nucleic acid in which hydrogen bond to one another, a (adenine) is complementary to t (thymine) and g (guanine) is complementary to c (cytosine).

■ **Complete Blood Count (CBC)**
breakdown of the various cells in a sample of blood into white cells, red blood cells, platelets, etc.

■ **complex medium**
medium for growing bacteria that has some ingredients of unknown chemical composition.

■ **compliance**
how closely a particular protocol is followed. May be influenced by the willingness and/or ability of patients to conform to treatment by taking medications as prescribed and keeping necessary clinic appointments. Often the resources available to the

patient, and the resources and flexibility of the provider will have as great an implication for compliance as any specific patient behaviour.

- **compost**
organic residues which have been mixed, piled, and moistened, with or without addition of fertilizer and lime, and generally allowed to undergo thermophilic decomposition until the original organic materials are substantially altered or decomposed.

- **compound microscope**
microscope that employs two magnifying lenses, an objective lens and an ocular lens. The lenses in combination visually enlarge an object by a factor equal to the product of each lens' magnification.

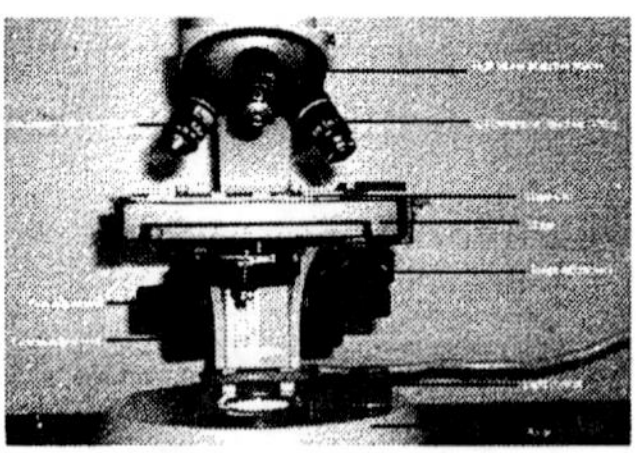

- **Computed Tomography (CAT/CT scan)**
a kind of computer aided imaging that assembles multiple X rays of 'slices' of the body to produce a three dimensional picture.

- **concomitant drugs**
drugs that are taken together at the same time. Certain concomitant medications may have adverse interactions.

- **concorde study**
joint French/British clinical trial of AZT in asymptomatic HIV positive individuals

- **condenser lens**
lens of a microscope that is used to focus the illumination, positioned between the light source and the specimen and does not effect the magnification.

- **conditional lethal mutant**
mutant which under some environmental conditions will grow but under other conditions will not grow.

condyloma(condyloma acuminatum).
a papilloma with a central core of connective tissue in a treelike structure covered with epithelium, usually occurring on the mucous membrane or skin of the external genitals or in the perianal i.e. tissue surrounding the anus region. Although the lesions are usually few in num-

ber, they may aggregate to form large cauliflower like masses. Caused by the human papilloma virus (HPV), it is infectious and autoinoculable i.e. capable of being transmitted by inoculation from one part of the body to another. Also called acuminate or venereal warts.

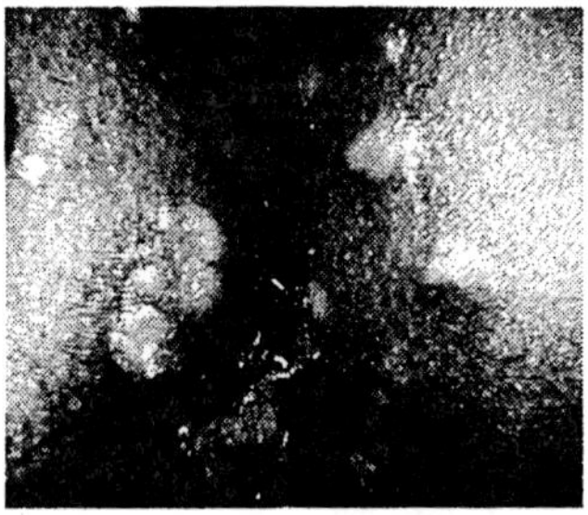

■ **confidence interval**
the range of values that includes, with a stated probability (e.g. 95%), the actual population descriptor of interest.

■ **confocal scanning laser microscope**
type of microscope that focuses a laser beam to illuminate a given point on one vertical plane of a specimen. After successive regions and planes have been scanned, a computer can construct a three dimensional image of a thick structure.

■ **congenital**
condition existing from the time of birth.

■ **conidia**
asexual spores borne on hyphae, produced by fungi and bacteria of the genus *streptomyces.*

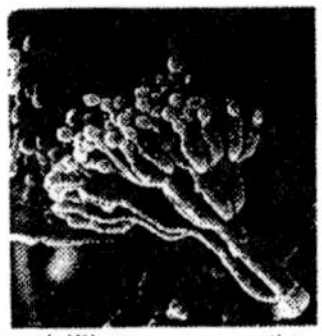

penicillium conidiophore

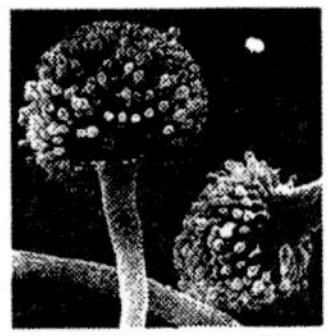

aspergillus conidiophore

■ **conidiophore**
aerial hypha bearing conidia.

■ **conidium (pl. conidia)**
nonmotile, asexual spore resulting from mitotic nuclear division and formed from the ends or sides of a hypha; produced in abundant numbers by the asexual phase of soil fungi in the phyla ascomycota and basidiomycota.

■ **conidobolus sp.**
can cause a chronic inflammatory disease of the nasal mucosa (entomophthoromycosis).

■ **conjugation**
mechanism of gene transfer in bacteria that involves cell to cell contact.

- **conjugative plasmid**
plasmid that carries the genes for sex pili and can transfer copies of itself to other bacteria during conjugation.

- **conjugative plasmid**
self transmissible plasmid, a plasmid that encodes all the functions needed for its own intercellular transmission by conjugation.

- **conjunctivitis**
inflammation of the protective membrane surrounding the eye.

- **connective tissue**
tissue that surrounds other more highly ordered tissues and organs, blood, cartilage and bone.

- **consensus sequence**
common theme of nucleotides that characterise a stretch of DNA that has a certain function.

- **consortium**
two or more members of a natural assemblage in which each organism benefits from the other. The group may collectively carryout some process that no single member can accomplish on its own.

- **constant region**
that part of the antibody molecule that does not vary in amino acid sequences among molecules of the same immunoglobulin class.

- **constitutive enzyme**
enzyme always synthesised by the cell regardless of environmental conditions.

- **consumption**
stage of biogeochemical recycling in which consumer organisms metabolise the organic materials made by producers.

- **contact dermatitis**
T-cell mediated inflammation of the skin occurring in sensitised individuals as a result of contact with the particular antigen, a form of delayed hypersensitivity.

- **contagious**
any infectious disease that is capable of being transmitted by casual contact from one person to another. Casual contact can be defined as normal day to day contact between people at home, school, work or in the community. A contagious infection e.g., a common cold can be communicable by casual

contact, an infectious infection, on the other hand, is communicable by intimate contact such as sex. AIDS is infectious, not contagious.

■ **contagious diseases**
diseases that are highly communicable and are spread from one host to another very readily.

■ **continuous culture**
method used to maintain cells in a state of uninterrupted growth by continuously adding nutrients and removing waste products, a type of open system.

■ **contraindication ('to indicate against')**
specific circumstance when the use of certain treatments could be harmful.

■ **control**
standard against which, experimental observations are evaluated. In clinical trials, one group of patients is given an experimental drug, while another group i.e., the control group is given either a standard treatment for the disease or a placebo.

■ **controlled**
constrained, monitored or watched.

■ **controlled clinical trial**
clinical trial involving one or more test treatments, at least one control treatment, and concurrent enrolment, treatment, and follow up of all patients in the trial.

■ **convalescence**
period of recuperation and recovery from an illness.

■ **convergent evolution**
process of evolution when two genetically different organisms develop similar environmental adaptations.

■ **cooperative clinical trial**
term frequently used to denote a multi centre trial.

■ **coordinating centre**
centre in the structure of a study that is responsible for receiving, editing, processing, analysing, and storing data generated in a study and that, in addition, has responsibility for coordination of activities required for execution of the study.

■ **core protein**
as related to HIV an integral protein of the HIV virus.

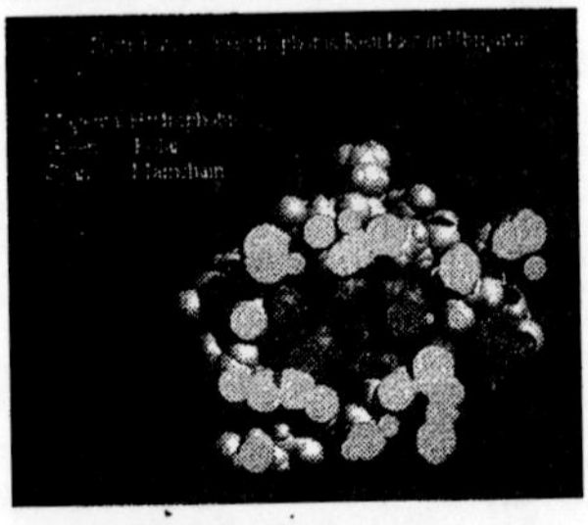

■ **co repressor**
molecule that binds to an inactive repressor and, as a consequence, enables it to function as a repressor.

■ **correlates of immunity/ protection**
immune responses that protect an individual from a certain disease. The precise identities of the correlates of immunity in HIV are unknown.

■ **correlation(Pearson r)**
a statistical technique used to assess the magnitude and the direction of the relationship between two variables. Values of the Pearson r can range between 1 and + 1. The continuum of 1 to 0 indicates the degree of strength of an inverse relationship. The continuum of 0 to + 1 indicates the degree of strength of a positive relationship. A Pearson r of 0 indicates no linear relationship. For example, bicycle helmet use and bicycle accident head injury are negatively correlated; asbestos exposure and cumulative incidence of mesothelioma are positively correlated.

■ **cortex**
exterior or surrounding portion of an organ.

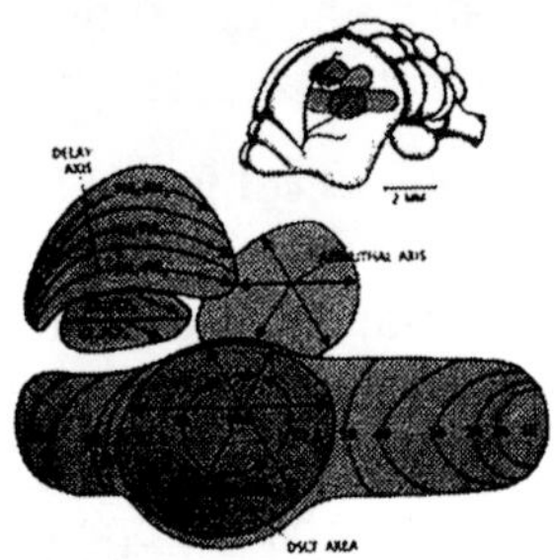

■ **corticosteroids**
any of a number of steroid substances obtained from the cortex of the adrenal gland or manufactured synthetically. Corticosteroids are immunosuppressive and people with HIV should be cautious about taking them for longer than a few weeks. Steroids appear to be an effective adjunct to standard PCP treatments in people with moderate to severe PCP.

■ **counterstain**
in a differential staining procedure, the stain applied to im-

part a contrasting colour to bacteria that do not retain the primary stain.

■ **covalent**
non-ionic chemical bond formed by a sharing of electrons between two atoms.

■ **covalent bond**
strong chemical bond formed by the sharing of electrons between atoms.

■ **creatinine**
protein found in muscles and blood and excreted by the kidneys in the urine. The level of creatinine in the blood and urine provides a measure of kidney function.

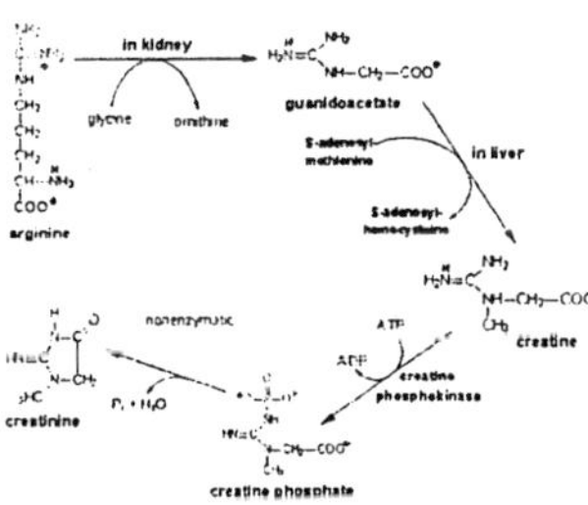

■ **creatinine kinase (creatinine phospho kinase)**
enzyme found in the muscles. High levels in the blood indicate breakdown of muscle tissue. In aids, may be diagnostic of myopathy.

■ **critical items**
medical instruments such as needles and scalpels that come into direct contact with body tissue.

■ **cross contamination**
transfer of pathogens from one item to another.

■ **crossed treatments**
two or more study treatments that are used in sequence e.g., as in a crossover design or in combination e.g., as in a factorial treatment structure.

■ **cross feeding**
specific type of syntrophy where two populations cooperate to metabolise a compound.

■ **crossover**
treatment crossover. A patient who does not comply to assigned treatment and begins to adhere to one of the other treatments. Patient may be a drop in or drop out, depending on the direction of the crossover.

■ **crossover design**
crossover treatment design. Patients are given treatments in sequence, and crossover is determined by time, not clinical outcomes.

■ **cross sectional study**
study that surveys a range of people to determine the prevalence of characteristics including disease, risk factors associated with disease, or previous exposure to a disease causing agent.

■ **croup**
acute obstruction of the larynx occurring mainly in infants and young children, often resulting from respiratory syncytial or other viral infection

■ **crown gall tumour**
tumour on a plant caused by agrobacterium sp.

■ **cryotherapy**
the use of intense cold as a treatment, as in freezing off warts.

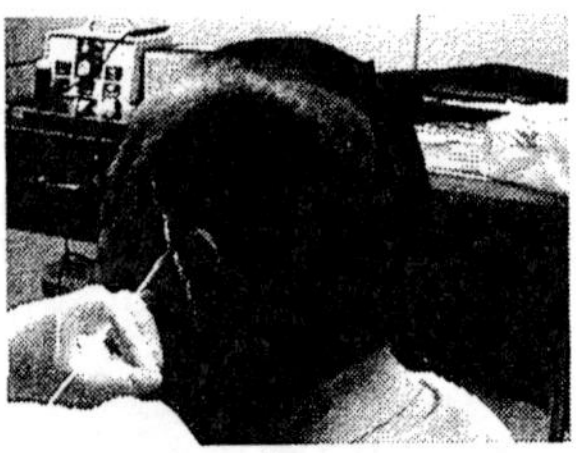

■ **cryptococcal meningitis**
life threatening infection of the membranes i.e. meninges that line the brain and the spinal cord. Cryptococcal disease is caused by a fungus (cryptococcus neoformans). Most people have been exposed to this organism, which is found in soil contaminated by bird droppings, but it usually does not cause disease in healthy people. The majority of people with cryptococcal meningitis have immune systems that are damaged by disease, such as aids, or suppressed by drugs. The organism can infect almost all organs of the body, although it most commonly causes disease of the meninges, skin or lungs.

■ **cryptococcosis**
infectious disease seen in HIV infected patients due to the fungus cryptococcus neoformans, which is acquired via the respiratory tract. It can spread from the lungs to the brain, the central nervous system, the skin, skeletal system and urinary tract.

■ **cryptococcus neoformans**
fungus, pathogenic in the immune suppressed, which is acquired via the respiratory tract. Cryptococcosis most frequently causes meningitis, with symptoms of headache and stiff neck.

■ **cryptosporidiosis**
opportunistic infection caused by the protozoan parasite cryptosporidium parvum.

- **cryptosporidium parvum**
waterborne enterocyte protozoan, *c. Parvum* is often deposited in water supply by wild or domestic animals. *C parvum* has caused at least one large epidemic of diarrhoeal disease through contamination of a municipal water supply.

- **cryptostroma corticale**
conidia dimensions 4 6.5 x 3.5 4 microns. Found on the bark of maple and sycamore trees and on stored logs.

- **CSF**
abbreviation for colony stimulating factor.

- **CT**
abbreviation for Computed Tomography. Radiography using x rays creates a three dimensional image of a body structure by computer, using a series of plane cross sectional images made along an axis. Also referred to as CAT scan.

- **culture**
process of growing bacteria or other micro-organisms in the laboratory, so that organisms can be identified.

- **cunninghamella sp.**
can cause disseminated and pulmonary infections in immune compromised hosts.

- **curd**
coagulated milk proteins, produced during cheese making. reported to be allergenic. It may cause corneal infections, mycetoma and infections in immune compromised hosts.

- **cutaneous**
of, pertaining to or affecting the skin.

- **cut point**
point or value in an ordered sequence of values that is used to separate those values into two subparts.

- **cyanobacterium**
prokaryotic, oxygenic phototrophic bacterium containing chlorophyll *a* and phycobilins, formerly the 'blue green algae.'

- **Cyclic AMP activating protein (CAP)**
protein that binds to camp to promote gene transcription.

- **cyclic photophosphorylation**
type of photophosphorylation in which electrons are returned directly to the chlorophyll; used to synthesise atp without generating reducing power.

■ **cyst**
dormant resting protozoan cell characterised by a thickened cell wall.

■ **cysticercus(pl. Cysticerci)**
cyst like larval form of tapeworms.

■ **cystitis**
inflammation of the urinary bladder.

■ **cytochrome**
1. iron containing porphyrin ring (e.g., heme) complexed with proteins which act as electron carriers in an electron transport chain.
2. proteins that carry electrons usually as members of electron transport chains.

■ **cytokine**
1. immune system proteins involved in the normal regulation of the immune response. A chemical messenger protein released by certain white blood cells, including macrophages, monocytes or lymphocytes, the cytokines include the interferons, the interleukins, tumor necrosis factor, and many others. Cytokines produced by lymphatic cells are also called 'lymphokines'.
2. low molecular weight regulatory proteins made by cells that affect the behaviour of other cells, attach to specific cytokine receptors and are essential for communication between cells.

■ **cytolytic**
having a destructive effect on cells, causing them to erupt or burst open.

■ **cytomegalovirus (CMV)**
herpes virus, a common cause of opportunistic diseases in people with AIDS and others with suppressed immune system. While CMV can infect most organs of the body, people with aids are most susceptible to CMV retinitis (disease of the eye) and Colitis (disease of the colon).

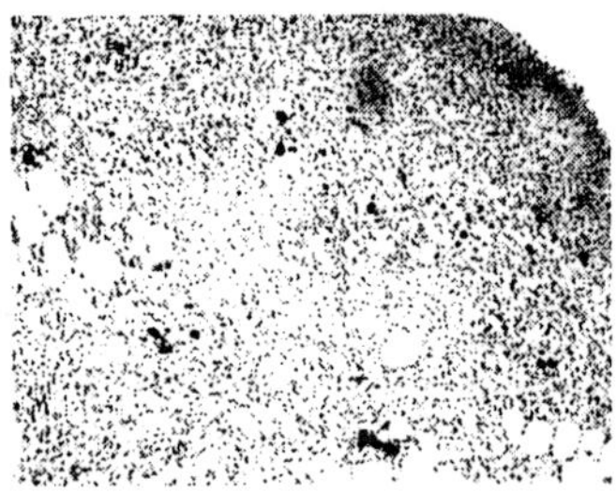

■ **cytomegalovirus (CMV) retinitis**
most adults in the US have been infected by cytomegalovirus, although the virus usually does not cause disease

in healthy people. Because the virus remains in the body for life, it can cause disease if the immune system becomes severely damaged by disease or suppressed by drugs. CMV retinitis is an eye disease common among people who are infected with HIV. Without treatment, people with CMV retinitis can lose their vision. CMV infection can affect both eyes and is the most common cause of blindness among people with aids.

■ **cytometry**
counting of cells, especially blood cells, using a cytometer i.e. a standardised, ruled glass slide or small glass chamber of known volume.

■ **cytopathic effect**
observable change in a cell in vitro produced by viral action such as lysis of the cell.

■ **cytopenia**
lack of specific cellular components in the blood signifying deficiency in the cellular elements of the blood.

■ **cytoplasm**
all of the substance of a cell other than the nucleus.

■ **cytoplasmic membrane**
flexible structure immediately surrounding the cytoplasm of all cells.

■ **cytoskeleton**
dynamic filamentous network that provides structure and shape to eukaryotic cells.

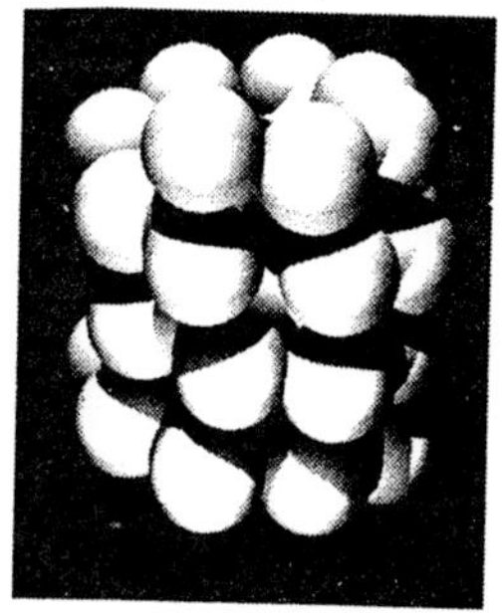

■ **cytotoxic**
kills cells.

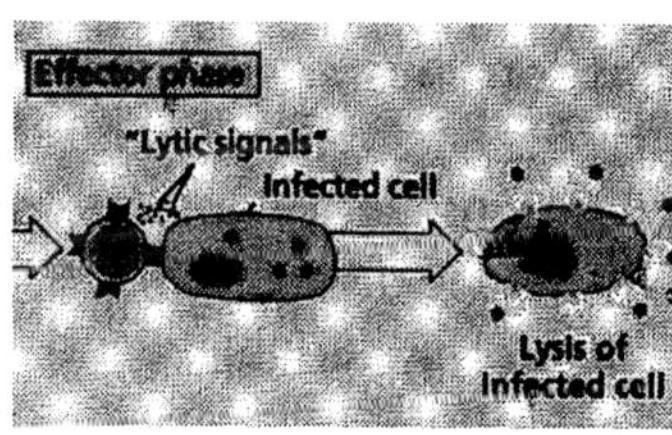

■ **Cytotoxic T Lymphocyte (CTL)**
lymphocyte that is able to kill foreign cells that have been marked for destruction by the cellular immune system.

■ **d4t**
also known as stavudine and zerit. d4t is a dideoxynucleoside

pyrimidine analog (2'3' didehydro 3' deoxythymidine). Like other nucleoside analogs, d4t inhibits HIV replication by inducing premature viral DNA chain termination. d4t has been approved for patients with advanced HIV infection intolerant to or failing other antiretroviral drugs.

■ **dapsone**

antibiotic active against *pneumocystis carinii*, leprosy, and other pathogens, and to a lesser degree against *toxoplasma gondii* and mac. Often used as a second line PCP prophylaxis in those unable to tolerate trimethoprim sulphamethoxazole.

■ **dark reactions**

process of carbon fixation in photosynthetic organisms, the ATP used to drive the process is obtained in the light reactions, the dark reactions are called the light independent reactions.

■ **dark repair**

enzymes of DNA repair that do not depend on visible light.

■ **dark field microscope**

type of microscope that directs light toward the specimen at an angle, so that only light scattered by the specimen enters the objective lens; material in the specimen stands out as bright objects against a dark background.

■ **data (pl. of datum)**

factual information, such as measurements, observations, or statistics used as a basis for reasoning, discussion or calculation.

■ **Data And Safety Monitoring Board (DSMB)**

standing committee responsible for periodically reviewing accumulated data for evidence of adverse or beneficial treatment effects during the trial and for initiating recommendations for modification of a study treatment, including termination of the treatment when appropriate.

■ **data collection visit**

any visit by a patient to a study clinic that is used for data collection in the trial.

■ **data dredging**

term used to characterise analyses that are done on an ad hoc basis, without benefit of pre stated hypotheses.

■ **data editing**

process of reviewing data for the purpose of detecting deficiencies or errors in the way they are collected or recorded.

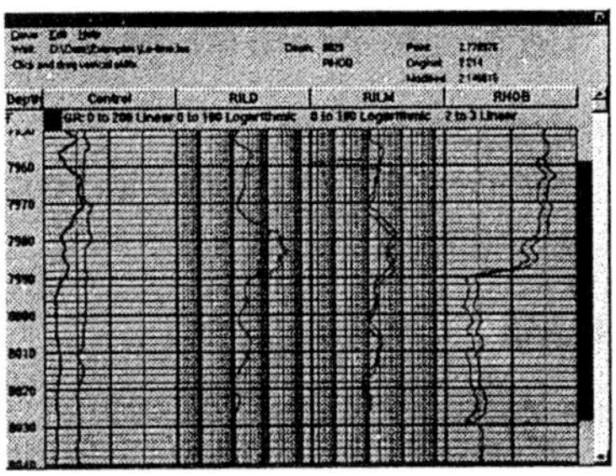

■ **data entry**

process of keying data, as contained on completed data forms, in order to render information into an arrangement more suitable for storage and subsequent use, usually for tabulations and analyses, especially on a computer.

■ **data field**

space on a data form or in an electronic record designated to contain, or that actually contains, alphabetic or numeric characters of information recorded in response to a specific data item on the form.

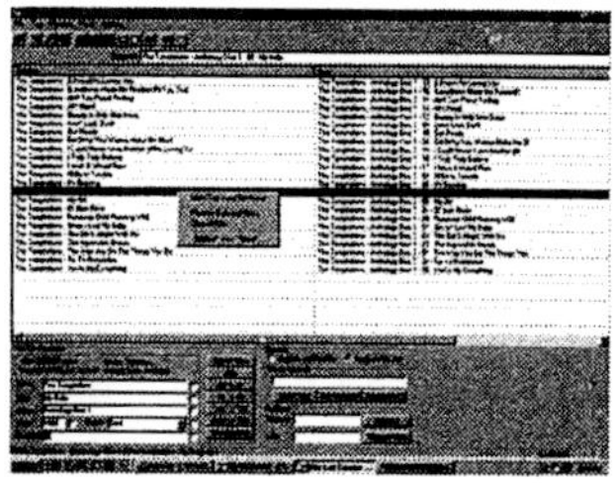

■ **data file**

collection of data records. The collection may be of paper records or of electronic records that are arraved in some way.

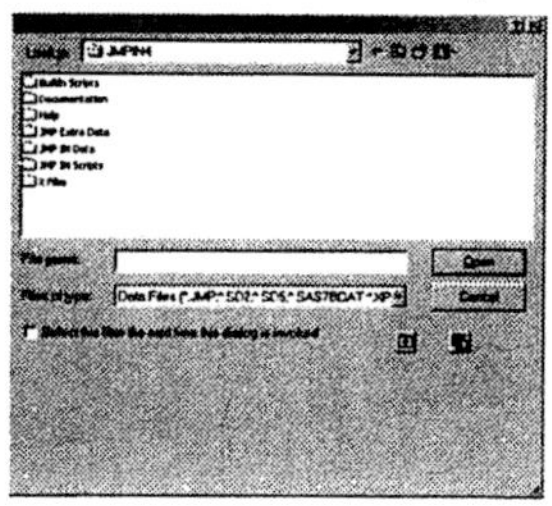

■ **data item**

question or statement appearing on a data form.

■ **data (interval)**

data classified into equal intervals without an absolute zero point, e.g., IQ of 120 is 60 points higher than an IQ of 60, but this does not necessarily indicate twice as much intelligence. Temperature is another example.

■ **data (nominal)**

data classified into unordered categories, e.g., male/female, diabetes/no diabetes, mammogram yes/mammogram no.

■ **data (ordinal)**
data classified into ordered categories, e.g., intensity of pain (+/++/+++/++++), severity of disease (mild/moderate/severe/fatal).

■ **database**
a collection of data files that are organised in a specified manner, used in the analysis of trials.

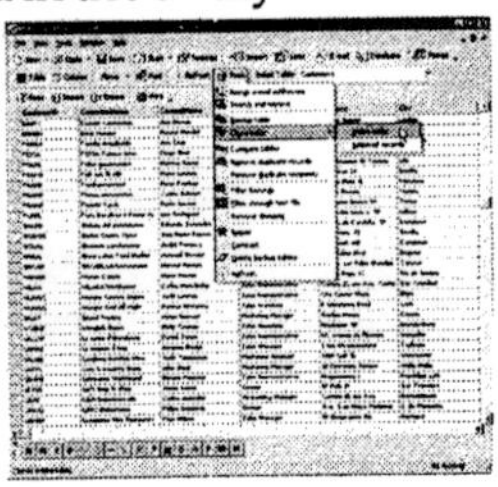

■ **datum**
singular of data.

■ **dc**
discontinuation (of treatment)

■ **ddc**
dideoxycytidine (zalcitabine, HIVid), a nucleoside analog drug that inhibits the replication of HIV.

■ **ddi**
dideoxyinosine (didanosine, videx), a nucleoside analog drug that inhibits the replication of HIV.

■ **death phase**
stage in which the number of viable bacteria in a population decreases at an exponential rate.

■ **deca**
prefix meaning ten times, as in decagram, or ten grams.

■ **decarboxylation**
removal of carbon dioxide from a chemical.

■ **deci**
prefix meaning one tenth, as in decigram, or a tenth of a gram.

■ **decimal reduction time**
time required for 90% of the organisms to be killed under specific conditions, d value.

■ **decomposer**
heterotrophic organism that breaks down organic compounds.

■ **decomposition**
chemical breakdown of a compound into simpler compounds, often accomplished by microbial metabolism.

■ **decontamination**
treatment to reduce the number of disease causing organisms to a level that it is considered safe.

■ **deficit**
lack, or shortfall.

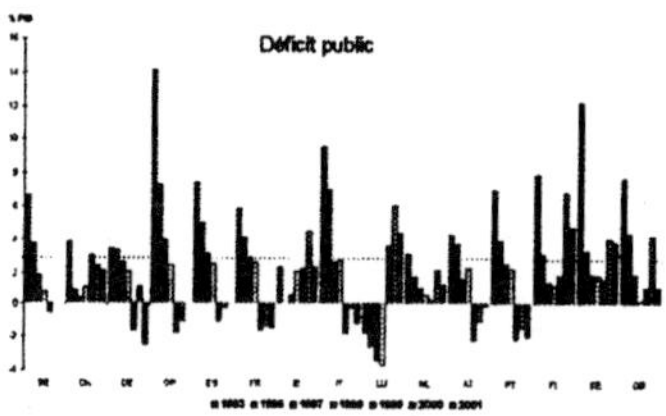

■ **defined medium**
medium whose exact chemical composition is quantitatively known.

■ **degeneration**
deterioration, change from a higher to lower form, especially as in change to less functional or healthy tissue.

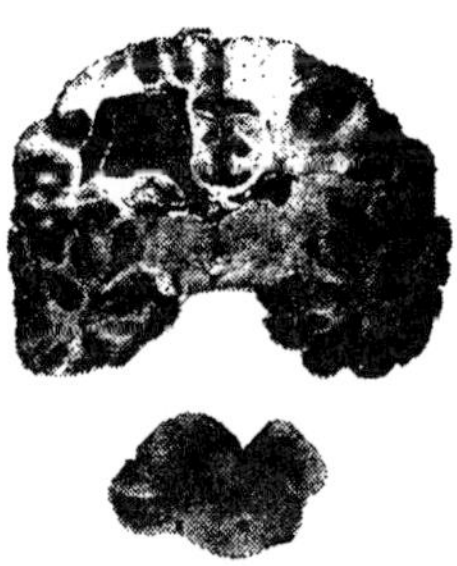

■ **degradation**
process whereby a compound is usually transformed into simpler compounds.

■ **degranulation**
release of mediators from granules in the cell, as histamine release from mast cells.

■ **dehydration synthesis**
chemical reaction in which water is removed with the result that two molecules are joined together.

■ **dehydrogenation**
oxidation reaction in which both an electron and an accompanying proton are removed.

■ **delayed hypersensitivity**
hypersensitivity caused by cytokines released from sensitised T lymphocytes; reactions occur within 48 to 72 hours after exposure of a sensitised individual to antigen.

■ **delayed type hypersensitivity (DTH)**
cell mediated immune response that produces a cellular infiltrate and oedema, redness and induration i.e. hardness between 48 and 72 hours after exposure to an antigen. DTH response is the basis for PPD testing of tuberculosis exposure.

■ **deletion**
elimination of a gene from a chromosome, either in nature or in the laboratory.

■ **demarcate**
to separate or to indicate the interface between two areas.

■ **dementia**
chronic intellectual impairment i.e. loss of mental capacity with organic origins, that affects a person's ability to function in a social or occupational setting.

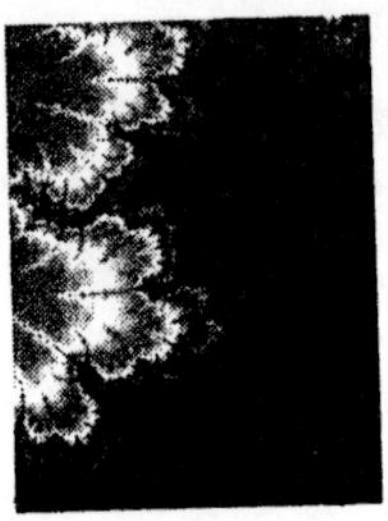

■ **demyelination**
destruction, removal or loss of the myelin sheath of a nerve or nerves.

■ **denaturation**
disruption of the three dimensional structure of a protein molecule.

■ **dendrite**
any of the usual branching protoplasmic processes that direct impulses towards the body of a nerve cell.

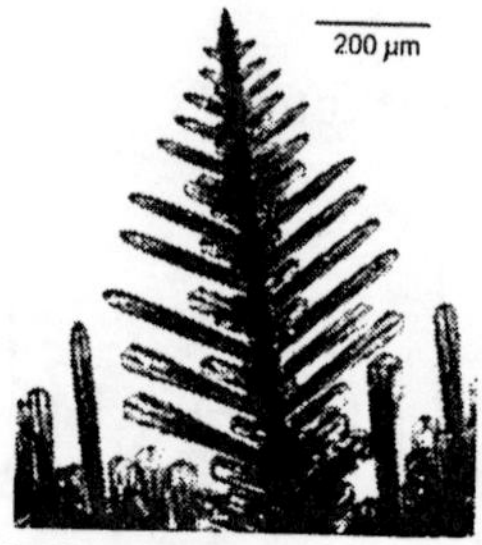

■ **dendritic cells**
cells with a branched morphology, some of which are related to macrophages, some are antigen presenting cells.

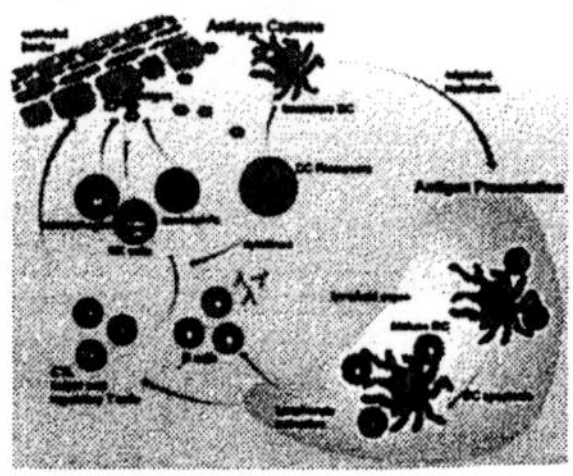

■ **denitrification**
bacterial conversion of nitrate to gaseous nitrogen by anaerobic respiration.

■ **dental plaque**
a biofilm on teeth.

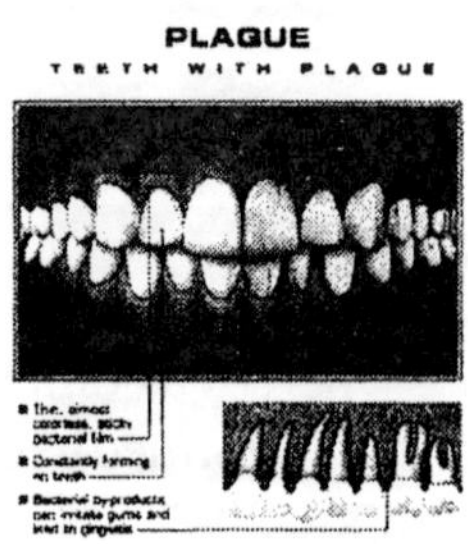

■ **deoxyribonucleic acid (DNA)**
macromolecule in the cell that carries the genetic information.

■ **depth filter**
type of filter with complex, tortuous passages that allow the suspending fluid pass through while retaining micro-organisms.

■ **derepressible enzyme**
enzyme that is produced in the absence of a specific inhibitory compound acting at the transcriptional level.

■ **dermal**
relating to the skin.

■ **dermatophytes**
certain mould like fungi that live on the skin and can be responsible for disease of the hair, nails and skin.

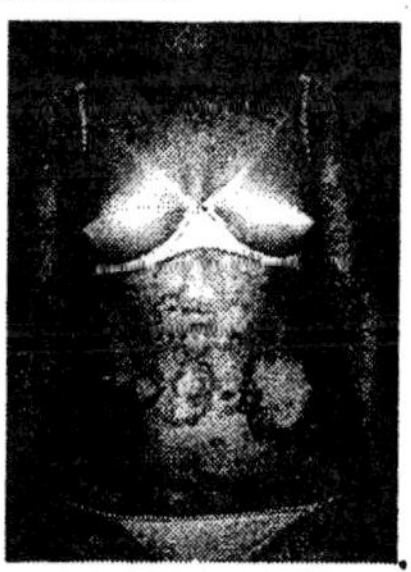

■ **descriptive study**
type of study that seeks to characterise a disease outbreak by determining the characteristics of the persons involved and the place and time of the outbreak.

■ **desquamating**
shedding or losing skin, particularly as in grade 3 and 4 rashes

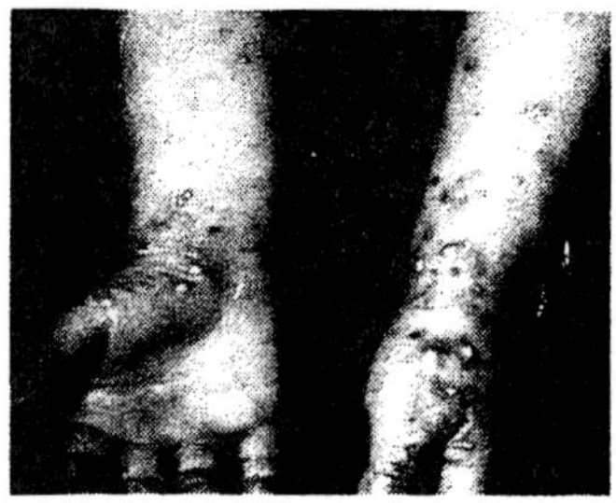

■ **diagnosis**
determination of the presence of a specific disease or infection, usually accomplished by evaluating clinical symptoms and laboratory tests.

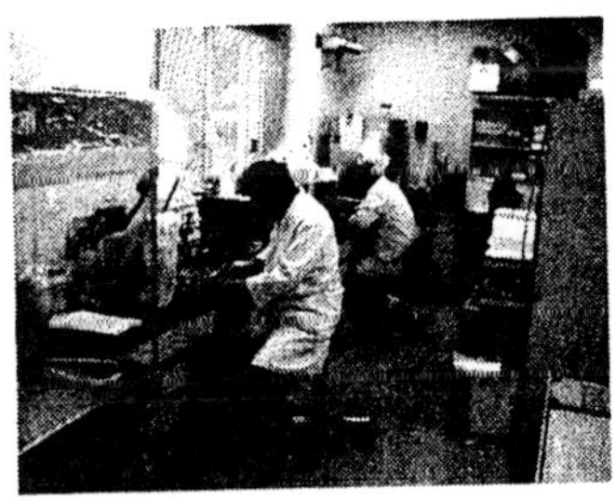

■ **diapedesis**
movement of leukocytes from blood vessels into tissues in response to a chemotactic stimulus during inflammation.

■ **diarrhoea**

uncontrolled, loose and frequent bowel movements. Almost all people with aids develop diarrhoea at some time in the course of their disease. Severe or prolonged diarrhoea can lead to weight loss and malnutrition. The excessive loss of fluid that may occur with aids related diarrhoea can be life threatening. There are many possible causes of diarrhoea in people who have aids. The most common infectious organism causing aids related diarrhoea include cytomegalovirus (CMV), the parasites cryptosporidium, microsporidia and giardia lamblia, and the bacterium mycobacterium avium inracellulare (MAC). Other bacteria and parasites that cause diarrhoeal symptoms in otherwise healthy people may cause more severe, prolonged or recurrent diarrhoea in people with HIV or aids.

■ **diatom**

alga with siliceous cell walls that persist as a skeleton after death. Any of the microscopic unicellular or colonial alga constituting the class bacillariophyceae.

■ **diatomaceous earth**

sedimentary soil composed largely of the skeletons of diatoms, contains large amounts of silicon.

■ **diauxic growth**

two step growth frequency observed when bacteria are growing in media containing two carbon sources.

■ **diazotroph**

organism that can use dinitrogen as its sole-nitrogen source.

■ **dichotomous key**

flow chart of tests used for identifying an organism that give either a positive or negative result.

■ **didanosine (DDI)**

a nucleoside analogue reverse transcriptase inhibitor, didanosine is in the same family of antiviral drugs as AZT. It's primary toxicities are pancreatitis and neuropathy.

■ **dideoxynucleotide (DDNTP)**

nucleotide that lacks the 3' OH group, the portion required for the addition of subsequent nucleotides during DNA synthesis.

■ **differential media**
culture media that contain ingredients such as sugars and ph indicators used to distinguish among organisms based on their metabolic traits.

■ **differential medium**
cultural medium with an indicator, such as a dye, which allows various chemical reactions to be distinguished during growth.

■ **differential staining**
Type of staining procedure used to distinguish one group of bacteria from another by taking advantage of the fact that certain bacteria have distinctly different chemical structures in some of their components.

■ **differentiated**
a type of cell, which specialises in one specific task or has one specific purpose.

■ **diffusion**
to spread out evenly, as in a liquid.

■ **diffusion (nutrient)**
movement of nutrients in soil that results from a concentration gradient.

■ **di hydrofolate reductase (DHR)**
the bacterial (or protozoal) enzyme targeted by trimethoprim sulphamethoxazole. DHR is necessary for pneumocystis or toxoplasmosis to survive.

■ **dikaryon**
two nuclei present in the same hyphal compartment, they constitute a homokaryon when both nuclei are genetically the same or a heterokaryon when each nucleus is genetically different from the other.

■ **diluent**
sterile solution used to make the dilutions.

■ **dilution plate count method**
method for estimating the viable numbers of micro-organisms in a sample. The sample is diluted serially and then transferred to agar plates to permit growth and quantification of colony forming units.

■ **dimorphic**
able to assume two forms, as the yeast and mould forms of pathogenic fungi.

■ **dinitrogen fixation**
conversion of molecular dinitrogen to ammonia and subsequently to organic combi-

nations or to forms useful in biological processes.

- **diphtheroids**
gram positive cells that are club shaped and arranged to form v shapes and palisades, the typical microscopic morphology of *corynebacterium*.

- **diplococci**
cocci that typically occur in pairs

- **diploid**
in eukaryotes, an organism or cell with two chromosome complements, one derived from each haploid gamete.

- **diplopia**
double vision.

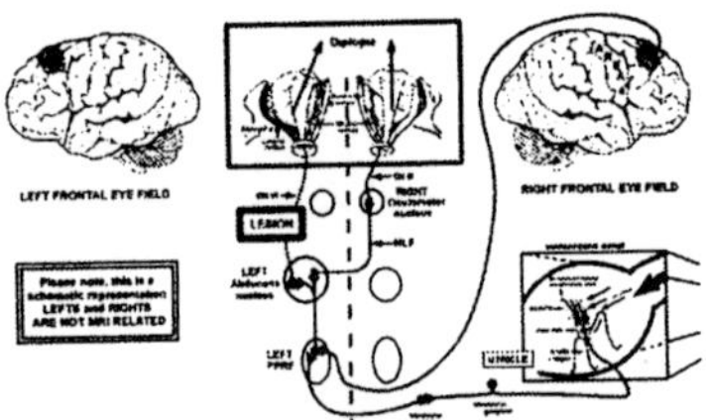

Lesion of the LEFT Abducens nerve = atrophy of the LEFT lateral rectus. LEFT eye deviated medially. Diplopia

- **direct count**
method of estimating the total number of micro-organisms in a given mass of soil by direct microscopic examination.

- **direct microscopic count**
method of determining the number of bacteria in a measured volume of liquid by counting them microscopically using special glass slides.

- **direct patient contact**
patient contacts that are initiated by the study clinic for the purpose of patient recruitment or data collection and that are directed at specified patients without any reliance on interviewing persons, agencies, institutions or generalized advertising campaigns to make contacts.

- **direct selection**
technique of selecting mutants by plating organisms on a medium on which the desired mutants but not the parent will grow.

- **directly observed therapy**
method used to ensure that patients comply with their antimicrobial therapy, health care workers routinely visit patients in the community and watch them take their drugs.

- **disaccharide**
carbohydrate molecule consisting of two monosaccharide molecules

■ **discrete variable**
variable is capable of assuming only certain values over a defined range.

■ **disease**
process resulting in tissue damage or alteration of function, producing body changes noticeable by physical examination or laboratory tests.

■ **disinfectant**
agent that kills micro-organisms.

■ **disinfection**
process of reducing or eliminating pathogenic micro-organisms or viruses in or on a material so that they are no longer a hazard.

■ **disseminated**
spread throughout the body.

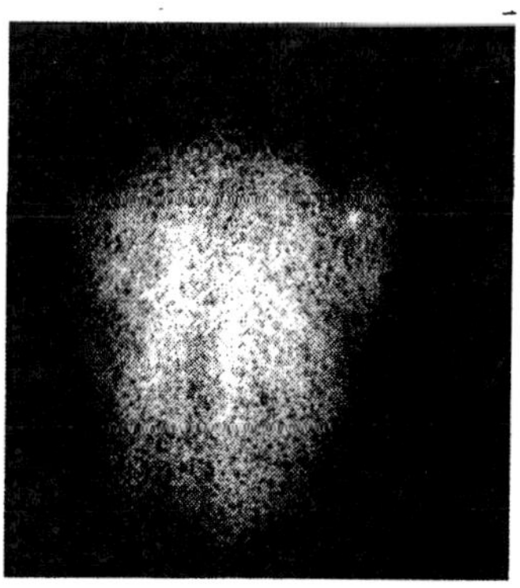

■ **disseminated intravascular coagulation**
devastating condition in which clots form in small blood vessels, leading to failure of vital organs.

■ **dissimilatory nitrate reduction to ammonium (DNRA)**
use of nitrate by organisms as an alternate electron acceptor in the absence of oxygen resulting in the reduction of nitrate to ammonium.

■ **distribution (normal Gaussian distribution)**
a symmetrical distribution which has a shape defined by its mean and standard deviation. Mean=median=mode. Often called the bell shaped curve.

■ **division**
taxonomic rank that groups similar classes, also called a phylum. A collection of similar divisions comprises a kingdom.

■ **DNA**
abbreviation for deoxyribonucleic acid.

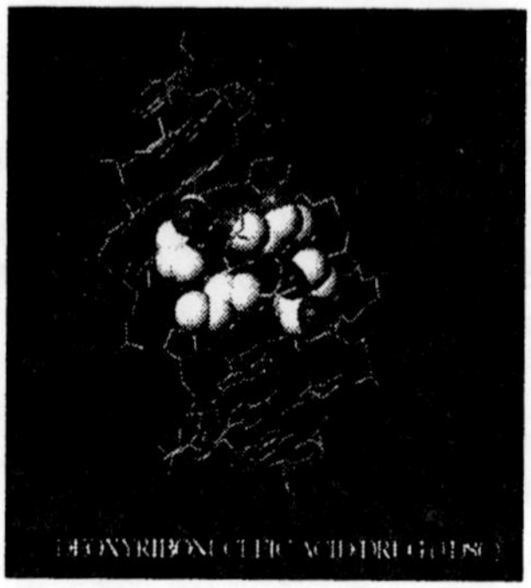

■ **DNA chip**
silicon chip of less than an inch in diameter that can carry an array of hundreds of thousands of oligonucleotides.

■ **DNA fingerprinting**
the use of characteristic patterns in DNA to match a specimen to a probable source.

■ **DNA gyrase**
enzyme that helps relieve the tension in DNA caused by the unwinding of the two strands of the DNA helix.

■ **DNA library**
collection of cloned DNA fragments which in total contain genes from the entire genome of an organism; also called a gene library.

■ **DNA ligase**
enzyme that joins short fragments of DNA.

■ **DNA polymerases**
enzymes that synthesise DNA, they use one strand as a template to generate the complementary strand.

■ **DNA probe**
a piece of DNA, labelled in some manner, which is used to identify the presence of similar DNA by hybridising to it.

■ **DNA replication**
duplication of a DNA molecule.

■ **DNA mediated transformation**
process of gene transfer in which DNA is transferred as a 'naked' molecule.

■ **dolipore septum**
specialised cross-wall separating compartments of a hypha of fungi in the phylum basidiomycota; consisting of a central pore covered with perforated membranes on both sides (called a parenthosome).

■ **domain**
region of a gene or gene product.

- **donor**
  refers to the cell that donates DNA in DNA transfer.

- **dormant**
  at rest, clinically silent.

- **dosage**
  a specific quantity of a biologically active compound.

- **dose ranging**
  establishment of the optimal dosage of a new drug by repeated trials of varying dosages

- **dose ranging study**
  a clinical trial in which two or more doses of an agent (such as a drug) are tested against each other to determine which dose works best and is least harmful.

- **dose response relationship**
  relationship between the dose of some agent (such as a drug), or the extent of exposure, and a physiological response. A dose response effect means that as the dose increases so does the effect.

- **double blind**
  procedure in a clinical trial for issuing and administering treatment assignments by code number in order to keep study patients and all members of the clinic staff, especially those responsible for patient treatment and data collection, from knowing the assigned treatments.

- **double blinded clinical trial**
  clinical trial with double blinded administration of the study treatments.

- **double diffusion in gel**
  qualitative precipitation reaction in which antigen and antibody diffuse toward each other, making a line of precipitation in the area of optimal proportions.

- **double blind**
  type of study where neither the physicians nor the patients know who is receiving the actual treatment.

- **double blind study**
  clinical trial design in which neither the participating individuals nor the study staff know which patients are receiving the experimental drug and which are receiving placebo or another therapy. Double blind trials are thought to produce objective results, since the doctor's and patient's expectations about the experimental drug do not affect the outcome.

■ **doubling time**
time needed for a population to double in number or biomass.

■ **downstream**
direction toward the 3' end of an RNA molecule or the analogous (+) strand of DNA.

■ **dreschlera sp.**
conidia dimensions 40 120 x 17 28 microns .Found on grasses, grains and decaying food. It can occasionally cause a corneal infection of the eye .

■ **dronabinol (marinol)**
a synthetic form of the active ingredient in marijuana, used to increase hunger and ameliorate nausea in persons with severe involuntary weight loss.

■ **droplet transmission**
transmission of infectious agents through inhalation of respiratory droplets

■ **drop out**
patient enrolled in a clinical trial who is either unwilling or unable to return to the study clinic for regular follow up visits.

■ **drug trial**
clinical trial in which the test treatments are drugs.

■ **drug drug interaction**
a modification of the effect of a drug when administered with another drug. The effect may be an increase or a decrease in the action of either substance, or it may be an adverse effect that is not normally associated with either drug.

■ **durham tube**
small inverted tube placed in a broth of sugar containing media that is used to detect gas production by a micro-organism.

■ **dysentery**
condition characterised by cramps, abdominal pain and bloody diarrhoea.

■ **dysmenorrhea**
difficult and painful menstruation.

■ **dyspepsia**
digestive upset.

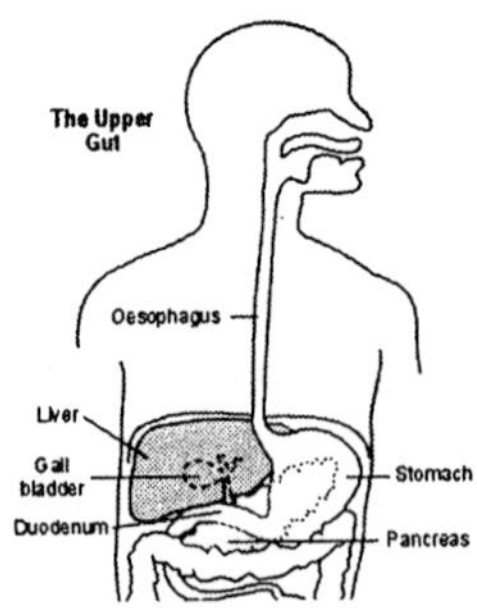

■ **dysphagia**
difficulty in swallowing.

■ **dysplasia**
abnormal development of tissue. In disease, the alteration of size, shape and organisation of adult cells.

■ **dyspnea**
difficult or laboured breathing.

■ **dysregulation**
refers to interruption or interference of normal process.

■ **e test**
modification of the disk diffusion test that utilises a strip impregnated with a gradient of concentrations of an anti-microbial drug.

■ **early stopping**
condition or provision incorporated into the design of a clinical trial that enables investigators to terminate patient recruitment or treatment if data accumulated during the trial strongly indicate an adverse or beneficial treatment effect.

■ **eclipse period**
time during which viruses exist within the host cell separated into their protein and nucleic acid components.

■ **ecology**
science which studies the interrelations among organisms and between organisms and their environment.

■ **ecosystem**
an environment and the organisms that inhabit it.

■ **ectomycorrhiza (EM)**
mycorrhizal type in which the fungal mycelia extend inward, between root cortical cells, to form a network (Hartig net) and outward into the surrounding soil. Usually the fungal hyphae also form a mantle on the surface of the root.

■ **eczema**
condition characterised by a blistery skin rash, with weeping of fluid and formation of crusts, usually due to an allergy.

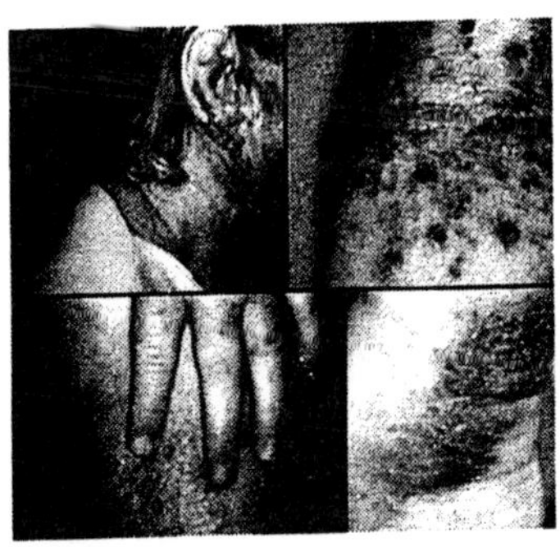

■ **ed50**
short for 'effective dose 50', the dosage of a drug or poison that kills, or stops replication in 50% of the organisms it is tested against. Often applies to doses of drug against micro-organisms.

■ **edaphic**
of or pertaining to the soil.

■ **edema**
swelling.

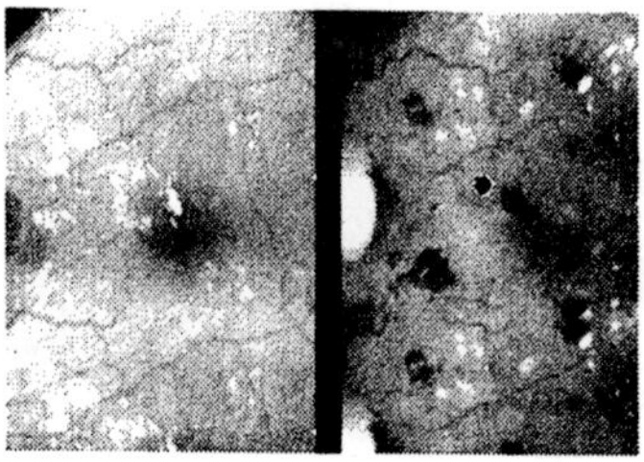

■ **effector**
regulatory molecule that binds to the allosteric site of an enzyme, the binding alters the shape of the enzyme, altering its affinity for the substrate.

■ **efficacy**
(of a drug or treatment). The maximum ability of a drug or treatment to produce a result regardless of dosage. A drug passes efficacy trials if it is effective at the dose tested and against the illness for which it is prescribed. In the procedure mandated by the food and drug administration, phase II clinical trials gauge efficacy, phase III trials confirm it.

■ **eh**
potential generated between an oxidation or reduction half reaction and the H electrode in the standard state.

■ **electrochemical gradient**
a separation of charged ions across the membrane.

■ **electron**
negatively charged component of an atom which orbits the nucleus.

■ **electron acceptor**
substance that accepts electrons during an oxidation reduction reaction. An electron acceptor is an oxidant.

■ **electron donor**
substance that donates electrons in an oxidation reduction reaction. An electron donor is a reductant.

■ **electron microscope**
microscope that uses electrons instead of light and can magnify images in excess of 100,000x.

■ **electron microscopy**
imaging method, which uses

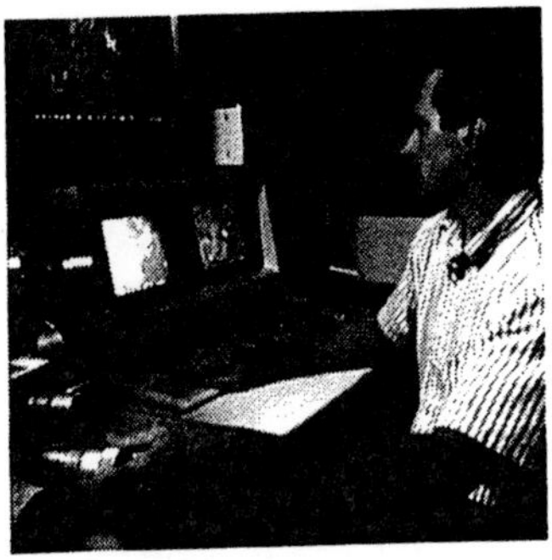

a focused beam of electrons to enlarge the image of an object on a screen or photographic plate.

- **electron transport chain**
  series of electron carriers that transfer electrons from donors to acceptors such as oxygen.

- **electrophilic compounds**
  chemicals that attack or are drawn to regions in other chemicals in which electrons are readily available, oxidising agents act as electrophilic compounds.

- **electrophoresis**
  separation of charged molecules, such as nucleic acids, in an electrical field.

- **electroporation**
  process of treating cells with an electric current to introduce DNA into them.

- **elementary body**
  small dense appearing infectious form of *chlamydia* specie that is released upon death and rupture of the host cell.

- **elephantiasis**
  massive enlargement of the legs and/or external genitalia due to lymphatic obstruction, caused by the inflammatory response to larval roundworms such as *wuchereria bancrofti.*

- **ELISA**
  abbreviation for Enzyme Linked Immunosorbent Assay.

- **eluviation**
  removal of soil material from a layer of soil as a suspension .

- **embden meyerhof pathway**
  metabolic pathway that oxidises glucose to pyruvate, generating ATP and reducing power, also known as glycolysis and the glycolytic pathway.

- **emerging diseases**
  diseases that have increased in incidence in the past two decades.

■ **empirical**
based on experimental data, not on a theory.

■ **encephalitis**
inflammation of the brain.

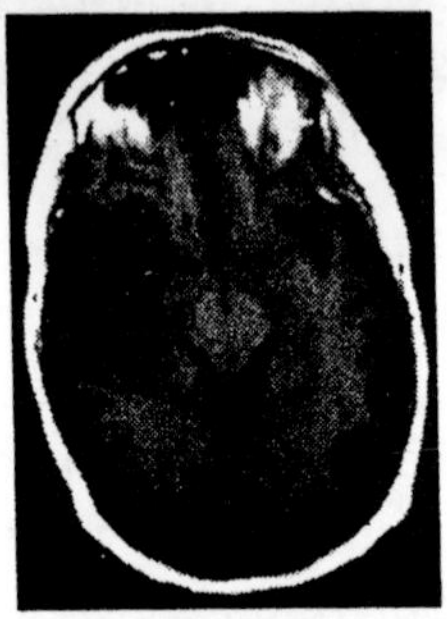

■ **encephalopathy**
lesions in the brain, or general degeneration of brain matter

■ **end product repression**
inhibition of gene activity by the end product of a biosynthetic pathway.

■ **endemic**
pertaining to diseases associated with particular locales or population groups.

■ **endemic**
constantly present in a population.

■ **endergonic**
chemical reaction that requires a net input of energy because the products have more free energy than the reactants.

■ **endergonic reaction**
chemical reaction that proceeds with the consumption of energy.

■ **endocarditis**
inflammation of the heart valves or lining of the heart chambers.

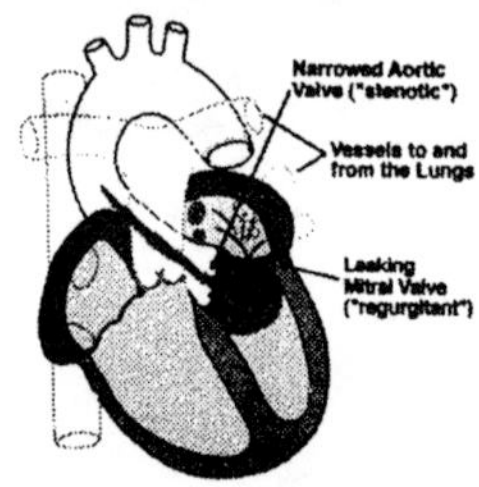

■ **endocrine**
relating to the internal secretion of hormones into systemic circulation.

■ **endocrine glands**
the organs in the body that produce hormones. They are ductless glands that empty hormonal secretions directly into the bloodstream.

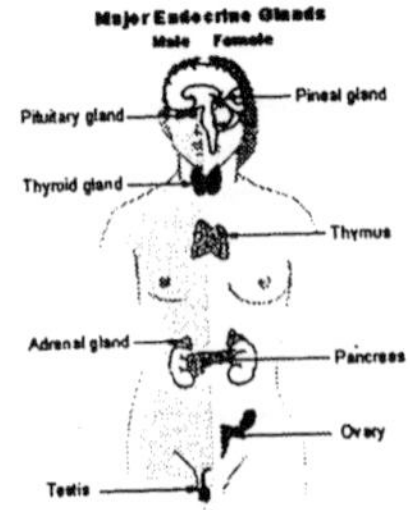

■ **endocytosis**
process in which cells take in fluids or other large molecules.

■ **endoenzyme**
enzyme that operates along the internal portions of a polymer.

■ **endogenous**
relating to or produced by the body.

■ **endomycorrhiza**
mycorrhizal association with intracellular penetration of the host root cortical cells by the fungus as well as outward extension into the surrounding soil.

■ **endonuclease**
endoenzyme that cleaves phosphodiester bonds within a nucleic acid molecule.

■ **endophyte**
organism growing within a plant. The association may be symbiotic or parasitic.

■ **endoplasmic reticulum**
internal membrane of a eukaryotic cell to which ribosomes are attached.

■ **endoscopy**
viewing the inside of a body cavity with a device using flexible fibre optics.

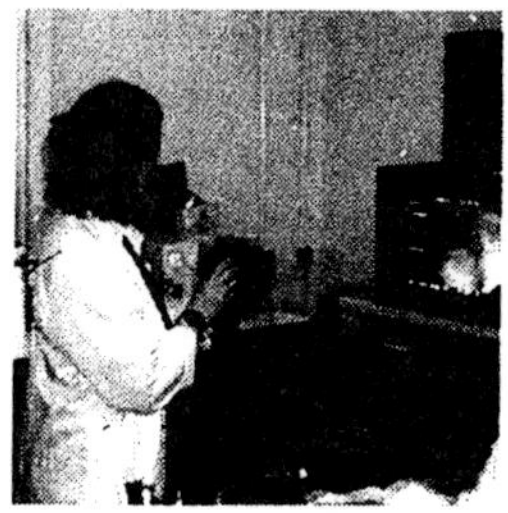

■ **endosome**
vesicle formed when a cell takes up material from the surrounding environment using the process of endocytosis.

■ **endospore**
kind of resting cell, characteristic of a limited number of bacterial species, highly resistant to heat, radiation and disinfectants.

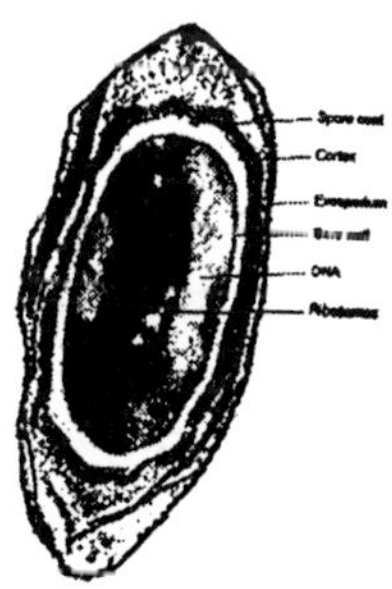

■ **endosymbiont**
micro-organism that resides within another cell, providing a benefit to the host cell.

■ **endosymbiont theory**
theory that the ancestors of mitochondria and chloroplasts were bacteria that had been residing within other cells in a mutually beneficial partnership.

■ **endotoxin**
toxin present inside a bacterial cell.

■ **endpoint**
primary or secondary outcome variable used to judge the effectiveness of a treatment this term is confusing because it often incorrectly implies that patients in a study are no longer followed after they experience an endpoint. This is obviously true where the event is death, but need not be so for nonfatal events. In fact, the design of the trial may require continued treatment and follow up of patients over the entire course of the trial, regardless of the number of nonfatal 'endpoints' observed.

■ **end stage disease**
final period or phase in the course of a disease leading to a person's death.

■ **energy**
capacity to do work.

■ **energy source**
compound that is oxidised by a cell to release energy, also called an electron donor.

■ **enrichment culture**
culture method that provides conditions to enhance the growth of one particular organism in a mixed population.

■ **enteral**
within or by way of the intestines or gastrointestinal tract.

■ **enteric**
pertaining to the intestines.

■ **enteric bacteria**
general term for a group of bacteria that inhabit the intestinal tract of humans and other animals. Among this group are pathogenic bacteria such as *salmonella* and *shigella*.

■ **enterics**
common name for members of the family *enterobacteriaceae*.

■ **enteritis**
inflammation of the intestine.

■ **enterotoxin**
poisonous substance, usually of bacterial origin, that acts on

the intestinal lining cells to cause diarrhoea and vomiting.

- **entner doudoroff pathway**
  pathway that converts glucose to pyruvate and glyceraldehyde 3 phosphate by producing 6 phosphogluconate and then dehydrating it.

- **entropy**
  degree of disorder in a system.

- **env**
  gene of HIV that codes for the protein gp160, the precursor of the envelope proteins gp120 and gp41.

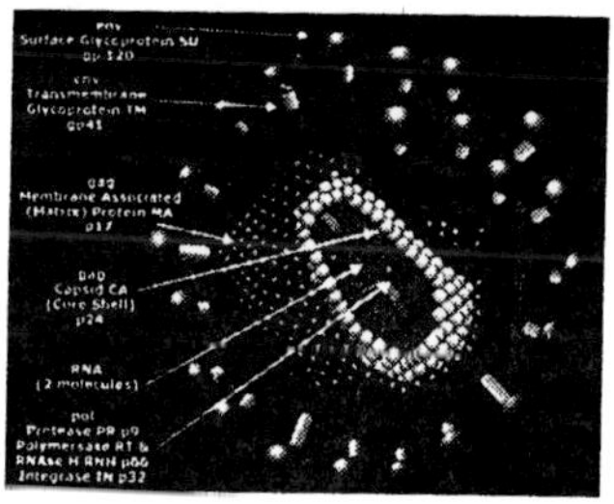

- **envelope**
  structure that surrounds the cytoplasm of the cell, includes the capsule, cell wall and cytoplasmic membrane.

- **enveloped viruses**
  viruses that have a double layer of lipid surrounding their nucleocapsid.

- **enzyme**
  protein catalyst.

- **Enzyme Linked Immunosorbent Assay (ELISA)**
  technique used for detecting and quantifying specific antigens or antibodies by using an antibody labelled with an enzyme.

ELISA testing of western flower thrips for INSV
(red color is a postive result)

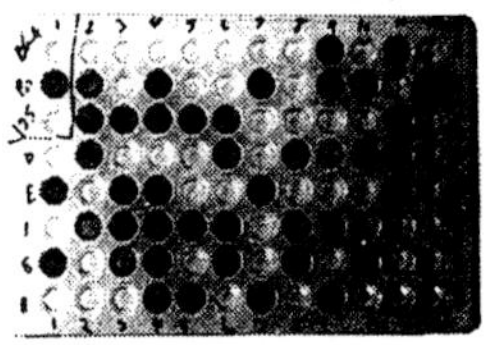

- **enzyme substrate complex**
  transient form that occurs in an enzyme mediated reaction, as the enzyme converts a substrate into a product.

- **eosinophil**
  a type of white blood cell, called granulocyte, that can digest micro-organisms. The granules can be stained by the acid dye, eosin, for microscopic examination.

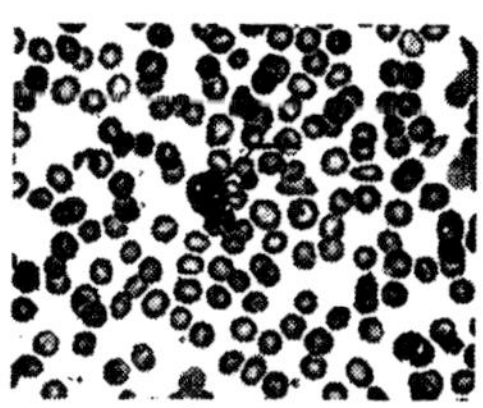

■ **epicoccum sp.**
conidia dimensions 15-25 microns. A common allergen, it is found in plants, soil, grains, textiles and paper products.

■ **epidemic**
a disease or other occurrence whose incidence is higher than expected within a region or population.

■ **epidemiologic surveillance**
the ongoing and systematic collection, analysis and interpretation of data about a disease or health condition. As part of a surveillance system to monitor the HIV epidemic in the us, the local health departments, blood collection agencies and medical research institutions, conducts standardised HIV seroprevalence surveys in designated subgroups in the population. Collecting blood samples for the purpose of surveillance is called serosurveillance.

■ **epidemiology**
study of factors influencing the frequency and distribution of diseases.

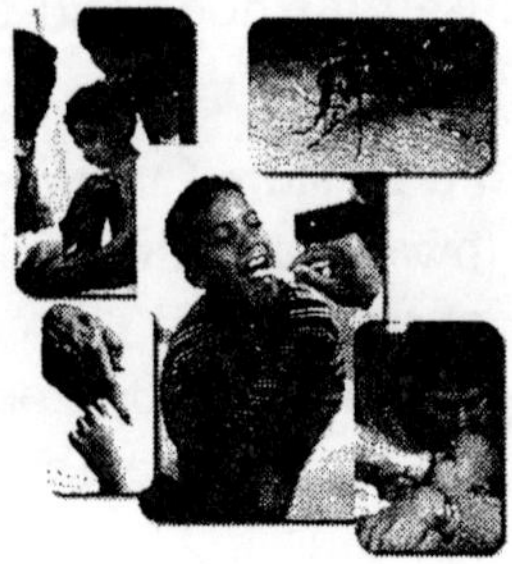

■ **epidermophyton sp.**
can cause infections of skin and nails.

■ **episome**
plasmid that replicates by inserting itself into the bacterial chromosome.

■ **epithelial**
cell linings covering most of the internal and external surface of the body and its organs.

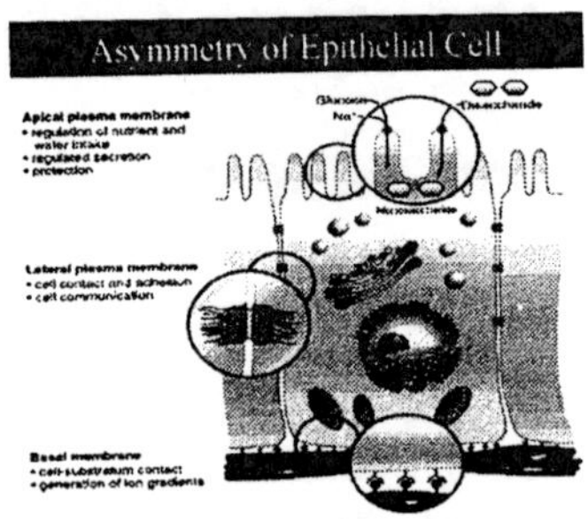

■ **epithelium**
covering of the internal and external organs of the body and also the lining of vessels, body

cavities, glands and organs. It consists of cells bound together by connective material and varies in the number of layers and the kinds of cells.

■ **epitope**
the region of an antigen to which the variable region of an antibody binds.

■ **epogen**
brand name of erythropoietin

■ **Epstein Barr Virus (EBV)**
herpes virus that causes infectious mononucleosis and hairy leukoplakia. EBV also has been associated with burkitt's lymphoma, a cancer of the lymph nodes and the nasopharynx, the part of the pharynx (throat) which lies above the soft palate.

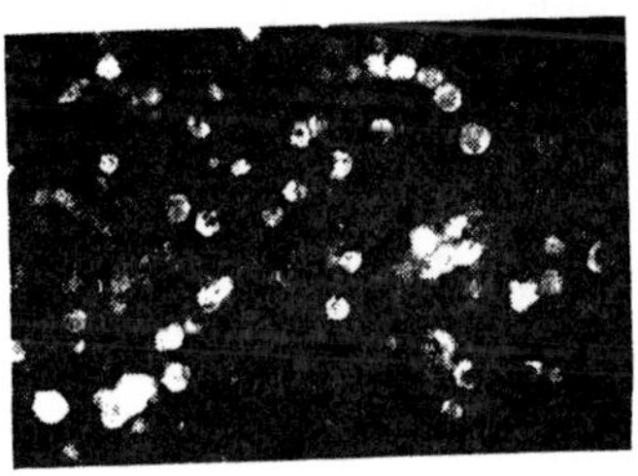

■ **equal allocation**
equal treatment allocation.

■ **equal treatment allocation**
scheme in which the assignment probability in the randomisation process for any one treatment is the same as for every other treatment in the trial. A process that ensures that approximately equal numbers of patients receive each treatment

■ **ergosterol**
sterol found in fungal cell membranes, the target of many antifungal drugs.

■ **ergot**
poisonous substance produced by the fungus that causes rye smut.

■ **ericoid mycorrhiza**
type of mycorrhiza found on plants in the ericales. The hyphae in the root are able to penetrate cortical cells (endomycorrhizal habit), however, no arbuscules are formed. Major forms are ericoid, arbutoid and monotropoid.

■ **erythema**
redness, usually of the skin.

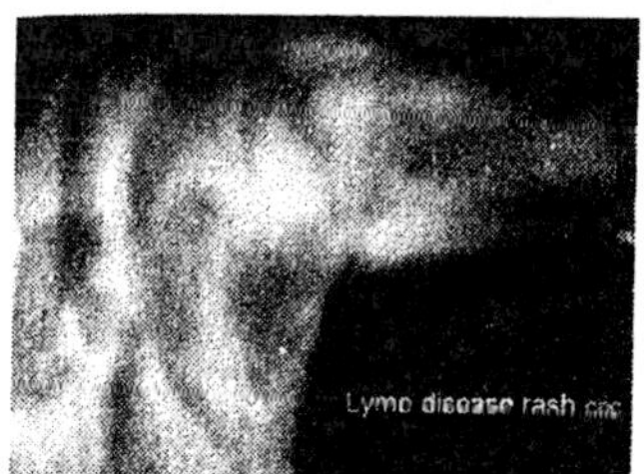

■ **erythema multiforme**
a skin disease characterised by

papular (small, solid, usually conic elevation of the skin) or vesicular lesions (blisters), and reddening or discolouration of the skin often in concentric zones about the lesion. Erythema multiforme has been associated with many infections, collagen disease, drug sensitivities, allergies and pregnancy. A severe form of this condition is Stevens Johnson syndrome.

- **erythema**
  redness or inflammation of the skin or mucous membranes.

- **erythematous**
  red or reddened.

- **erythrocytes**
  red blood cells.

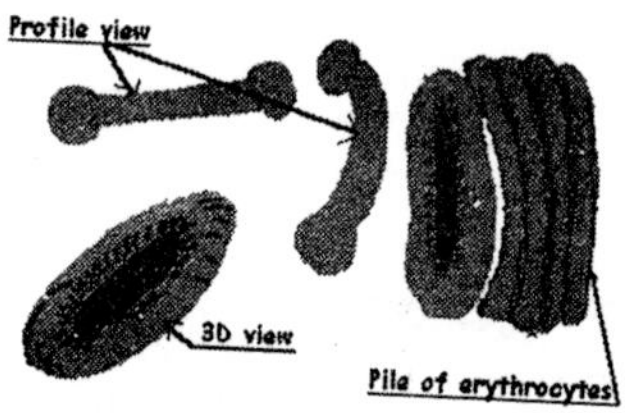

Erythrocytes

- **erythropoietin (EPO, procrit)**
  a recombinant version of a natural hormone that induces growth of red blood cells, erythropoietin is used in the treatment of anaemia.

- **e site (exit site)**
  site on the ribosome from which TRNA's exit after donating their amino acid to the adjacent TRNA

- **ester bond**
  covalent bond formed between a –COOH group and an –OH group with the removal of H_2O.

- **estimated sample size**
  number of patients required for a study, as derived from a sample size calculation or in some other way.

- **ethambutol**
  antimycobacterial drug that inhibits enzymes required for synthesis of mycobacterial cell wall components.

- **ethambutol (myambutol)**
  antibiotic used as a component in combination therapy to treat tuberculosis or *mycobacterium avium* complex.

- **ethidium bromide**
  mutagenic dye that binds to nucleic acid by intercalating between the bases, ethidium bromide stained DNA is fluorescent when viewed with UV light.

- **etiology**
  study or theory of factors which

cause disease.

eubacteria
old term for the Bacteria.

eukarya
name of the domain comprising eukaryotic organisms.

eukaryote
organism having a unit membrane bound nucleus and usually other organelles.

euryarchaeota
phylogenetic group of the domain Archaea.

eutrophic
having high concentrations of nutrients optimal, or nearly so, for plant or animal growth. Can be applied to nutrient or soil solutions and bodies of water.

eutrophication
nutrient enrichment leading to the overproduction of algae.

event
an occurrence, incident, or experience, especially one of some significance.

event driven data
data whose collection is triggered by clinically manifest occurrence, as opposed to on a particular schedule.

event rate
the number of events experienced by a specified number of patients in a specified unit of time.

exanthema
skin rash.

excision repair
mechanism of DNA repair in which a fragment of single stranded DNA containing mismatched bases is cut out.

exclusion/inclusion criteria
medical or social standards determining whether a person may or may not be allowed to enter a clinical trial. For example, some trials may not include people with chronic liver disease, or may exclude people with certain drug allergies, others may exclude men or women or only include people with a lowered T cell count.

exergonic
chemical reaction that releases energy because the starting compounds have more free energy than the products.

exergonic reaction
chemical reaction that pro-

ceeds with the liberation of energy.

■ **exobiology**
branch of biology concerned with the effects of extra-terrestrial environments on living organisms.

■ **exocytosis**
process by which eukaryotic cells expel material, membrane bound vesicles inside the cell fuse with the plasma membrane, releasing their contents to the external medium.

■ **exoenzyme**
enzyme that acts outside the cell that produces it.

■ **exoerythrocytic**
occurring outside the red blood cells, as the developmental cycle in malaria that occurs in the liver.

■ **exogenous**
developed or originating outside the body.

■ **exons**
portions of eukaryotic genes that are expressed, interrupted by introns.

■ **exotoxin**
soluble poisonous protein substance released by a micro-organism.

■ **expanded access**
general term for methods of distributing experimental drugs to patients who are unable to participate in ongoing clinical trials and have no other treatment options. Specific types of expanded access mechanisms include parallel track and compassionate use.

■ **experimental study**
type of study done to assess the effectiveness of measures to prevent or treat disease.

■ **explanatory trial**
trials that are designed to explain how a treatment works, in which patients are typically analysed by treatment received and not as assigned.

■ **exponential growth**
period of sustained growth of a micro-organism in which the cell number constantly doubles within a fixed time period.

■ **exponential phase**
stage of growth of a bacterial culture in which cells are multiplying exponentially; log phase.

■ **expression system**
in HIV vaccine production, cells

into which an HIV gene has been inserted to produce desired HIV proteins.

- **expression vectors**
  vectors that facilitate transcription and translation of cloned DNA.

- **external node**
  point on a phylogenetic tree that represents a named species that still exists.

- **external or temporary transmission**
  refers to transmission of viruses to plants by insects in which the virus is associated with the external mouth parts of the insect.

- **extracellular**
  outside the cells.

- **extracerebral**
  outside the brain or skull

- **extracorporeal**
  outside the body.

- **extramural**
  research that is conducted and supported by either contract or grant support.

- **extrapulmonary**
  outside the lungs.

- **extremophiles**
  organisms that live under extremes of temperature, barometric pressure or other environmental conditions.

- **extrinsic factors**
  environmental conditions such as the temperature and atmosphere that influence the rate of microbial growth.

- **exudate**
  low molecular weight metabolites that leak from plant roots into soil.

- **f– cell**
  recipient bacterial cell in conjugation.

- **f plasmid**
  plasmid found in donor cells of *E.coli* that codes for sex pilus biosynthesis.

- **f+ cell**
  donor bacterial cell in conjugation.

- **fab (fragment antigen binding) region**
  portion of an antibody molecule that binds to the antigen.

- **facilitated diffusion**
  transport process that enables movement of impermeable compounds from one side of

the membrane to the other by exploiting a concentration gradient, does not require expenditure of energy by the cell.

■ **factorial treatment structure**
treatment structure in which one study treatment is used in combination with at least one other study treatment in a trial, or where multiples of a defined dose of a specified treatment are used in the same trial.

■ **facultative**
flexible with respect to growth conditions, for example, able to live with or without O_2.

■ **facultative anaerobe**
organism that grows best in the presence of oxygen (O_2), but can grow in its absence.

■ **facultative organism**
organism that can carry out both options of a mutually exclusive process (e.g., aerobic and anaerobic metabolism).

■ **fad**
abbreviation for flavin adenine dinucleotide.

■ **fallopian tubes**
part of the female reproductive system. A pair of ducts opening at one end into the uterus and at the other end into the peritoneal cavity, over the ovary. Each tube serves as a passage through which the ovum (egg) is carried to the uterus and through which spermatozoa (sperm) move towards the ovary.

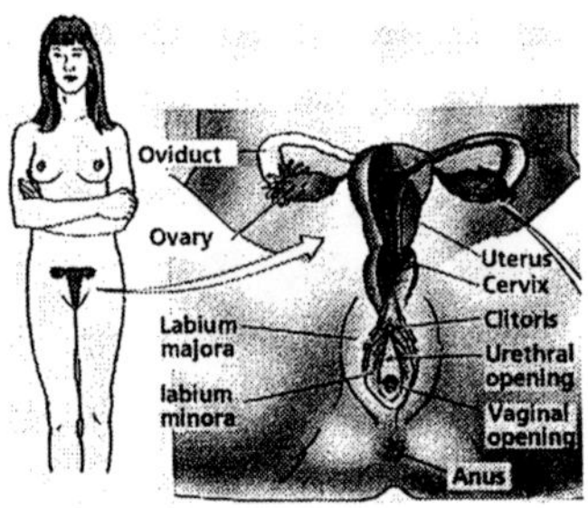

■ **false positive error**
probability of rejecting the null hypothesis of no treatment difference when there is no treatment difference, that is, falsely claiming a treatment difference. Also called type i error.

■ **famciclovir (famvir)**
drug chemically related to acyclovir, used in the treatment of herpetic diseases

■ **family**
taxonomic group between or-

der and genus.

- **fansidar**
  a combination of two antibiotics, pyrimethamine and sulphadoxine, fansidar was once used in the treatment of pcp. It proved highly toxic, however, with a high rate of allergic reactions and rash, including Stevens Johnson syndrome. Rarely used anymore.

- **fastidious**
  exacting, refers to organisms that require growth factors.

- **FC portion of antibody**
  crystallisable end of the constant region of an immunoglobulin molecule, responsible for binding to Fc receptors on cells, for initiating the classical pathway of complement activation and other biological functions.

- **feasibility study**
  preliminary study designed to determine the practicality of a larger study.

- **febrile**
  with a fever.

- **fecal coliforms**
  thermotolerant coliform bacteria.

- **faecal oral transmission**
  transmitting organisms that colonise the intestine by ingesting faecally contaminated material.

- **feedback inhibition**
  inhibition by an end product of the biosynthetic pathway involved in its synthesis.

- **feeding tolerance**
  lack of immune response to a specific antigen resulting from introducing the antigen orally.

- **fermentation**
  metabolic process in which the final electron acceptor is an organic compound.

- **fertility or f plasmid**
  plasmid found in donor cells of *E. Coli* which codes for the sex pilus and makes the cell F^+

- **fertilizer**
  any organic or inorganic material of natural or synthetic origin (other than liming materials) added to a soil to supply one or more elements essential to plant growth.

- **fever**
  increase in internal body temperature to 37.8 °C or higher.

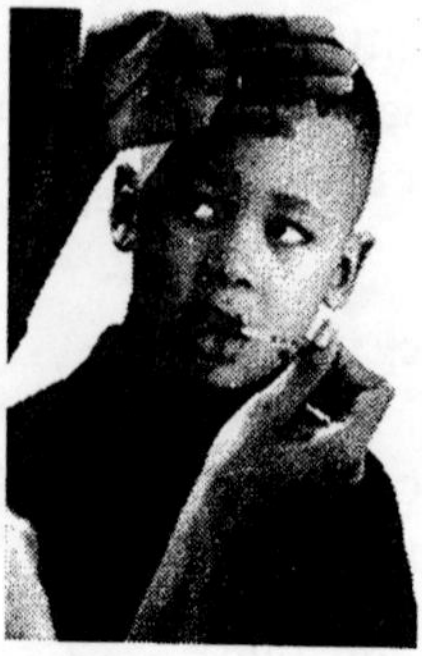

■ **fibronectin**

glycoprotein occurring on the surface of cells and also in a circulating form that adheres tightly to medical devices. Certain pathogens attach to it to initiate colonisation.

■ **field capacity**

content of water, on a mass or volume basis, remaining in a soil after being saturated with water and after free drainage is negligible.

■ **filamentous**

in the form of very long rods, many times longer than wide (for bacteria), in the form of long branching strands (for fungi).

■ **filgrastim (granulocyte colony stimulating factor)**

recombinant version of an endogenous cytokine that stimulates the production of white blood cells. Often used for treatment of neutropenia attendant upon chemotherapy, or treatment with AZT.

■ **filovirus**

thread like virus family which includes such viruses as ebola and marburg, very deadly.

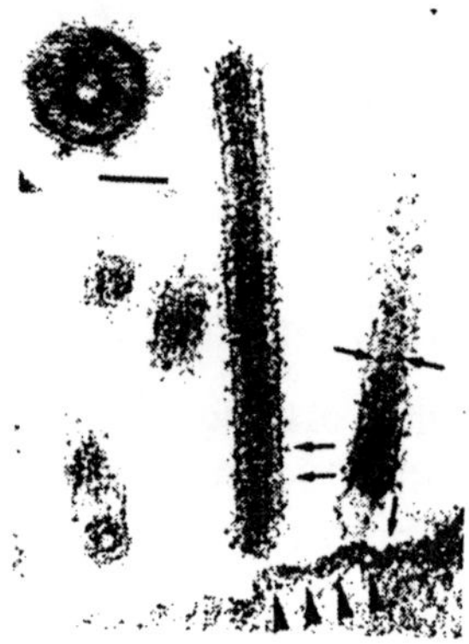

■ **filterable viruses**

old terminology for viruses.

■ **fimbria (pl. fimbriae)**

type of pilus that enables cells to attach to a specific surface.

■ **fimbria (pl. fimbriae)**

short filamentous structure on a bacterial cell, although flagella like in structure, generally present in many copies and not involved in motility. Plays a role in adherence to surfaces and in the formation of pellicles.

■ **final data analysis**
the term given to data analyses carried out at the end of the trial, normally in the termination stage, for describing results of the trial.

■ **first line antimicrobials**
in antimycobacterial drug therapy, the group of antimicrobials that is preferred because they are most effective as well as least toxic.

■ **first line treatment**
the preferred therapy for a particular condition (e.g., trimethoprim sulfamethoxazole (tmp smx) is the first line treatment for PCP).

■ **fission**
type of cell division in which overall cell growth is followed by formation of a cross-wall which typically divides the fully grown cell into two similar or identical cells.

■ **flagellate**
protozoan that moves by means of one to several flagella.

■ **flagellin**
protein subunits that make up the filament of flagella.

■ **flagellum (pl. flagella)**
whiplike tubular structure attached to a microbial cell responsible for motility.

■ **flavin adenine dinucleotide (FAD)**
a derivative of the vitamin riboflavin.

■ **flouroquinolones**
a family of antibiotics, including ciprofloxacin, ofloxacin, and sparfloxacin. Sometimes used as components of combination therapy for *mycobacterium avium* complex.

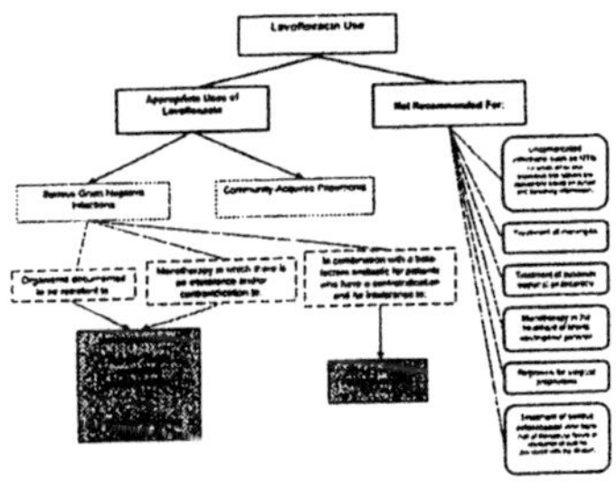

■ **flow cytometer**
instrument that counts cells in a suspension by measuring the scattering of light by individual cells as they pass by a laser.

■ **fluconazole**
an antifungal drug that is used to treat fungal infections in persons with HIV, including can-

dida, cryptococcus, histoplasmosis and others.

- **flucytosine (5 FC)**
  antifungal drug used as an adjunct to amphotericin for the treatment of cryptococcal meningitis.

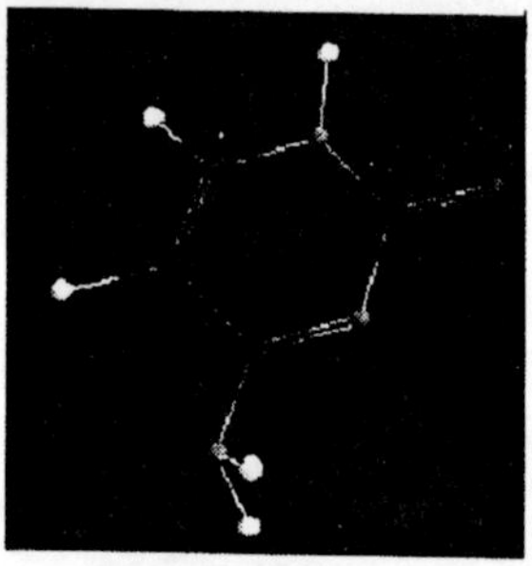

- **fluid mosaic model**
  model that describes the dynamic nature of the cytoplasmic membrane.

- **fluke**
  short, non segmented, bilaterally symmetrical flatworm

- **fluorescence microscope**
  special type of microscope used to observe cells that have been stained or tagged with fluorescent dyes.

- **fluorescence activated cell sorter**
  machine that sorts fluorescent labelled cells in a mixture by passing single cells in a stream past photo detectors.

- **fluorescent**
  able to emit light of a certain wavelength when activated by light of a shorter wavelength.

- **fluorescent antibody**
  antiserum conjugated with a fluorescent dye, such as fluorescein or rhodamine.

- **fluoroquinolones**
  group of antimicrobial drugs that interferes with nucleic acid synthesis.

- **fluxes**
  rate of emission, sorption or deposition of a material from one pool to another. For example, the exchange of methane between the land and the atmosphere is a flux, while the production of methane within the soil is not.

- **folate**
  a salt or ester of folic acid, a crystalline vitamin of the b complex. Drugs such as trimethoprim sulfa and trimetrexate work by 'starving' bacteria of foliate but do not starve the human body.

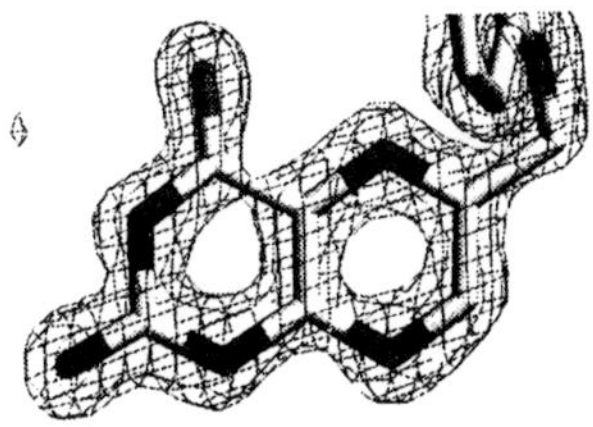

■ **folic acid**
crystalline vitamin of the b complex that is used especially in the treatment of nutritional anaemia. It occurs in green plants, fresh fruit, liver and yeast. Also called folacin, folate, and vitamin B9.

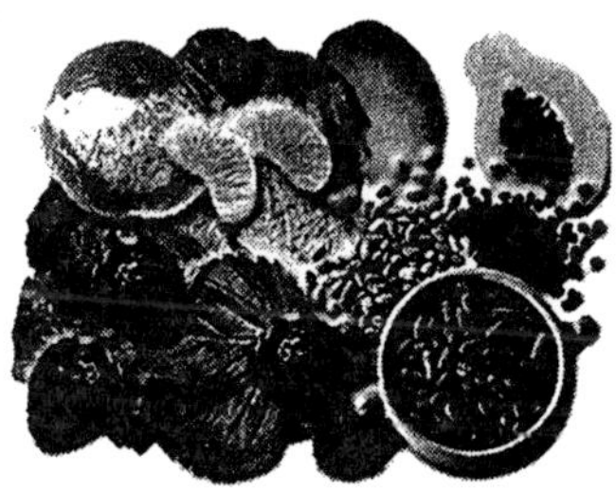

■ **folinic acid**
also called citrovorum factor. A metabolically active form of folic acid that has been used in cancer therapy to protect normal cells against methotrexate (a cancer chemotherapy agent). Also used to treat megaloblastic anemias.

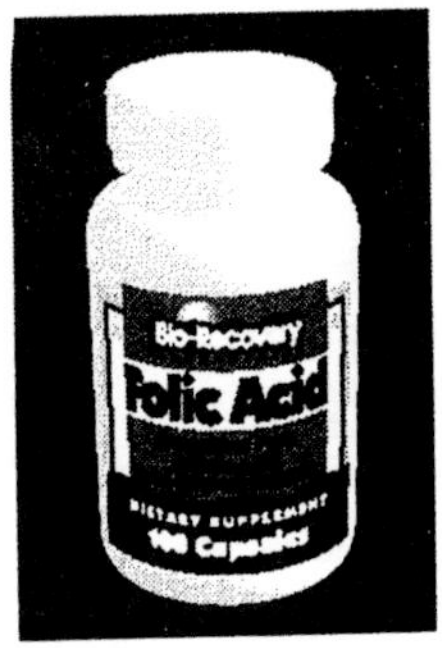

■ **follicle**
a small anatomical cavity or deep narrow mouthed depression, a small lymph node.

■ **follicular dendritic cells (FDC's)**
cells found in the germinal centres of lymphoid organs. FDC's have thread like tentacles that form a web-like network to trap invaders and present them to other cells of the immune system (for destruction).

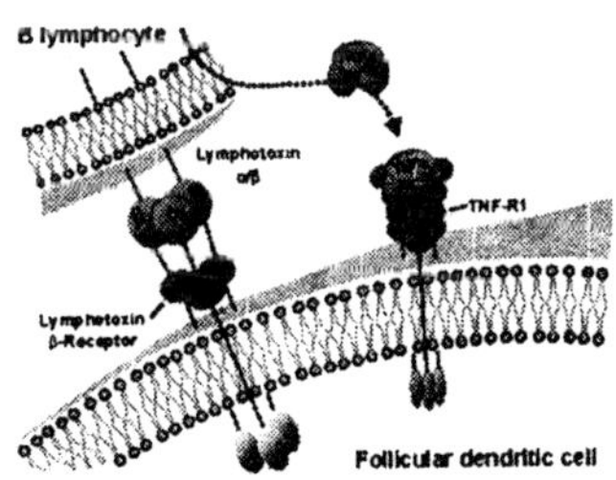

■ **folliculitis**
infection or inflammation of the follicle, at the root of a hair.

Folliculitis may be aseptic, as in eosinophilic folliculitis.

■ **follow up**
patient follow up.

■ **follow up data**
data collected on a patient, or a set of patients, after enrolment into a trial.

■ **follow up visit**
any patient clinic visit that takes place after the randomisation visit for study related purposes.

■ **fomite**
inanimate object that can harbour pathogenic micro-organisms and thus serve as an agent of transmission of an infection.

■ **food chain**
movement of nutrients from one life form to another as a result of the different feeding habits and dietary requirements of organisms in an ecosystem.

■ **food web**
diagram of the interconnections of nutrient flow through a food chain.

■ **foraminifera**
protozoa that have silicon or calcium in their cell walls.

■ **forespore**
portion of the endospore formed during the process of sporulation that will ultimately become the core of the endospore.

■ **foscarnet (foscavir)**
antiviral drug for the treatment of cytomegalovirus (CMV) retinitis and other diseases caused by cmv. It is also used to treat acyclovir resistant herpes virus infections. Adverse side effects may include kidney toxicity, muscle twitching, nausea and skin ulcers.

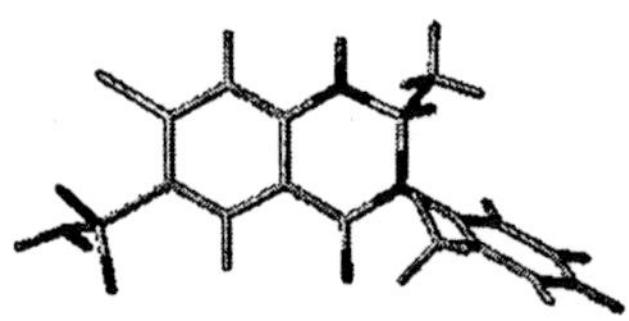

■ **fowl cholera**
worldwide septicemic illness of wild and domestic fowl, caused by *pasteurella ultocida*, focus of the discovery by Pasteur that an attenuated organism could be used as a vaccine.

■ **fragmentation**
form of asexual reproduction in which a filament composed of a string of cells breaks apart, forming multiple reproductive units.

■ **frame shift mutation**
mutation resulting from the addition or deletion of nucleotides.

■ **free energy**
amount of energy that can be gained by breaking the bonds of a chemical, does not include the energy that is always lost as heat.

■ **freeze etching**
process used to prepare specimens for transmission electron microscopy that allows the shape of underlying regions within structures of a cell to be viewed.

■ **fruiting body**
with respect to myxobacteria, a complex aggregate of cells, visible to the naked eye, produced when nutrients or water are depleted.

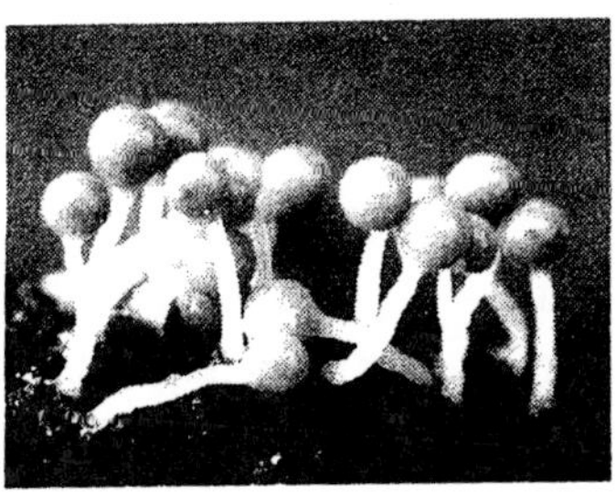

■ **frustule**
siliceous wall and protoplast of a diatom.

■ **fulminating**
serious acute, active infection.

■ **fulvic acid**
yellow organic material that remains in solution after removal of humic acid by acidification.

■ **functional antibody**
antibody that binds to an antigen and has an effect. For example, neutralising antibodies inactivate HIV or prevent it from infecting other cells.

■ **fundoscopic exam**
visual inspection of the interior of the eye. Often used to diagnose CMV retinitis.

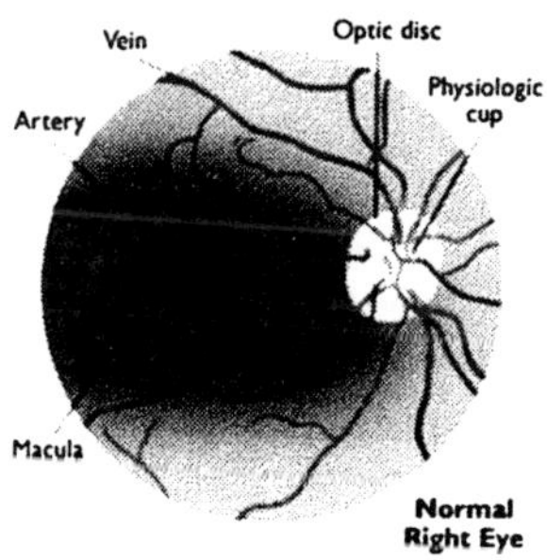

■ **fungemia**
the presence of fungus in the blood.

■ **fungicide**
kills fungi, used to describe the effects of some anti-microbial chemicals.

■ **fungistasis**
suppression of germination of fungal spores or other resting structures in natural soils as a result of competition for available nutrients, presence of inhibitory compounds or both.

■ **fungistatic**
able to inhibit the growth of fungi.

■ **fungizone**
brand name for amphotericin b.

■ **fungus (pl. fungi)**
nonphototrophic, eukaryotic micro-organisms that contain rigid cell walls.

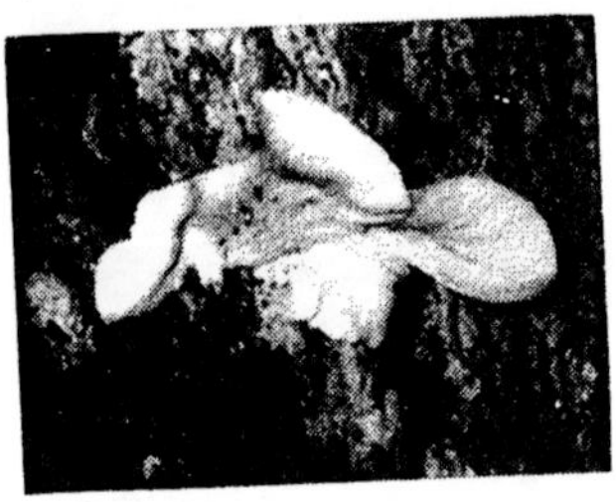

■ **furuncle**
a boil, a localised skin infection that penetrates into the subcutaneous tissue, usually caused by *s. Aureus.*

■ **fusiform**
spindle shaped, tapered at both ends.

■ **g + c content**
percentage of guanine plus cytosine in double stranded DNA, also called the GC content.

■ **gallium scan**
diagnostic procedure where mildly radioactive gallium particles are ingested, and then disease (often pneumocystis carinii pneumonia) is diagnosed by

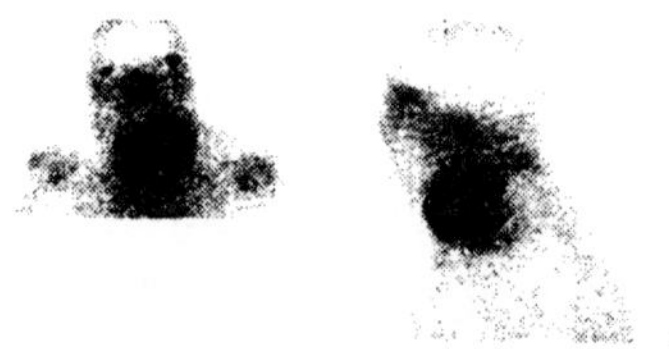

scanning the body for radioactive signature.

■ **GALT**
abbreviation for gut associated lymphoid tissue

■ **gametangium**
fungal structure that contains one or more gametes.

■ **gamete**
in eukaryotes, the haploid cell analogous to sperm and egg, which results from meiosis.

■ **gamma globulin**
portion of blood serum proteins that is separated by electrophoresis and contains most of the immunoglobulins of the

blood.

■ **gamma interferon**
a T cell derived stimulating substance that suppresses virus

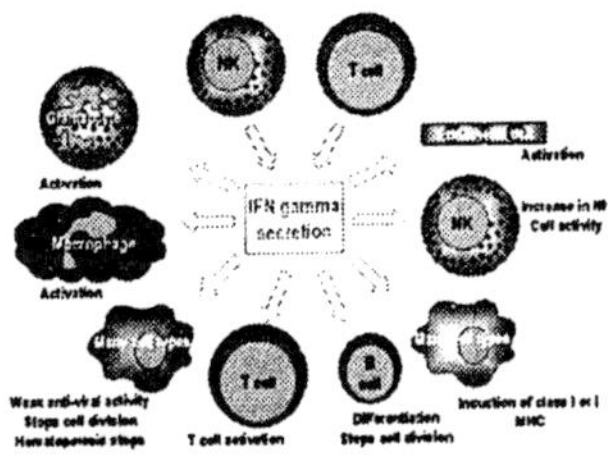

reproduction, stimulates other T cells and activates macrophage cells.

■ **ganciclovir (cytovene)**
antiviral drug to treat cytomegalovirus (CMV) retinitis and to prevent CMV disease in transplant patients at risk for CMV. It has also been used to treat CMV colitis, CMV esophagitis, aids related meningoencephalitis and aids related polyradiculopathy, generally administered intravenously. An oral form of the drug is under study for the treatment and prevention of CMV disease in people with HIV infection.

■ **ganglion**
mass of nervous tissue, composed principally of nerve cell bodies, usually lying outside the central nervous system.

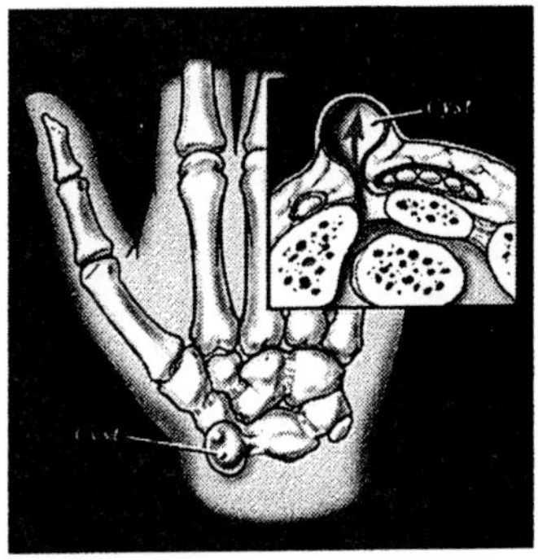

■ **gas chromatography**
technique of separating and identifying gaseous components of a substance.

■ **gas vesicles small**
rigid compartments produced by some aquatic bacteria that provide buoyancy to the cell. Gases, but not water, flow freely into the vesicles, thereby decreasing the density of the cell.

■ **gastric**
relating to the stomach.

■ **gastroenteritis**
inflammation of the stomach and/or intestines.

■ **gastrointestinal**
relating to the stomach and intestines.

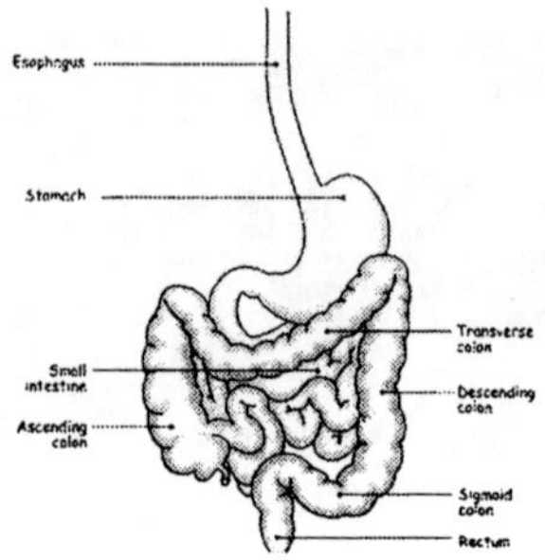

■ **gel**

inert polymer, usually made of agarose or polyacrylamide, that separates macromolecules such as nucleic acids or proteins during electrophoresis.

■ **gel electrophoresis**

technique that uses electric current to separate either DNA fragments or proteins according to size by drawing them through a slab of gel, which has the consistency of very firm gelatin.

■ **gene**

unit of dna that carries information for the bio synthesis of a specific product.

■ **gene cloning**

procedure by which genes are inserted into a replicon such as a plasmid or bacteriophage which is then introduced into cells where the replicon can replicate.

■ **gene library**

sum total of all of the genes of an organism that have been inserted into cloning vectors.

■ **gene probe**

strand of nucleic acid which can be labelled and hybridised to a complementary molecule from a mixture of other nucleic acids.

■ **general paresis**

group of symptoms arising from nervous system damage, usually occurring 10 to 20 years after contracting syphilis, often manifest by emotional instability, memory loss, hallucinations, abnormalities of the eyes, and paralysis.

■ **general secretory pathway**

primary mechanism bacterial cells use to secrete proteins; those destined for secretion are recognised by their characteristic sequence of amino acids that make up the amino terminal end.

■ **generalised transducing phage**

bacteriophage that is capable of transferring any part of the bacterial chromosome from one cell to another. (by contrast, a specialised transducing phage transfers only specific parts of the genome.)

- **generalised transduction**
transfer of any bacterial gene to other bacteria by phage.

- **generation time**
time needed for a population to double in number or biomass.

- **genetic code**
information for the synthesis of proteins contained in the nucleotide sequence of a DNA molecule (or in certain viruses, of an RNA molecule).

- **genetic engineering**
process of deliberately altering an organism's genetic information by changing its nucleic acid sequences.

- **genetic reassortment**
exchange of genetic information following two different segmented viruses infecting the same cell.

- **genetic recombination**
the joining together of genes from different organisms.

- **genetics**
the study of the function and transfer of genes.

- **genitourinary tract**
system of organs comprising the organs concerned with the production and excretion of urine and those concerned with reproduction. Also called genitourinary system, urogenital system, urogenital tract.

- **genome**
complete set of genetic information in a cell.

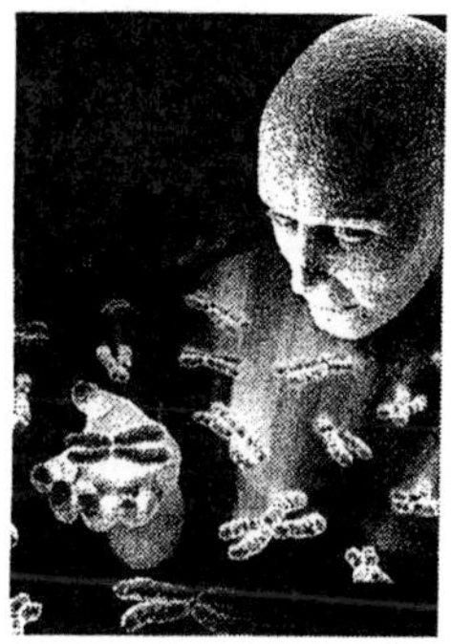

- **genome mining**
searching genomic databases. For example, companies might search genomic databases to locate orfs that may encode proteins of medical value.

- **genomics**
study and analysis of the nucleotide sequence of DNA.

- **genotype**
precise genetic constitution of

an organism.

■ **genus (pl. genera)**
the first name of the scientific name (binomial), the taxon between family and species.

■ **germicide**
agent that kills micro-organisms and inactivates viruses.

■ **germinal centres**
structures within lymphoid tissues that contain FDC's in which immune responses are initiated.

■ **germination**
sum total of the biochemical and morphological changes that an endospore or other resting cell undergoes before becoming a vegetative cell.

■ **giant cell**
very large cell with many nuclei, formed by the fusion of many macrophages during a chronic cell mediated response, found in granulomas.

■ **giardiasis**
common protozoal infection of the small intestine spread via contaminated food and water and direct person to person contact.

Giardiasis is caused by the protozoan Giardia lamblia

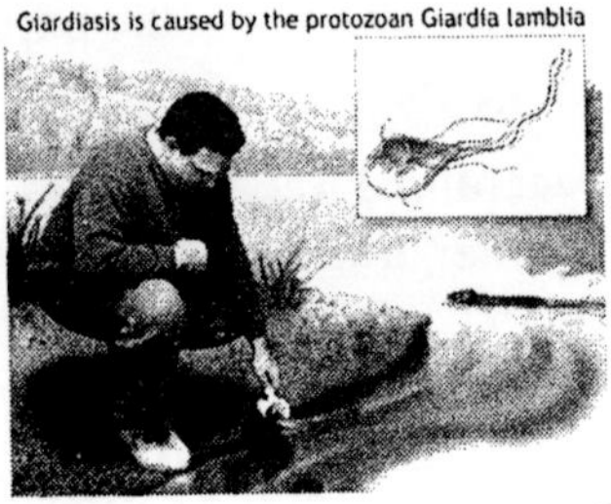

■ **giga**
prefix meaning a billion times.

■ **gingivitis**
inflammation of the gums.

■ **global regulation**
simultaneous regulation of numerous unrelated genes, global control.

■ **global repressor**
regulatory protein involved in the control of several different biosynthetic or degradative pathways.

■ **glucose salts**
type of chemically defined medium that contains only glucose and certain inorganic salts, supports the growth of *e. Coli.*

■ **glycan chain**
high molecular weight linear polymer of alternating subunits of *n* acetylglucosamine and *n* acetylmuramic acid that serves as the backbone of the pepti-

doglycan molecule.

- **glycocalyx**
gel like layer that surrounds some cells and generally functions as a mechanism of either protection or attachment.

- **glycogen**
polysaccharide composed of glucose molecules.

- **glycolipids**
lipids that have various sugars attached.

- **glycolysis**
reactions of the embden meyerhof (glycolytic) pathway in which glucose is oxidised to pyruvate.

- **glycoprotein**
protein molecule coated with sugars.

- **glycoproteins**
proteins with covalently bonded sugar molecules.

- **glycosidase**
enzyme that hydrolyses a glucosidic linkage between two sugar molecules.

- **goblet cells**
mucus secreting epithelial cells.

- **golgi apparatus**
series of membrane bound flattened sacs within eukaryotic cells that serve as the site where macromolecules that are synthesised in the endoplasmic reticulum are modified before they are transported to other destinations.

- **gonorrhea**
sexually transmitted disease, inflammation of genital mucous membranes caused by the bacteria *gonococcus*.

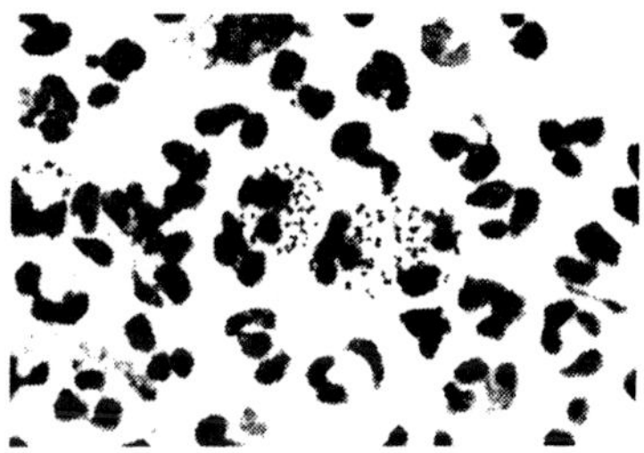

- **Gp120**
another protein on the outer shell, or envelope, of HIV. Gp120 is the portion of HIV that binds to a helper t cell's surface protein, cd4. The 120 refers to its molecular weight.

- **gp160**
the 'precursor' protein to both Gp41 and Gp120. Gp160 is cleaved by viral enzymes into the two surface proteins at a late stage of viral assembly.

■ **gp160**
glycoprotein 160, a precursor of HIV envelope proteins Gp41 and Gp120.

■ **gp41**
a protein on the outer shell, or envelope, of HIV. Gp41 is the portion of HIV, pierces a helper t cell's surface protein, cd4, allowing viral entry. The '120' refers to its molecular weight.

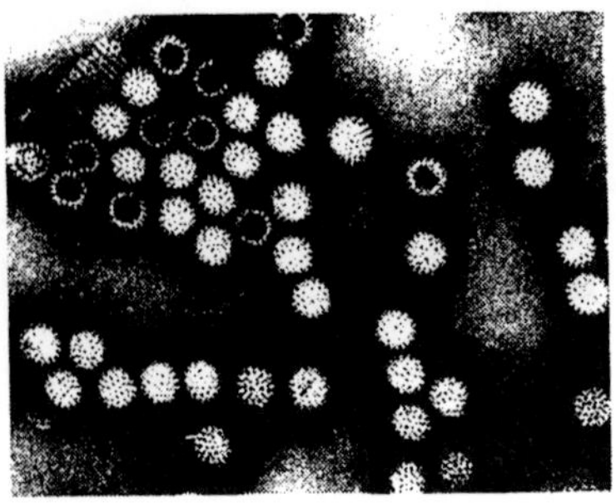

■ **gram**
a metric unit of weight measure. There are approximately 454 grams to a pound.

■ **Gram Stain**
staining technique that divides bacteria into one of two groups, Gram positive or Gram negative, on the basis of colour. Among eubacteria, the staining reaction correlates well with cell wall structure.

■ **Gram Negative**
bacteria that lose the crystal violet in the Gram stain procedure and therefore stain pink, the cell wall of these organisms is composed of a thin layer of peptidoglycan surrounded by an outer membrane.

■ **Gram Positive**
bacteria that retain the crystal violet stain in the Gram stain procedure and therefore stain purple, the cell wall of these organisms is composed of a thick layer of peptidoglycan.

■ **granulation tissue**
new tissue formed during healing of an injury, consisting of small, red, translucent nodules containing abundant blood vessels.

■ **granulocyte**
a cell type of the immune system filled with granules of toxic chemicals that enable them to digest micro-organisms. Basophils, neutrophils, and eosinophils are examples of granulocytes.

■ **granulocytopenia**
a lack or low level of granulocytes in the blood. Often used

interchangeably with neutropenia.

■ **granuloma**
found in a chronic cell mediated response, collections of lymphocytes and stages of macrophages, an attempt by the body to wall off and contain persistent organisms and antigens.

■ **gravitational water**
portion of total soil water, potential due to differences in elevation.

■ **griseofulvin**
antifungal medication that appears to interfere with the action of tubulin, a necessary factor in nuclear division.

■ **groschung catheter**
indwelling line used for administering medication and total parenteral nutrition over long durations.

■ **groundwater**
portion of the water below the surface of the ground at a pressure equal to or greater than atmospheric.

■ **group translocation**
type of transport process that chemically alters a molecule during its passage through the cytoplasmic membrane.

■ **growth**
in microbiology, an increase in both cell number and cellular constituents.

■ **growth curve**
growth pattern observed when cells are grown in a closed system, consists of four stages lag phase, log phase (or exponential phase), stationary phase and death phase.

■ **growth factor**
organic compound necessary for growth because it is an essential cell component or precursor of such components and cannot be synthesised by the organism itself. Usually required in trace amounts.

■ **growth rate**
rate at which growth occurs, usually expressed as the generation time.

■ **growth yield coefficient**
quantity of biomass carbon formed per unit of substrate carbon consumed.

■ **guillian barre syndrome**
acute febrile (i.e. with fever) polyneuritis.

■ **gumma**
localised area of chronic inflammation and necrosis in tertiary syphilis often manifest as a swelling

■ **gut associated lymphoid tissue (GALT)**
part of the mucosa associated lymphoid tissue, found in the intestines including Peyer's patches, the appendix and some lymph nodes.

■ **haart**
highly active anti retroviral therapy, a cocktail of medications that act at different sites during replication of human immunodeficiency virus.

■ **habitat**
place where an organism lives.

■ **hairy leukoplakia**
whitish patch, usually appearing on the tongue of individuals with severe immunodeficiency, thought to be caused by reactivation of latent epstein barr virus (EBV) infection.

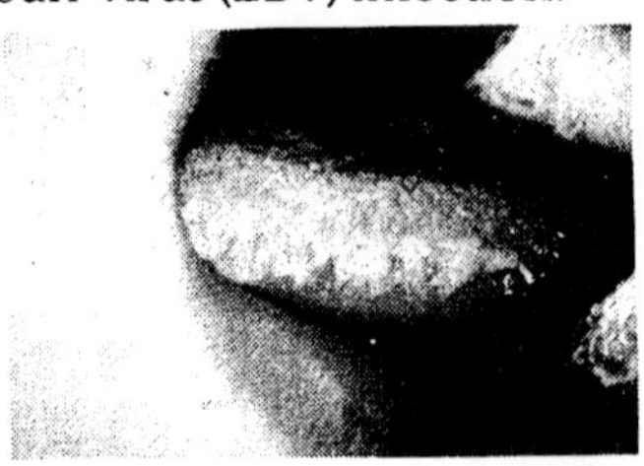

■ **half life**
amount of time required for half of a given substance to be eliminated from the body.

■ **halogen**
elements Flourine, Chlorine, Bromine, Iodine, and those part of group vii a of the periodic table.

■ **halophile**
organism that prefers or requires a high salt (NaCl) medium.

■ **haphazard**
process occurring without any apparent order or pattern. Distinct from random, in that there is no mathematical basis for characterising a haphazard process.

■ **haploid**
condition in which each type of chromosome is represented only once.

■ **hapten**
substance that can combine with specific antibodies but cannot incite the production of those antibodies unless it is attached to a large carrier molecule.

■ **hard endpoint**
outcome measure that is not subject to serious errors of interpretation or measurement. Usually death, infection or some other explicit clinical event.

■ **haustoria**
specialised hypha of parasitic fungi that can penetrate plant or animal cell walls.

■ **heavy metals**
those metals which have densities > 5.0 mg/m^3. These include the metallic elements cu, Fe, Mn, Mo, Co, Zn, Cd, Hg, Ni, and Pb. Al and se have densities < 5 but are also considered heavy metals.

■ **helicase**
enzyme that unwind the DNA helix ahead of the replication fork.

■ **helminth**
parasitic worm.

■ **helper T lymphocytes**
CD4+ lymphocytes that provide assistance needed for other cells such as B lymphocytes and macrophages to carry out their functions. T helper cells usually act by producing cytokines.

■ **helper suppresser ratio**
ratio of helper (cd4+) t cells to suppresser (cd8+) t cells.

■ **hemagglutination**
clumping of red blood cells.

■ **haematocrit**
laboratory measurement that determines the percentage of packed red blood cells in a given volume of blood.

■ **haematologic**
pertaining to, or involving the blood, or it's constituent cells.

■ **haematoma**
bruise.

■ **haematopoietic**
pertaining to the formation of blood cells.

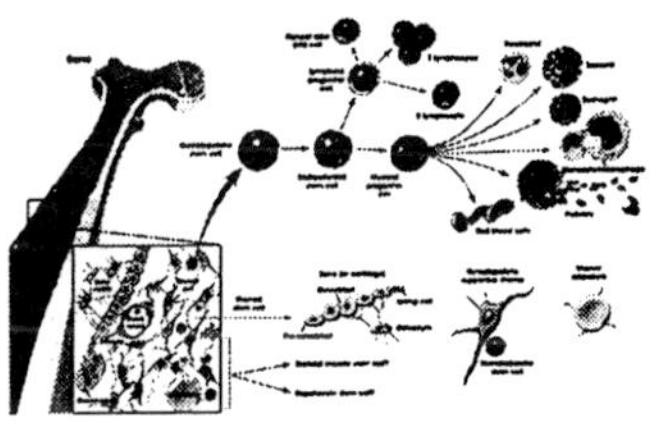

■ **haematopoietic stem cells**
bone marrow cells that give rise to all blood cells.

■ **haematotoxic**
poisonous to the blood or bone marrow.

■ **hemiparesis**
paralysis of only one side of the body.

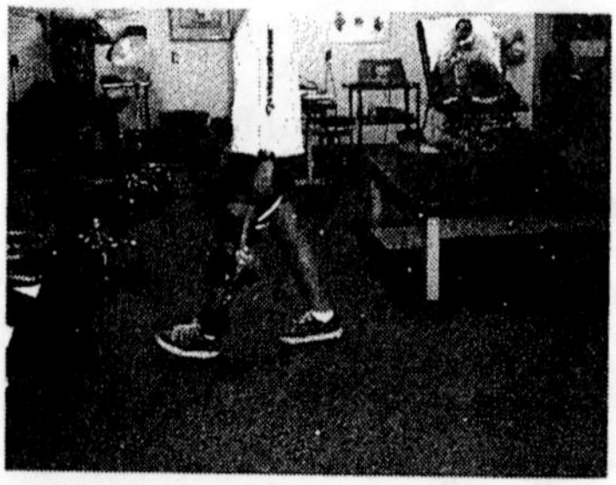

■ **haemoglobin**
component of red blood cells that carries oxygen.

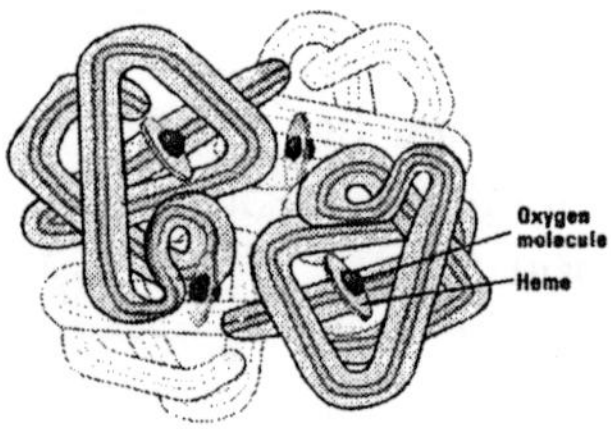

■ **haemolysis**
rupture of red blood cells.

■ **Haemolytic Disease of the Newborn (HDN)**
disease of the foetus or newborn caused by transplacental passage of maternal antibodies against the baby's red blood cells, resulting in red cell destruction, usually anti Rhesus (Rh) antibodies are involved and the disease is called Rh disease; also called erythroblastosis fetalis.

■ **haemolytic uremic syndrome**
serious condition characterised by red cell breakdown and kidney failure, a sequel to infection by certain shiga toxin producing strains *shigella dysenteriae* and *escherichia coli.*

■ **haemophilia**
inherited disease that prevents the normal clotting of blood.

■ **haemorrhagic fever**
condition characterised by non stop internal or external bleeding resulting from a viral infection which has caused blood vessel damage.

■ **haeparin**
chemical that prevents blood from clotting.

■ **hepatic**
pertaining to the liver.

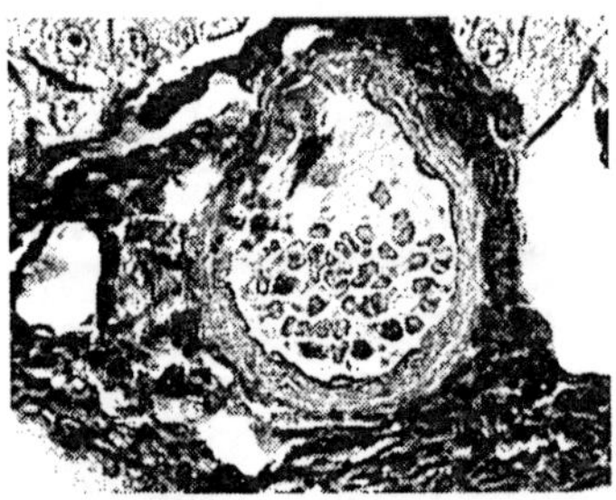

■ **hepatitis b**
viral liver disease that can be

acute or chronic and even life threatening, particularly in people with poor immune resistance. Like HIV, sexual contact, contaminated needles or contaminated blood or blood products can transmit the hepatitis b virus. Unlike HIV, it is also transmissible through close casual contact.

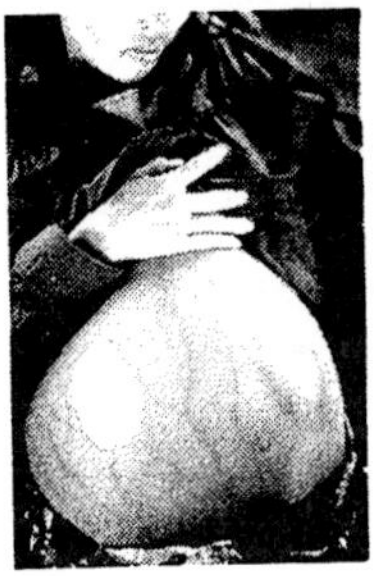

■ **hepatitis b virus**

formerly called serum hepatitis virus because it can be transmitted from the blood of an infected individual.

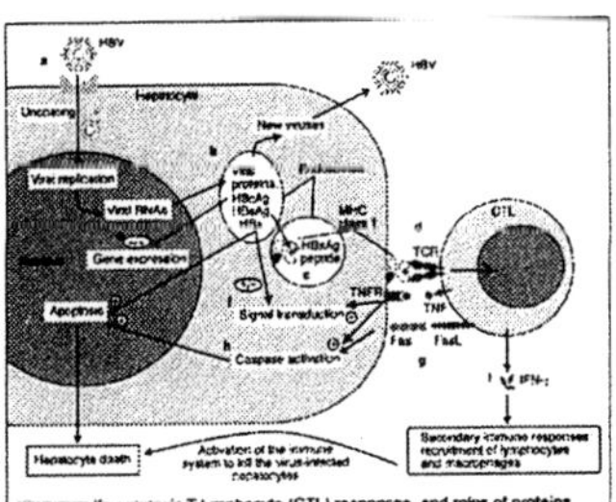

Virus-specific cytotoxic T lymphocyte (CTL) responses and roles of proteins of hepatitis B virus

■ **hepatitis c**

recently recognised viral disease that causes inflammation of the liver, and may cause severe, life threatening liver damage. Hepatitis c was formerly called 'non a/non b' hepatitis.

MODEL OF THE HUMAN HEPATITIS C VIRUS

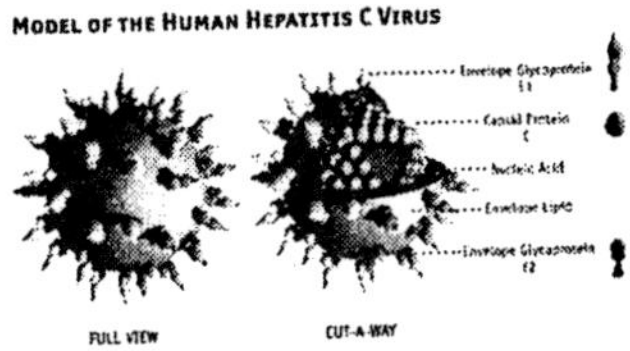

■ **hepatitis**

inflammation of the liver caused by certain viruses and other factors such as alcohol abuse, some medications and trauma. Although many cases of hepatitis are not a serious threat to health, the disease can become chronic and can sometimes lead to liver failure and death. There are four major types of viral hepatitis (a) hepatitis a, caused by infection with the hepatitis a virus, (b) hepatitis b, caused by infection with the hepatitis b virus (HBV), which is most commonly passed on to a partner during intercourse, especially during anal sex, as well as through sharing drug needles, (c) non a, non b hepatitis, caused by the hepatitis c virus, which appears to be spread through sexual contact as well as through sharing drug needles (another type of non a, non b hepatitis is caused by the hepatitis e virus, principally spread through contaminated water) (d) delta hepatitis occurs only in people who are already infected with HBV and is caused by the HDV virus, most cases of delta hepatitis occur among people who are frequently exposed to blood and blood products such as people with haemophilia.

■ **hepatltls**
inflammation of the liver caused by any of several causes. Often accompanied by jaundice, enlarged liver, fever, fatigue and nausea, and abnormal liver function blood tests.

■ **hepatomegaly**
enlargement of the liver.

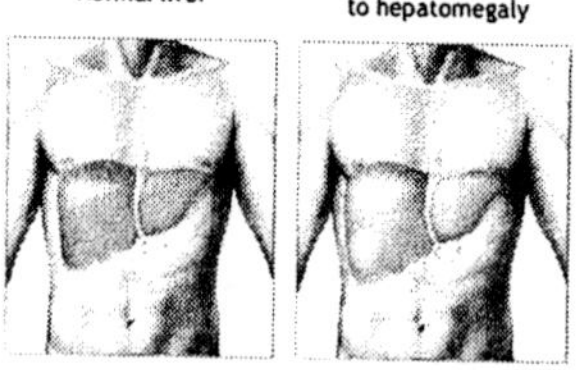

■ **hepatosplenomegaly**
enlargement of the liver and spleen.

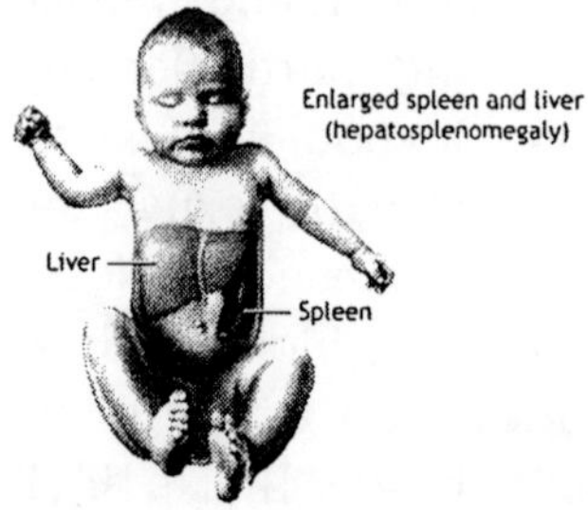

■ **herd immunity**
phenomenon that occurs when a critical concentration of immune hosts prevents the spread of an infectious agent.

■ **hereditary material**
material responsible for the transmission of qualities from ancestor to descendant through genes.

■ **hermaphroditic**
having both male and female reproductive structures in the same organism.

■ **Herpes Simplex Virus 1 (HSV 1)**
a virus that can cause painful 'cold sores' or blisters on the lips ('fever blisters') or in the mouth or around the eyes. The symptomatic disease stage occurs at unpredictable intervals of weeks, months or years. The latent (inactive) virus can reactivate due to emotional stress, physical trauma, other infections, or sup-

pression of the immune system. HSV 1 responds well to treatment with acyclovir.

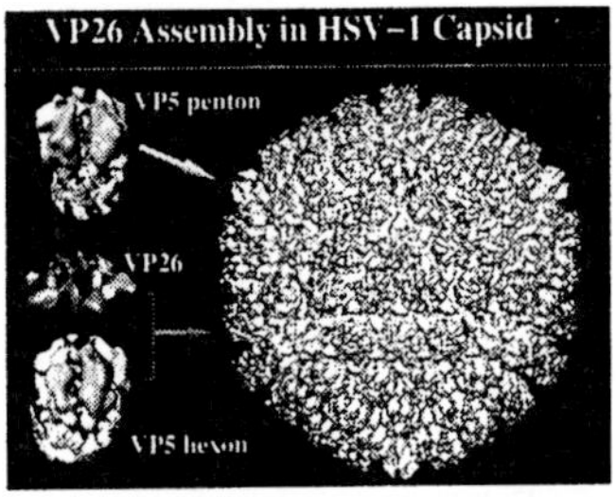

- **Herpes Simplex Virus 2 (HSV 2)**
  virus closely related to HSV 1 that causes similar lesions. However, HSV 2 is usually transmitted sexually, and its lesions generally are in the anogenital area.

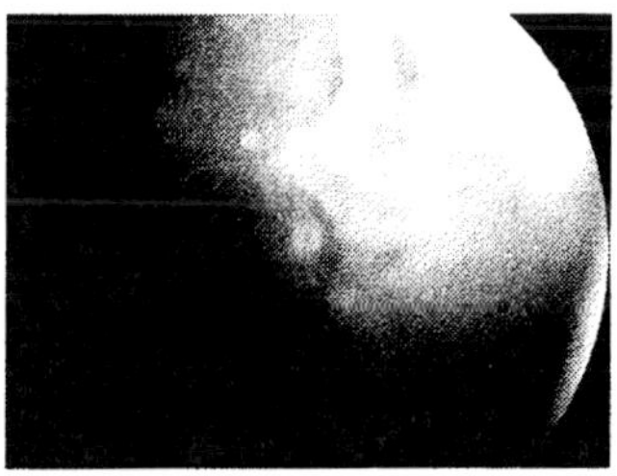

- **Herpes Varicella Zoster virus (HVZ/VZV)**
  varicella virus causes chicken pox in children and may reappear in adulthood as herpes zoster. Herpes zoster, also called shingles, consists of very painful blisters on the skin that follow nerve pathways.

- **herpes virus**
  a family of viruses including herpes simplex 1 and 2, herpes zoster, epstein barr virus, cytomegalovirus, and the newly discovered kaposi's sarcoma associated herpes virus.

- **herpes zoster**
  another name for shingles; a disease which results from reactivation of the herpes virus causing chickenpox.

- **heterocyst**
  differentiated cyanobacterial cell that carries out dinitrogen fixation.

- **heterofermenters**
  bacteria that produce various substances such as ethanol, CO_2, lactic and other acids from glucose.

- **heterokaryon**
  hypha that contains at least two genetically dissimilar nuclei.

- **heterophile antibody**
  antibody that reacts with the red blood cells of another animal.

- **heterothallic**
  hyphae that are incompatible with each other each requiring contact with another hypha of

compatible mating type which, upon fusion, forms a dikaryon or a diploid.

- **heterotroph**
  organism that obtains carbon from an organic compound such as glucose.

- **heterotrophic nitrification**
  biochemical oxidation of ammonium to nitrite and nitrate by heterotrophic micro-organisms.

- **HFR cells (high frequency of recombination cells)**
  rare cells in the F^+ population that can transfer their chromosome to an F^- cell.

- **hickman catheter**
  indwelling line used for administering medication and total parental nutrition over long durations.

- **high copy number plasmid**
  plasmid whose numbers in the cell range from 50 to 500.

- **High Efficiency Particulate Air (HEPA) filters**
  special filters that remove from air nearly all particles, including micro-organisms, that have a diameter greater than 0.3 mm.

- **high energy phosphate bond**
  bond that joins a phosphate group to a molecule and releases a relatively high amount of energy when hydrolysed, denoted by the symbol ~

- **high level disinfectant**
  chemical used to destroy all viruses and vegetative cells, but not endospores.

- **high temperature short time method (HTST)**
  most common pasteurisation protocol, using this method, milk is pasteurised by holding it at 72°c for 15 seconds.

- **histamine**
  substance found in basophil and mast cell granules that upon release can cause dilation and increased permeability of blood vessel walls and other effects, a mediator of inflammation.

- **histocompatibility antigens**
  cell surface molecules involved in the immunological rejection of transplanted tissues and organs and in recognition between cells during the immune response; also called major his-

tocompatibility (MHC) antigens, and in people, the human leukocyte antigens (HLA).

■ **histocompatibility testing**
method of matching the self antigens on the tissues of a transplant donor with those of a recipient. The closer the match, the better the chance that the transplant will not be rejected.

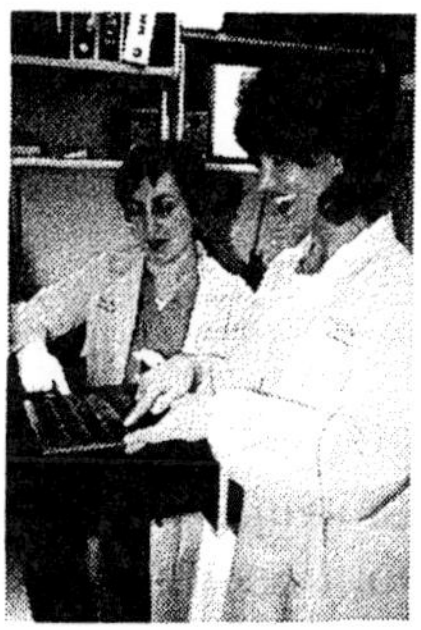

■ **histoplasmosis**
fungal infection, commonly of the lungs, caused by the fungus histoplasma capsulatum. This fungus is commonly found in bird and/or bat droppings in the caribbean. Breathing in the spores of the fungus spreads it. The most definitive test for the fungus has been from fungal stains and bone marrow cultures. Blood testing has proved to be less reliable. In areas where h. Capsulatum is prevalent, 80 percent or more of the population has been exposed to infection through breathing in airborne spores produced by the fungus. People with severely damaged immune systems, such as those with aids, are vulnerable to a very serious disease known as progressive disseminated histoplasmosis. In geographic areas where the fungus is common, people with aids are at high risk for disseminated histoplasmosis.

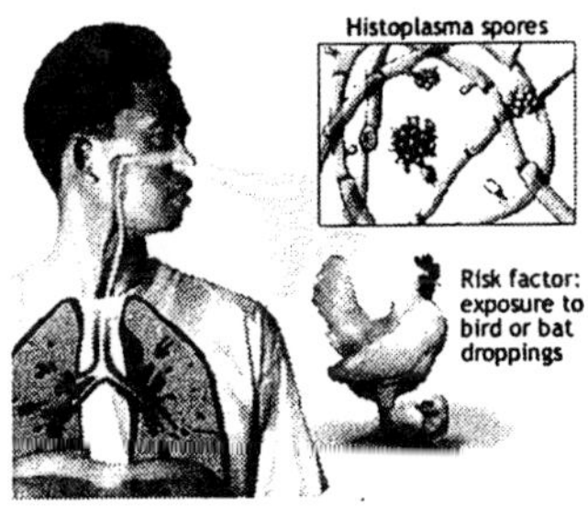

■ **histoplasmosis**
a fungal disease resulting from infection with *Histoplasma capsulatum*.

■ **historical control group**
group of patients (may be loosely or explicitly defined) considered to have the same disease or condition as the study group, but who were diagnosed and treated in a pe-

riod of time prior to that of the study group and who received the conventional form of therapy for that time. Historical control groups are generally only useful for evaluations of treatments involving rare diseases with highly predictable outcomes and where it is considered impractical or unethical to carry out a controlled clinical trial.

■ **HIV disease**
characterised by a gradual deterioration of immune function. During the course of infection, crucial immune cells called cd4+ t cells are disabled and killed, and their numbers progressively decline. Cd4+ t cells play a crucial role in the immune response, signalling other cells in the immune system to perform their special functions.

■ **HLA**
abbreviation for human leukocyte antigen.

■ **holomorph**
whole fungus consisting of all sexual and asexual stages in its life cycle.

■ **homofermenters**
bacteria that convert glucose into lactic acid as the end product of fermentation.

■ **homokaryon**
fungal hypha in which all nuclei are genetically identical.

■ **homologous**
with respect to DNA, stretches that have similar or identical nucleotide sequences and probably encode similar characteristics.

■ **homologous recombination**
genetic recombination between the same genes.

■ **homologous**
similar in appearance or structure, but not necessarily function.

■ **homoserine lactone (HSL)**
freely diffusible molecule that is used by bacteria to sense the density of cells within their population.

■ **homothallic**
hyphae that are self compatible in that sexual reproduction occurs in the same organism by meiosis and genetic recombination; fusion of hypha results in a dikaryon or diploid.

■ **hook**
curved structure that connects the filament of the flagella to the cell surface.

■ **hops**
flowers of the vine like hop plant, they are added to impart a desirable bitter flavour to beer and contribute antibacterial substances.

■ **horizontal evolution**
with respect to antimicrobial resistance, the acquisition of resistance through gene transfer.

■ **horizontal gene transfer**
transmission of DNA from one species to another, also called lateral gene transfer.

■ **horizontal transmission**
transfer of a pathogen from one person to another through contact, ingestion of food or water or via a living agent such as an insect is called.

■ **hormone**
active regulatory chemical substance formed in one part of the body and carried by the blood to another part of the body, where it signals the coordination of cellular functions.

■ **host**
cell or organism that supports the growth of a parasite or virus.

■ **host factors**
body's potent mechanisms for containing HIV, including immune system cells called cd8+ t cells, which may prove more effective than any antiretro viral drug in controlling HIV infection.

■ **host range**
refers to the range of cell types that a pathogen can infect.

■ **hot virus**
virus that has the potential to spread rapidly and therefore must be handled with extreme care. Examples include the ebola virus and hantavirus.

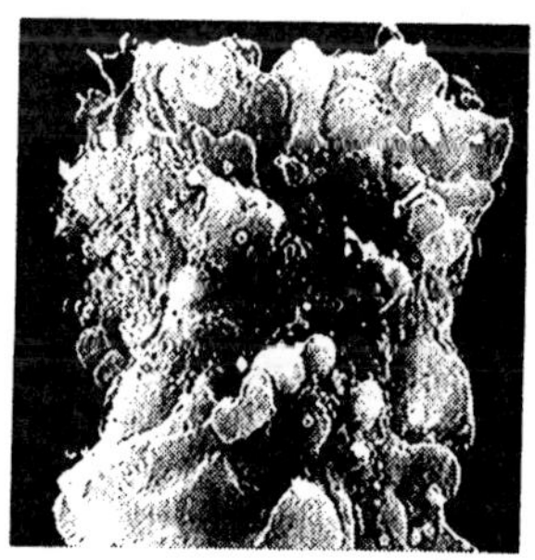

■ **HTST**
abbreviation for high temperature short time pasteurisation.

■ **human immunodeficiency virus or HIV infection**
infection with the retrovirus that causes the acquired immunodeficiency syndrome (AIDS).

■ **human immunodeficiency virus type 1 (HIV 1)**
the probable cause of aids. A human retrovirus of the lentivirus family, notable for long duration of asymptomatic infection, often followed by progressive deterioration of cell mediated immune function, and eventual opportunistic infection and neoplasm. The median time for an HIV infected individual to develop full clinical aids is probably over ten years. (formerly called HTLV iii or LAV).

■ **human immunodeficiency virus type 2 (HIV 2)**
virus closely related to HIV 1 that has been found to cause immune suppression. It is most common in Africa.

■ **human leukocyte anitgens (HLA)**
markers that identify cells as 'self' and prevent the immune system from attacking them.

■ **human papilloma virus (HPV)**
virus that is the cause of warts of the hands and feet, as well as lesions of the mucous membranes of the oral, anal and genital cavities. More than 50 types of HPV have been identified, some of which are associated with cancerous and pre-cancerous conditions. The virus can be transmitted through sexual contact and is a precursor to cancer of the cervix. There is no specific cure for an HPV infection, but the virus often can be controlled by podophyllin (medicine derived from the roots of the plant podophyllum peltatum) or interferon, and the warts can be removed by cryosurgery, laser treatment or conventional surgery.

■ **humatin**
brand name of paromomycin.

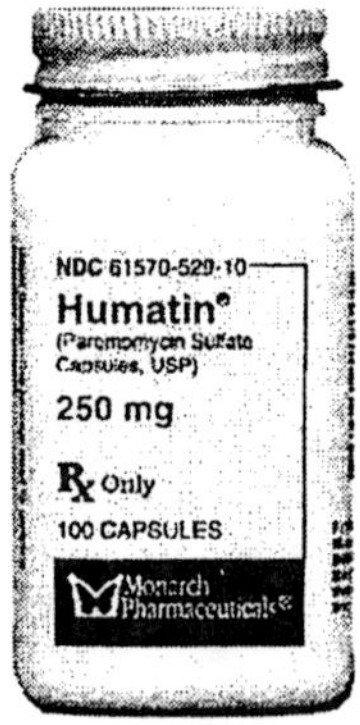

■ **humic acid**
dark coloured organic material extracted from soil by various reagents (e.g., dilute alkali) and that is precipitated by acid (ph 1 to 2).

■ **humic substances**
series of relatively high molecular weight, brown to black substances formed by secondary synthesis reactions. The term is generic in a sense that it describes the coloured material or its fractions obtained on the basis of solubility characteristics, such as humic acid or fulvic acid.

■ **humification**
process whereby the carbon of organic residues is transformed and converted to humic substances through biochemical and chemical processes.

■ **humeral immune response**
immune response that is mediated by b cells and involves production of antibodies. Humeral immunity (also known as th-1 immune response) is associated with the production of the cytokines interleukin 4 and interleukin 10.

■ **humeral immunity**
the branch of the immune system that relies primarily upon antibodies.

■ **humus**
total of the organic compounds in soil exclusive of undecayed plant and animal tissues, their 'partial decomposition' products, and the soil biomass. The term is often used synonymously with soil organic matter.

■ **hybrid**
offspring produced from mating plants or animals from different species, varieties or genotypes.

■ **hybridisation**
annealing of two complementary strands of DNA from different sources to create a hybrid double stranded molecule.

■ **hybridoma**
hybrid cell produced by the fusion of an antibody producing lymphocyte with a tumour cell. Hybridomas are used in the production of monoclonal antibodies

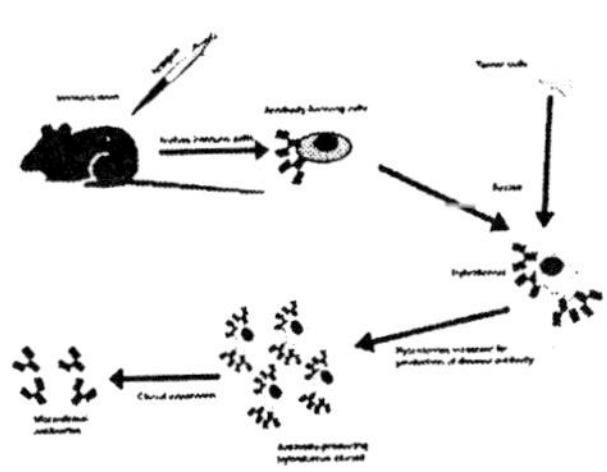

■ **hydrogen bond**
chemical bond between a hydrogen atom of one molecule and two unshared electrons of another molecule.

■ **hydrogenation**
reduction reaction in which an electron and an accompanying proton is added to a molecule.

■ **hydrogen oxidising bacterium**
facultative lithotrophs that, in the absence of an oxidisable organic source, oxidise h_2 for energy and synthesise carbohydrates with carbon dioxide as their source of carbon.

■ **hydrolysis**
chemical reaction in which a molecule is broken down as H_2O is added.

■ **hydrophilic**
water loving, soluble in water.

■ **hydrophobic bonds**
weak bonds formed between molecules as a result of their mutual repulsion of water molecules.

■ **hygroscopic water**
water adsorbed by a dry soil from an atmosphere of high relative humidity.

■ **hymenium**
layer of hyphae which are fertile in producing asci (fungi in the phylum Ascomycota) or basidia (fungi in the phylum Basidiomycota) from the process of meiosis.

■ **hypergammaglobulinemia**
abnormally high levels of antibodies in the blood, common in persons with HIV.

■ **hyperimmune globulin**
immunoglobulin prepared from the sera of donors with large amounts of antibodies to certain diseases, such as tetanus, used to prevent or treat the disease.

■ **hyperparasite**
parasite that feeds on another parasite.

■ **hyperplasia**
excessive cell growth.

■ **hypersensitivity**
abnormal sensitivity, medically, when the body responds in an exaggerated manner to a foreign agent, allergy.

■ **hypertension**
high blood pressure.

■ **hyperthermophiles**
organisms that have an opti-

mum growth temperature between 70° c and 110°c.

■ **hypervariable regions**
small areas in the fab portion of the immunoglobulin light and heavy polypeptide chains that binds the antigenic epitope.

■ **hypha (pl. hyphae)**
threadlike structure that characterises the growth of most fungi and some bacteria such as members of the genus *streptomyces.*

■ **hypogammaglobulinemia**
abnormally low levels of immunoglobulins.

■ **hyposensitisation (desensitisation)**
form of therapy for immediate ige mediated allergies in which extremely small but increasing amounts of antigen are injected regularly over a period of months, directing the response from ige to igg.

■ **hypothesis (alternative HA)**
investigator's initial supposition that the study will demonstrate that 'something is going on'; i.e., results observed are more than the outcome of chance. Common examples include that there is a difference in outcome measures between groups, correlation between factors of interest, or association between exposure and disease, i.e., observations are the result of real differences or correlations.

■ **hypothesis (null HO)**
the investigator's initial supposition that the study will demonstrate that 'nothing is going on', i.e., results observed are the outcome of chance. Common examples include that there is no difference in outcome measures between groups, no correlation between factors of interest, or no association between exposure and disease, i.e., observations are the result of random variation.

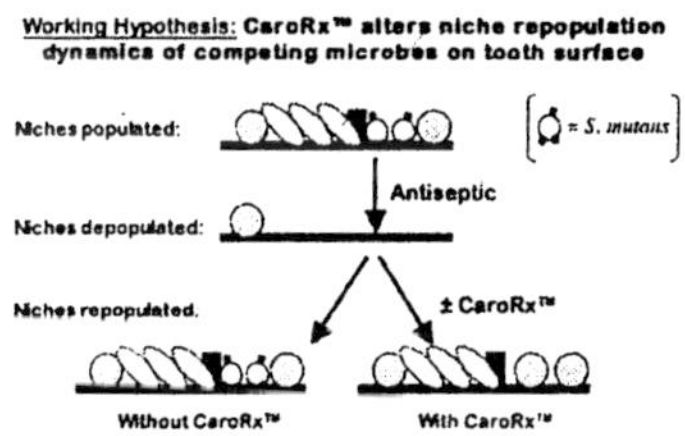

■ **hypoxia**
reduction of oxygen supply to tissue.

■ **id**
identification.

■ **icosahedral**
in virology, refers to a virus with a icosahedral capsid,

which has the shape of a regular polyhedron having 20 equilateral triangular faces and 12 corners.

■ **idiopathic**
without a known cause.

■ **idiotypes**
the unique and characteristic parts of an antibody's variable region, which can themselves serve as antigens.

■ **ifn**
abbreviation for interferons

■ **illness**
period of time during which symptoms and signs of disease occur.

■ **illuviation**
deposition of soil material removed from one horizon to another in the soil.

■ **immobilisation**
conversion of an element from the inorganic to the organic form in microbial or plant biomass.

■ **immune complex**
clusters formed when antigens and antibodies bind together.

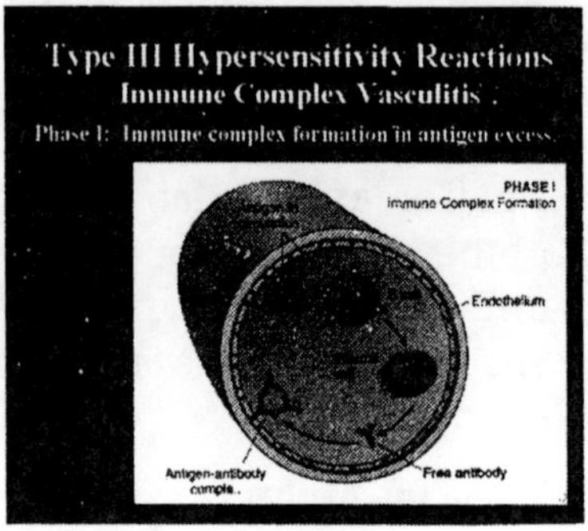

■ **immune deficiency**
breakdown or inability of certain parts of the immune system to function, thus making a person susceptible to certain diseases that they would not ordinarily develop.

■ **immune response**
activity of the immune system against foreign substances.

■ **immune serum globulin (immunoglobulin g)**
portion of pooled plasma from many donors, containing a wide variety of antibodies, used to provide passive protection.

■ **immune system**
the complex functions of the body that recognise foreign agents or substances, neutralise them, and recall the response later when confronted with the same challenge.

- **immune thrombocytopenic purpura (ITP)**
  HIV related loss of platelets in the blood. Its exact cause is unclear.
- **immunity**
  protection against infectious agents and other substances.
- **immunoassay**
  tests using immunological reagents such as antigens and antibodies.
- **immunoblot (western blot)**
  detection of proteins immobilised on a filter by complementary reaction with specific antibody.
- **immunocompetent**
  having a normally functioning immune system.
- **immunocompromised**
  having a deficient or damaged immune response.

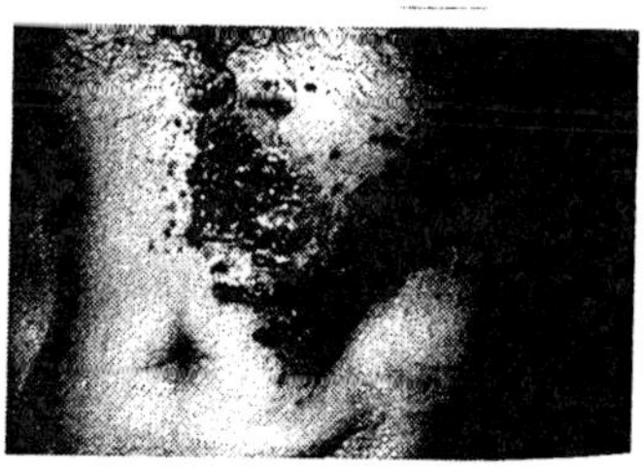

- **immunodeficiency**
  inability to produce a normal immune response to antigen.
- **immunodiffusion tests**
  precipitation reactions carried out in agarose or other gels.
- **immunoelectrophoresis**
  technique for separating proteins by subjecting the mixture to an electric current followed by diffusion and precipitation in gels using antibodies against the separated proteins.
- **immunofluorescence**
  technique used to identify particular antigens microscopically in cells by the binding of a fluorescent antibody to the antigen.
- **immunogen**
  antigen that can induce an immune response.
- **immunogenicity**
  ability of an antigen or vaccine to stimulate an immune response.
- **immunoglobulin**
  glycoprotein molecules that react specifically with the substance that induced their formation, antibodies.
- **immunological tolerance**
  state of specific unresponsiveness, failure to respond to a specific antigen, such as self antigen.

■ **immunology**
the study of immunity, or protection against infectious and other agents, and conditions arising from the mechanisms involved in immunity, such as hypersensitivities.

■ **immunomodulator**
any substance that influences the immune system.

■ **immunostimulant**
any agent or substance that triggers or enhances the body's defence, also called immunopotentiators.

■ **immunosuppression**
nonspecific suppression of acquired immune responses.

■ **immunotherapeutic**
aiming at reconstituting an impaired immune system.

■ **immunotherapy**
treatment aimed at reconstituting an impaired immune system.

■ **immunotoxin**
plant or animal toxin (i.e., poison) that is attached to a monoclonal antibody and used to destroy a specific target cell.

■ **in utero**
latin for 'in the uterus', or womb.

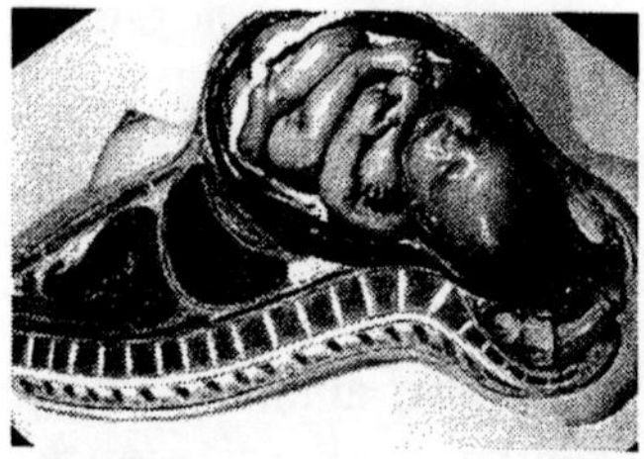

■ **in vitro**
in a test tube or other container as opposed to inside a living plant or animal.

■ **in vivo**
inside a living plant or animal as opposed to a test tube or other container.

■ **inactivated vaccine**
dead micro-organisms used as antigens to produce immunity.

■ **inactive control treatment**
control treatment that is not considered to have any pharmacological or physiological effect; a placebo treatment or sham procedure.

■ **inapparent (subclinical) infections**
infections in which symptoms do not occur or are mild enough to go unnoticed.

■ **incidence rate**
number of new cases of a disease within a specific time pe-

riod in a given population.

■ **incidence**
number of new cases occurring in a given population over a certain period of time.

■ **inclusion body**
microscopically visible structure within a cell representing the site at which an infecting virus replicates, can occur within the nucleus or the cytoplasm

■ **inclusion/exclusion criteria**
medical or social standards determining whether a person may or may not be allowed to enter a clinical trial. For example, some trials may not allow people with chronic liver disease or with certain drug allergies, others may exclude men or women, or only include people with a lowered t cell count.

■ **incubation period**
time interval between the initial infection and appearance of the first clinical symptom or sign of disease.

Pathways of Entry and Exit for Viral Pathogens

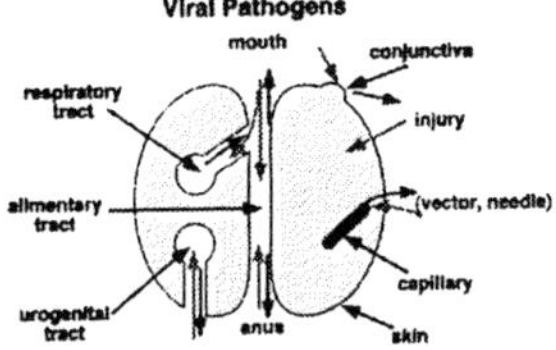

■ **index case**
first identified case of a disease in an epidemic.

■ **indication**
sign or symptom. Also called 'label indication'.

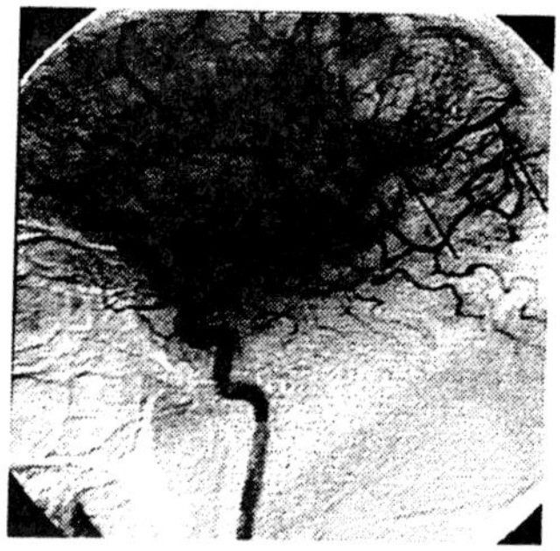

■ **indicator medium**
agar medium containing a component that is changed in a recognisable way by a particular species of micro-organism that helps identify the organism.

■ **indirect contact**
means of transmitting infectious disease by coughing or sneezing, through food and water, insect bites, and other indirect contact.

■ **indirect selection**
technique for isolating mutants and identifying organisms unable to grow on a me-

dium on which the parents do grow; often involves replica plating.

■ **indolent**
at rest, or in a quiescent state.

■ **induced**
with respect to gene expression, a gene product that is synthesised only under certain conditions.

■ **induced mutation**
mutation that results from the organism being treated with an agent that alters its DNA.

■ **induced sputum**
test where saline mist is breathed to induce a cough. Resultant sputum is then cultured or stained to look for micro-organisms, often *pneumocystis carinii.*

■ **inducer**
substance that activates transcription of certain genes.

■ **inducible enzyme**
enzyme synthesised only when a substrate on which it can act is present.

■ **induction**
the initiation of a particular therapy.

■ **induction**
process by which a prophage is excised from the host cell DNA, activation of gene transcription.

■ **infection**
growth of an organism within another living organism.

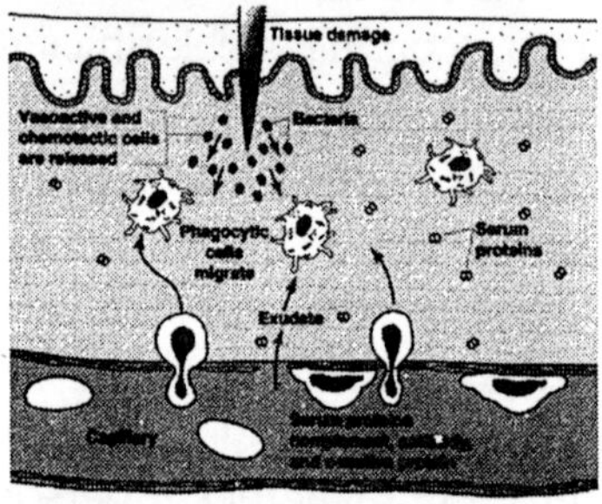

■ **infection thread**
cellulosic tube in a root hair through which rhizobia can travel to reach and infect root cells.

■ **infectious disease**
disease caused by a microbial or viral infection.

■ **infectious dose**
number of micro-organisms or viruses sufficient to establish an infection.

■ **infective dose (ID)**
concentration of infective virions. Often expressed as ID_{50} in which 50 percent of the hosts are infected.

■ **infiltrates**
something seeping or filling in

a space or cavity.

■ **inflammation**
redness, swelling, soreness of tissues.

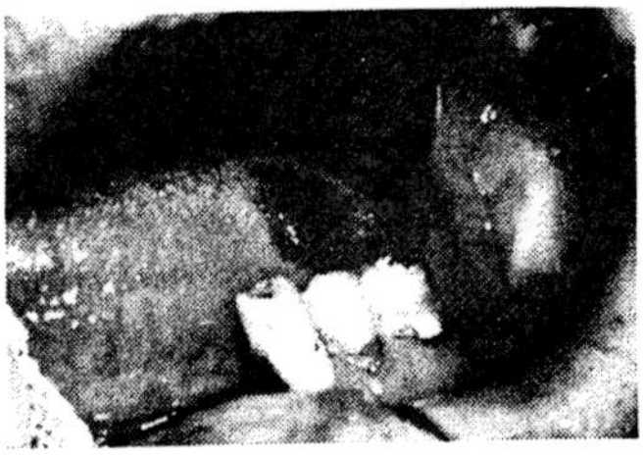

■ **informed consent**
voluntary consent given by a patient to participate in a study after being informed of its purpose, method of treatment, procedure for assignment to treatment, benefits and risks associated with participation, and required data collection procedures and schedule.

■ **infrared (IR)**
portion of the electromagnetic spectrum with wavelengths from about 0.75 μm to 1 mm.

■ **infusion**
administration of treatment in a dilute form by slow injection into a vein.

■ **inhibition**
prevention of growth or function.

■ **initiation complex**
complex of ribosomal subunit, a TRNA that carries f met, and elongation factors, that comes together at a start codon on mrna and begins the process of translation.

■ **injection drug user (IDU, IVDU, AVDA)**
also known as intravenous drug user (IVDU), or intravenous drug abuser (IVDA). None of these terms are very precise, often IVDU will be used to describe someone who injects sub q, and the distinction between 'user' and 'abuser' is a controversial and emotionally charged one. Nevertheless, a working definition for an IDU is anyone who regularly injects any substances, whether pharmaceutically or illicitly made, not under medical prescription and supervision.

■ **innate immunity**
non-specific immunity that is not acquired or affected by prior contact with the infectious agent or other material involved and is not mediated by lymphocytes.

■ **innate resistance**
resistance of an organism to an

antimicrobial medication due to the inherent characteristics of that type organism, also called intrinsic resistance.

■ **inner membrane**

in prokaryotic cells, the cytoplasmic membrane of gram negative bacteria and in eukaryotic cells, the membrane on the interior side of an organelle that has a double membrane.

■ **inoculate**

to treat with micro-organisms for the purpose of creating a favourable response. For example, treatment of legume seeds with rhizobia to stimulate N_2 fixation.

■ **inoculation**

introduction of a substance (inoculum; e.g., a vaccine, serum or virus) into the body to produce or to increase immunity to the disease or condition associated with the substance.

■ **inoculum**

material used to introduce a micro-organism into a suitable situation for growth.

■ **insert**

DNA that is (or will be) joined to a vector to create a recombinant DNA molecule.

■ **inserted repeat**

sequence of nucleotides on one strand of DNA that is identical to DNA on another strand when both are read in the same direction i.e., 5' to 3', associated with transposable elements.

■ **insertion**

genetic mutation in which one or more nucleotides are added to DNA.

■ **insertion mutation**

mutation resulting from the integration of a transposon into a gene.

■ **insertion sequence (IS element)**

simplest type of transposable element.

■ **insterstitial**

space or gap in a tissue in the context of 'interstitial infiltrates', means between the air passage in a lung

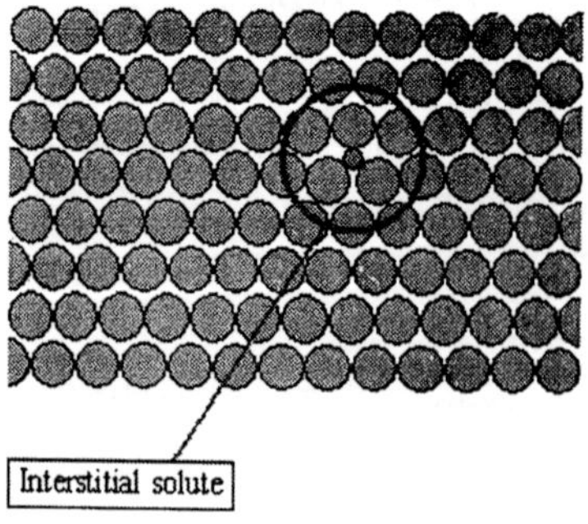

■ **Institutional Review Board (IRB)**
committee of physicians, statisticians, community advocates, and others which ensures that a clinical trial is ethical and that the rights of the study participants are protected.

■ **Insulin Dependent Diabetes Mellitus (IDDM)**
diabetes caused by autoimmune destruction of pancreatic cells by cytotoxic T cells.

■ **integrase**
HIV enzyme that governs the insertion of HIV's proviral genetic material into the host genome. Integrase is a target for a new generation of HIV drugs.

■ **integration**
process by which a dna molecule becomes incorporated into another genome.

■ **intent to treat**
analysis of clinical trial results that includes all data from patients in the groups to which they were randomised (i.e., assigned through random distribution) even if they never received the treatment.

■ **interaction**
situation in which the magnitude of the test control treatment difference for the outcome of interest depends upon the value assumed by a third factor, such as age or prior disease state of the study patients.

■ **interaction effect**
treatment interaction effect.

■ **intercalating agents**
agents that insert themselves between two nucleotides in opposite strands of a dna double helix.

■ **intercurrent**
occurring at the same time, or accompanying.

■ **interference microscope**
type of light microscope that employs special optical devices to cause the specimen to appear as a three dimensional image. An example is the Nomarski differential interference contrast microscope.

■ **interferon**
general term used to describe a family of 20-25 proteins that cause a cell to become resistant to a wide variety of viruses. Cells infected by almost any virus produce them.

■ **interim analysis**
any data analysis done before the trial is finished, for whatever reason, but usually concerned with assessments of treatment effects.

■ **interim result**
any test control treatment difference observed during the trial.

■ **interleukin**
chemical hormone messenger (cytokine) secreted by and affecting many different cells in the immune system.

■ **interleukin 6 (IL 6)**
cytokine whose production affects many different cells in the immune system.

■ **interleukin 1 (IL 1)**
natural cytokine released by monocytes, macrophages, t cells and other immune cells that fights infection.

■ **interleukin 10 (IL 10)**
cytokine released by lymphocytes (the th-2 subset of t helper lymphocytes) that enhances the humeral response, increasing antibody production.

■ **interleukin 12 (IL 12)**
cytokine that induces the production of natural killer and other cytotoxic immune cells. IL 12 is associated with a cell mediated or th-1 immune response. A recombinant IL 12 is under study as a treatment for HIV disease (immuno-modulator).

■ **interleukin 4 (IL 4)**
cytokine released by lymphocytes (the th-2 subset of t helper lymphocytes) that enhances the humeral response, increasing antibody production.

■ **intermediate filaments**
component of the eukaryotic cell cytoskeleton.

■ **intermediate level disinfectant**
type of chemical used to destroy all vegetative bacteria including mycobacteria, fungi, and most, but not all, viruses.

■ **internal node**
branch point on a phylogenetic tree that represents an ancestor to modern organisms.

■ **interstitial**
relating to or situated in the small, narrow spaces between tissues or parts of an organ.

■ **intolerant**
unable to take a drug because of toxicity.

■ **intracellular**
inside the cell.

■ **intradermal**
within the layers of the skin.

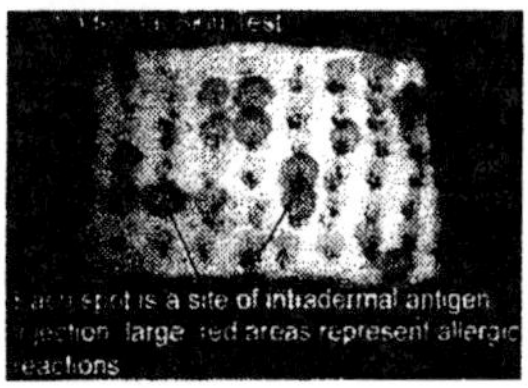

■ **intralesional**
injected directly into a lesion

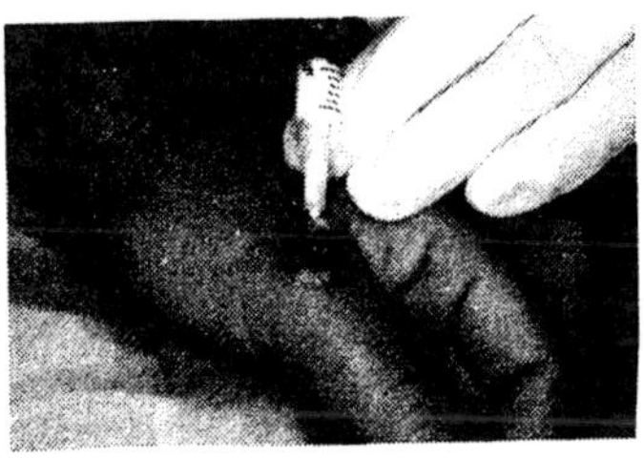

■ **intramural**
research that is done by one or more institute.

■ **intramuscular**
into the muscle, frequently in reference to injections.

■ **intranuclear inclusion body**
structure found within the nucleus of cells infected with certain viruses such as the cytomegalovirus.

■ **intrapartum**
during childbirth.

■ **intrathecal**
injected into the fluid surround ing the spinal cord.

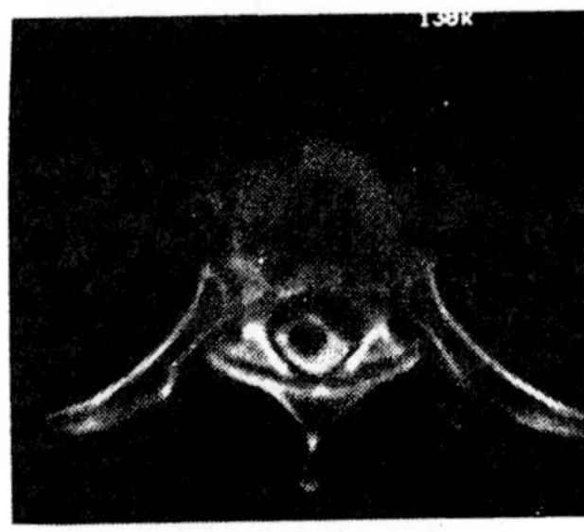

■ **intravenous (IV)**
within or into the veins. Intravenous drugs are injected directly into the veins.

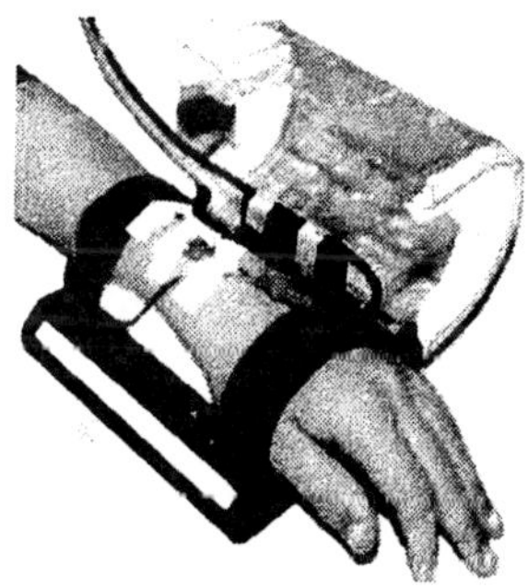

■ **intravitreal**
within the eye.

■ **intrinsic resistance**
resistance of an organism to an antimicrobial medication due to inherent characteristics of

that type of organism also called innate resistance.

- **intron**
part of the eukaryotic chromosome that does not code for a protein, removed from mrna before the mrna is translated.

- **investigational**
under study.

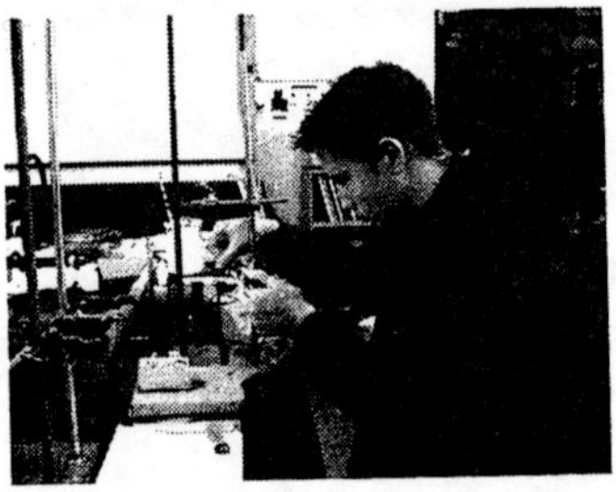

- **Investigational New Drug (IND)**
status of an experimental drug that it can be tested in people.

- **invirase**
brand name for saquinavir

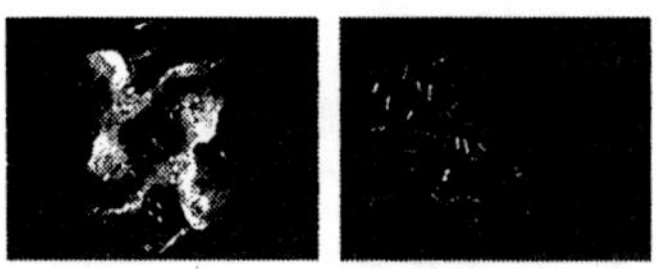

Vereinfachte Darstellung der beiden Ketten (rot und grün) der HIV-Protease mit Saquinavir im aktiven Zentrum (gelb)

- **ion**
charged atom or molecule

- **ionic bond**
bond formed by the attraction of positively charged atoms or molecules to negatively charged ones

- **ions**
atoms, groups of atoms, or compounds, that are electrically charged as a result of the loss of electrons (cations) or the gain of electrons (anions).

- **irrigation**
intentional watering of the soil.

- **IS**
abbreviation for insertion sequence.

- **isoenzyme (isozyme)**
when two different enzymes catalyse the same reaction(s), they are isoenzymes of each other. Isoenzymes could differ from each other in their primary structure or electrophoretic mobility.

- **isolate**
an individual (as a spore or a single organism), viable part of an organism (as a cell) or a strain that has been isolated (as from diseased tissue, contaminated water or the air). Also, a pure culture produced from such an isolate.

■ **isolation**
any procedure in which an organism present in a particular sample or environment, is obtained in pure culture.

■ **isomer**
molecule with the same number and types of atoms as another but differs in its structure.

■ **isometric**
relating to a shape characterised by equal sides

■ **isomorphous substitution**
substitution in a crystalline clay sheet of one atom by a similarly sized atom of lower valence.

■ **isoniazid**
an antibiotic that is one of the most common components in treatment for tuberculosis,

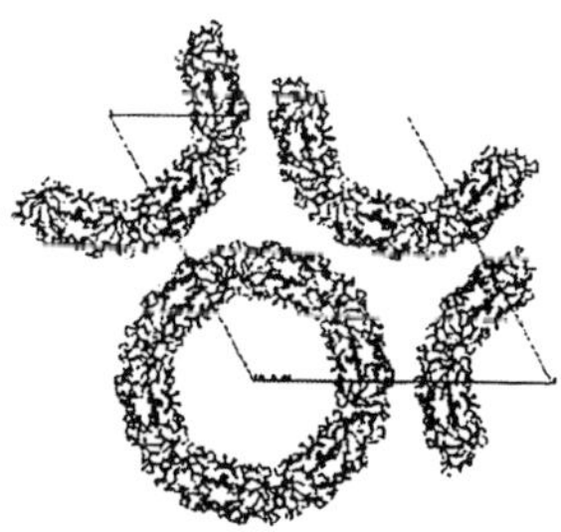

either alone or in combination.

■ **isosporiasis**
aprotozoal infection, isosporiasis is usually restricted to the lower gastrointestinal tract. Symptomatically similar to cryptosporidiosis, isosporiasis usually responds well to treatment.

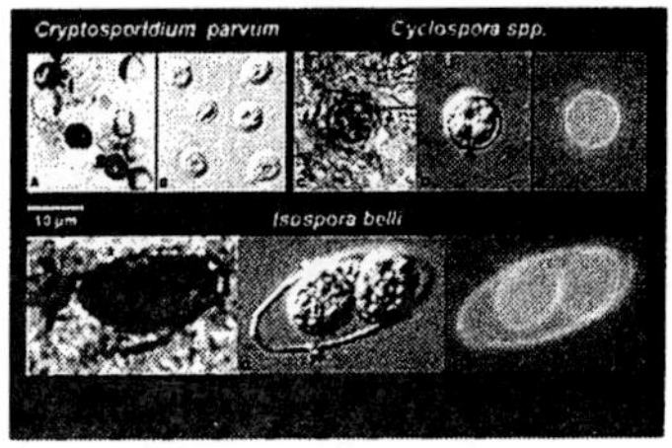

■ **isotonic**
refers to a solution whose salinity is the same as human blood.

■ **isotope**
form of an element that differs in atomic weight from the form most common in nature

■ **itraconazole (sporanox)**
an antifungal drug that is used to treat fungal infections in persons with HIV, including candida, cryptococcus, histoplasmosis and others.

■ **jarisch herxheimer reaction**
abrupt but transitory worsening of symptoms after starting effective antibacterial treatment, thought to be caused by substances released by the death of the bacteria.

■ **jaundice**
yellowish discolouration of the skin and eyes due to bile.

Usually associated with some form of liver damage or malfunction.

- **JC papovavirus**
suggested as a possible cause of progressive multifocal leukoencephalopathy.

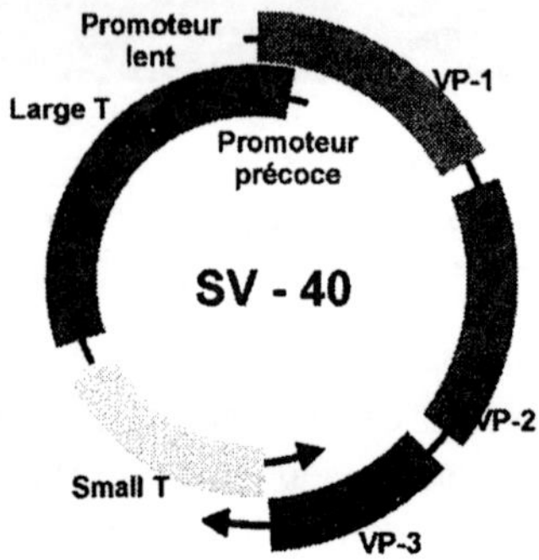

- **kaplan meier curve**
way of graphing patient progress (how many are still alive or free of infection) against time, a life table curve showing the percent of people free of a specific event at times following randomisation. The kaplan Meier method is especially well suited to situations with censored data, such as those encountered in clinical trials, where patients are enrolled over a period of time and followed to a common calendar time point.

- **kaposi's sarcoma**
previously uncommon form of cancer that attacks the connective tissue, bones, cartilage and muscles of the body. The cancer may spread and also attack the eyes. If the cancerous area is near the surface of the skin, lesions inches in length may develop. This disease was initially seen only in elderly men and natives of central Africa. Experimental work has shown that the aids related Kaposi's sarcoma and the central African variety respond differently to some types of medications. Radiotherapy and chemotherapy are usually recommended.

- **karnofsky score**
subjective score between 0 to 100, assigned by a physician to describe a patient's ability to perform common tasks.

- **karyogamy**
fusion in a cell of haploid (n) nuclei to form a diploid (2n).

- **ketaconazole (nizoral)**
antifungal drug that is used to treat fungal infections in persons with HIV, including candida, cryptococcus, histoplasmosis, and others.

- **killer t cells**
  killer cells infected with HIV or other viruses or transformed by cancer. Also known as cytotoxic t cells (or cytotoxic t lymphocytes).

- **kilo**
  prefix meaning a thousand time, as in kilogram, a thousand grams.

- **kinase**
  enzyme that mediates the addition of phosphorus to chemical groups. The AZT nucleoside must be phosphorylated to become a genetically active nucleotide.

- **kinetic energy**
  energy of motion.

- **kingdom**
  taxonomic rank that groups several phyla or divisions, a collection of similar kingdoms makes up a domain.

- **kirby bauer disk**
  diffusion test Procedure used to qualitatively determine the susceptibility of a given organism to a battery of different antimicrobial medications.

- **koch's postulates**
  group of criteria used to determine the cause fo an infectious disease by culturing the agent and reproducing the disease.

- **koplik's spots**
  lesions of the oral cavity caused by measles virus that resemble a grain of salt on a red base.

- **krebs cycle**
  metabolic pathway that incorporates acetyl COA, and generates CO_2 and reducing power; also called the tricarboxylic acid cycle (TCA cycle) and the citric acid cycle.

- **k strategy**
  ecological strategy where organisms depend on physiological adaptations to environmental resources. K strategists are usually stable and permanent members of the community.

- **kupffer cells**
  macrophages of the liver.

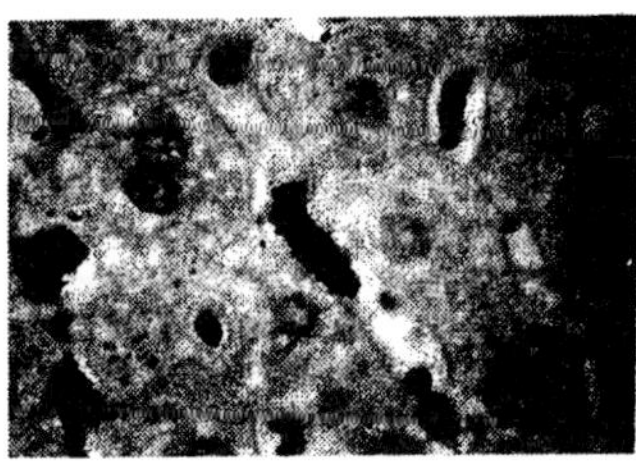

- **Lac operon**
  operon that encodes the proteins required for the degradation of

lactose, it has served as one of the most important models for studying gene regulation.

- **lactic acid bacteria**
  group of gram positive bacteria that generate lactic acid as a major end product of their fermentative metabolism.

- **lactoferrin**
  iron binding protein found in leukocytes, saliva, mucus, milk, and other substances; helps defend the body by depriving micro-organisms of iron.

- **lactose**
  disaccharide consisting of one molecule of glucose and one of galactose.

- **Lacz gene**
  gene used to visually determine whether or not a vector contains a fragment inserted into the multiple cloning site.

- **lag phase**
  period after inoculation of fresh growth medium during which population numbers do not increase.

- **lagging strand**
  strand of double stranded DNA that must be synthesised as a series of discontinuous fragments because of its 5' to 3' orientation with respect to the replication fork.

- **lagooning**
  sewage treatment method in which sewage is channelled into shallow lagoons, during which time it is stabilised by anaerobic and/or aerobic organisms.

- **Lai**
  group of closely related HIV isolates that includes the LAV, IIIB and BRU strains of HIV. Used in HIV vaccine development.

- **Lak cells**
  lymphocytes transformed in the laboratory into lymphokine activated killer cells, which attack tumour cells.

- **lamella (pl. lamellae)**
  thin layer, plate like arrangement or membrane.

- **laminar flow hood**
  biological safety cabinet in which laboratory personnel work with potentially dangerous airborne pathogens; a continuous flow of incoming and outgoing air is filtered through hepa filters to contain micro-organisms within the cabinet.

■ **lamivudine (3tc)**
nucleoside analogue drug, in the same family as AZT, that is used as an antiretroviral to treat HIV disease.

■ **lamprene**
brand name of clofazimine.

■ **lancefield grouping**
classification of b hemolytic streptococci based on serological identification

■ **langerhans cell**
type of dendritic cell found in the skin.

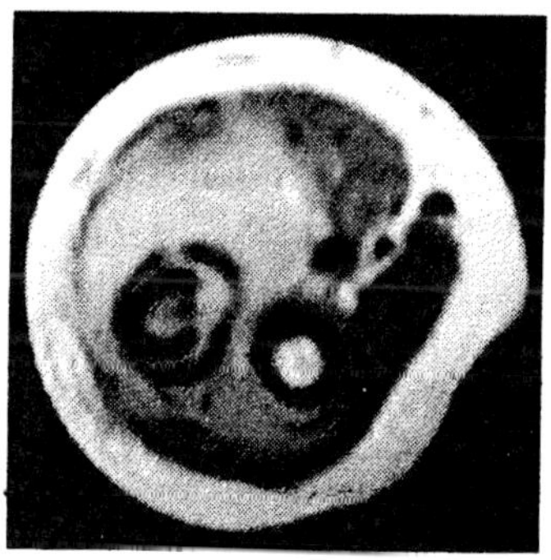

■ **langerhans cells**
antigen presenting dendritic cells of the skin, similar in some respects to macrophages.

■ **latency**
the period when an organism is in the body, shows no symptoms, but is in an inactive state (also known as incubation period).

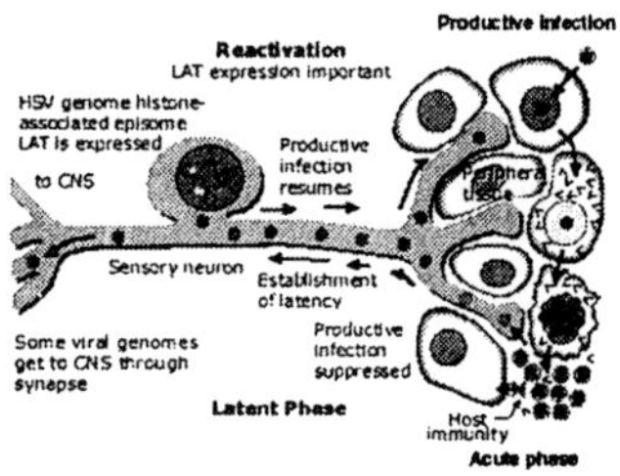

■ **latent infection**
infection in which the infectious agent is present but not active

■ **lateral**
to, or on the side.

■ **lateral gene transfer**
transfer of DNA from one prokaryotic species to another; also called horizontal gene transfer.

■ **LAV**
abbreviation for lymphadenopathy associated virus.

■ **laws of thermodynamics**
fundamental principles of energy relationships. The first of these laws states that the energy in the universe can never be created or destroyed. The second states that entropy always increases.

■ **ld50**

short for 'lethal dose 50'; the dosage of a drug or poison that is toxic to 50% of the organisms it is tested against. Often applies to does of drug against micro-organisms.

■ **leaching**

removal of valuable metals from ores by microbial action.

■ **leading strand**

strand of double stranded DNA that, because of its 5' to 3' orientation with respect to the replication fork, is synthesised continuously.

■ **leaky**

refers to a mutation in which the mutant gene codes for a protein that is partially functional.

■ **lecithin**

component of mammalian cell walls, attacked by the a toxin of *clostridium perfringens* and other lecithinases.

■ **lectin pathway**

pathway of complement activation non-specifically initiated by a host protein binding to mannose present in many bacterial cell walls.

■ **lectins**

plant proteins with a high affinity for specific sugar residues.

■ **leghemoglobin**

protein synthesised by leguminous plants that carries O_2 within a *rhizobium* harbouring nodule.

■ **legionella pneumophilae**

ubiquitous bacteria causing pneumonia, or 'legionnaire's disease'. Recognised fairly recently. Pneumophilae may be the cause of many pneumonias of indeterminate etiology. Most exposure is from tap water, often aerosolised by a showerhead or air conditioner

■ **legume**

any of a large family of dicotyledonous plants that bear nodules on the roots that contain nitrogen fixing bacteria, including important food and forage plants (peas, beans, and clovers).

■ **lentivirus**

sub family of retrovirii that is cytopathic and causes chronic diseases. HIV is a lentivirus.

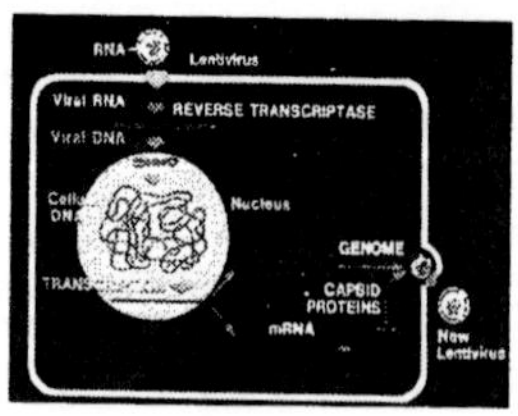

■ **leokocytosis**
abnormal high number of white blood cells in the circulating blood.

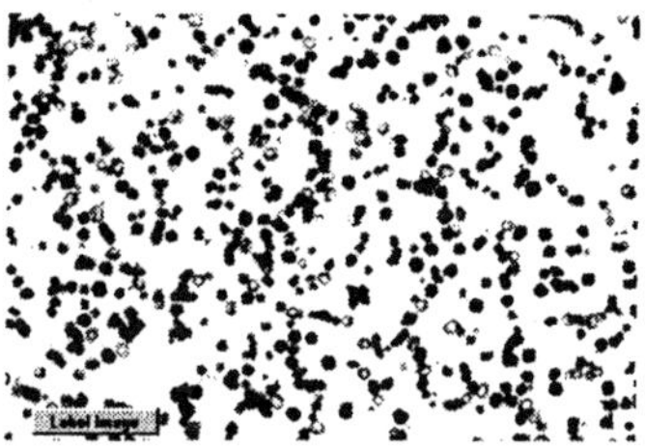

■ **lesion**
general term to describe an area of altered tissue (e.g., the infected patch or sore in a skin disease).

■ **lethal dose (LD)**
concentration of lethal virions. Often expressed as LD_{50}; the concentration of virus in which 50 percent of the hosts are killed

■ **leucovorin**
form of the b vitamin, foliate that is preferentially taken up by human cells. Leucovorin thereby protects from the effect of foliate antagonist antibiotics.

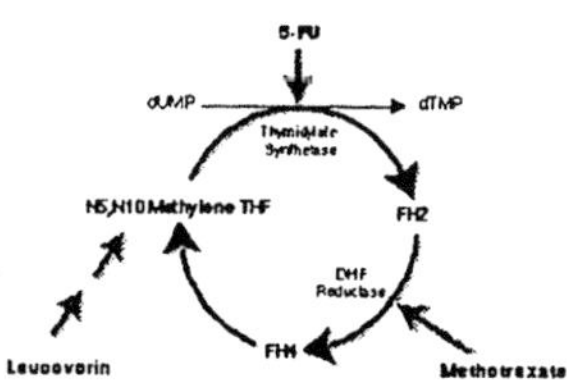

■ **leukemia**
cancer of the leukocytes (white blood cells).

■ **leukine**
brand name of sargramostim

■ **leukocidins**
substances that kill white blood cells.

■ **leukocytes**
white blood cells.

■ **leukopenia**
abnormally low number of white blood cells in the circulating blood.

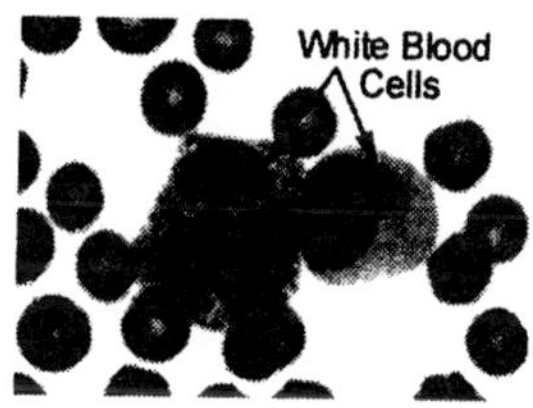

■ **leukotrienes**
substances active in inflammation, leading to chemotaxis and increased vascular permeability, produced by mast cells, basophils and macrophages.

■ **l forms**
bacterial variants that have lost the ability to synthesise the peptidoglycan portion of their cell wall.

■ **lichen**
fungus and an alga or a cyanobacterium living in symbiotic association.

■ **lifetable analysis**
method of analysis that relies on a count of the number of events observed and the time points at which those events occurred, relative to some zero point. The event may be death or some other event. In clinical trials, the time to an event for a patient is usually measured from the time of randomisation. Comparing event rates in the different treatment groups assesses treatment effects.

■ **ligand**
molecule, ion, or group bound to the central atom in a chelate or a coordination compound.

■ **light microscope**
microscope that uses visible light to illuminate objects.

■ **light reactions**
processes used by phototrophs to harvest energy from sunlight, the energy gathering component of photosynthesis, also called light dependent reactions.

■ **light repair**
process by which bacteria repair UV damage to their DNA only in the presence of light.

■ **light dependent reactions**
processes used by phototrophs to harvest energy from sunlight, the energy gathering component of photosynthesis.

■ **lime (agricultural)**
soil amendment containing calcium carbonate, magnesium carbonate or other materials to neutralise soil acidity and furnish calcium or magnesium or both for plant growth.

■ **lincosamides**
group of antimicrobials that interferes with protein synthesis.

■ **lipid**
a fatty and oily compound used by cells as energy reserves and material for structure.

■ **lipopolysaccharide (lps)**
molecule formed by bonding of lipid to polysaccharide, a part of the outer membrane of Gram negative bacteria.

■ **lipoprotein**
macromolecule formed by the bonding of lipid to protein

■ **liposome**

microscopic globules of fat used to encapsulate drugs, and ensure their delivery to the proper targets, reducing toxicity, and hopefully increasing activity.

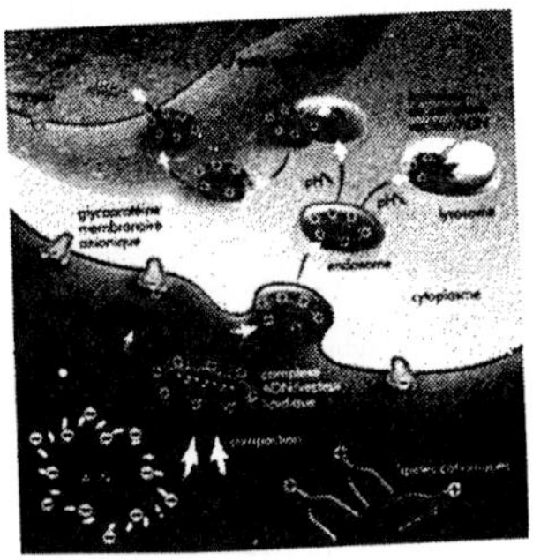

■ **lipoteicnoic acids**

component of the gram positive cell wall that is linked to the cytoplasmic membrane.

■ **lithoheterotroph**

organism that uses an inorganic compound for energy and an organic compound as a source of carbon.

■ **lithotroph**

organism that uses an inorganic substrate such as ammonia or hydrogen as an electron donor in energy metabolism. There are two types of lithotrophs are chemolithotroph and photolith-otroph.

■ **litter**

surface layer of the forest floor consisting of freshly fallen leaves, needles, twigs, stems, bark and fruits.

■ **liver function test (LFT)**

any of a number of tests that measure the health of the liver by checking the levels of various liver secreted chemicals in the blood.

■ **localised infections**

infections limited to one site in or on the body, as a furuncle.

■ **loci**

plural of locus, a place, usually, a specific site.

■ **log phase**

stage of growth of a bacterial culture in which the cells are multiplying exponentially.

■ **logarithm**

a number expressed as the exponent a certain base must be raised to so as to equal the original value. Usually logs are base 10, or calibrated to a special number 'e'(approximately 2.7 logarithms based on e are called natural logarithms.). For logs of base 10, 1 log is ten times, 2 logs is a hundred times, etc.

■ **long terminal repeat (LTR)**
genetic material at the beginning of the HIV genome that helps control replication.

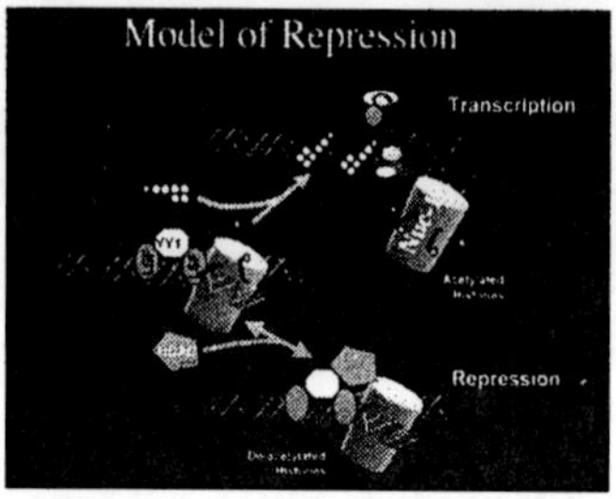

■ **long term non progressors**
individuals who are HIV infected for seven or more years, have stable cd4+ t cell counts of 600 or more cells per cubic millimetre of blood, no HIV related diseases and no previous antiretroviral therapy. Data suggest that this phenomenon is associated with the maintenance of the integrity of the lymphoid tissues and with less virus trapping in the lymph nodes than seen in other HIV infected individuals.

■ **lophotrichous**
having a tuft of polar flagella.

■ **lost to follow up**
patient who can no longer be followed for the outcome of interest, e.g., a patient who is unwilling or unable to return to the clinic for follow up examinations in the case of a clinical trial using an outcome measured at the clinic, or a patient who cannot be located for subsequent follow up in the case of a trial involving mortality or some other outcome that can be measured outside the clinic setting.

■ **lotrimin**
brand name of clotrimazole

■ **low copy number plasmid**
plasmid whose numbers in the cell are one or two copies

■ **lower limit of normal**
the bottom of the normal range for a particular laboratory helps assure between lab comparability.

■ **low level disinfectants**
type of chemical used to destroy fungi, enveloped viruses and vegetative bacteria except mycobacteria.

■ **LPS**
abbreviation for lipopolysaccharide.

■ **LTLT**
abbreviation for low temperature long time pasteurisation.

- **luciferase**
  enzyme that catalyses the chemical reactions that produce bioluminescence.

- **lumbar puncture**
  procedure in which fluid from the sub arachnoid space in the lumbar region is tapped for examination, also known as a spinal tap.

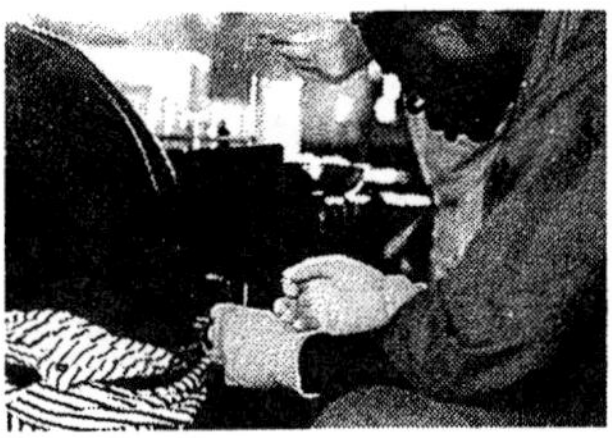

- **lumbar**
  of, relating to or constituting the loins or the vertebrae between the thoracic vertebrae and the sacrum region. The sacrum is the triangular bone made up of five fused vertebrae and forming the posterior section of the pelvis. The thorax is the part of the human body between the neck and the diaphragm, partially encased by the ribs and containing the heart and lungs; the chest.

- **luminescence**
  production of light.

- **luxury uptake**
  absorption by plants of nutrients in excess of their need for growth. Luxury contents accumulated during early growth may be used for later growth.

- **lymph**
  clear yellow liquid that flows within lymphatic vessels, generally contains lymphocytes and may contain globules of fat.

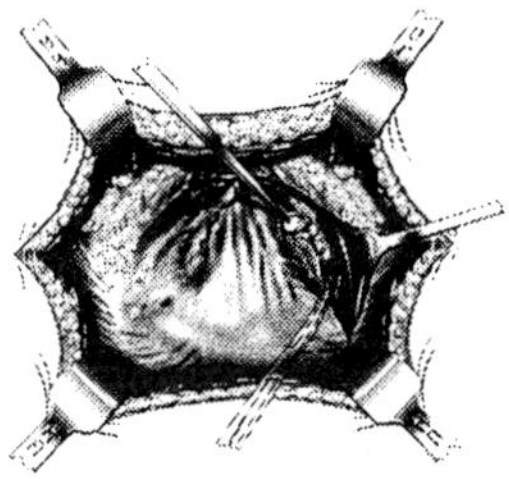

- **lymph nodes**
  small bean sized organs of the immune system, distributed widely throughout the body. Lymph fluid is filtered through the lymph nodes in which all types of lymphocytes take up temporary residence. Antigens, which enter the body, find their way into lymph or blood and are filtered out by lymph nodes or the spleen respectively, for attack by the immune system.

■ **lymphadenopathy**

swollen, firm and possibly tender lymph nodes. The cause may range from an infection such as HIV, the flu, mononucleosis, or lymphoma (cancer of the lymph nodes).

■ **lymphadenopathy syndrome (LAS)**

marked generalised enlargement of lymph nodes that often occurs at the end of the period of clinical well being in HIV disease.

■ **lymphatic vessels**

a body wide network of channels, similar to the blood vessels, which transport lymph to the immune organs and into the bloodstream.

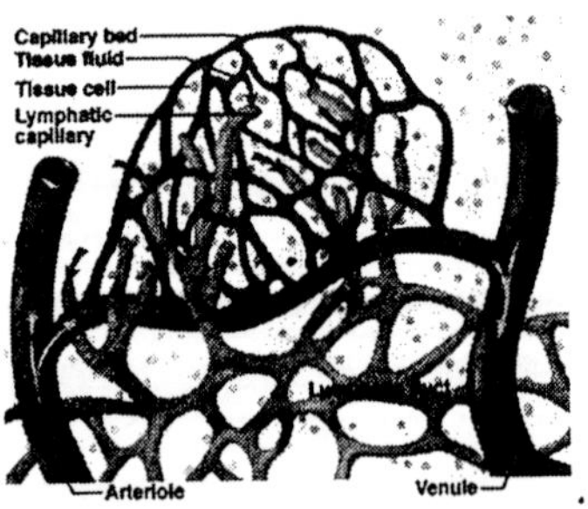

■ **lymphocyte**

white blood cells that mature and reside in the lymphoid organs, and are responsible for the acquired immune response.

■ **lymphoid interstitial pneumonitis (LIP)**

form of pneumonia that involves the lower lobes (of the lungs) with extensive alveolar infiltration by mature lymphocytes, plasma cells and histiocytes. Lip is associated with aids, dysproteinemia and other conditions

■ **lymphoid organs**

include tonsils, adenoids, lymph nodes, spleen and other tissues. Act as the body's filtering system, trapping invaders(i.e., foreign particles from bacteria, viruses, etc.) And presenting them to squadrons of immune cells that congregate there. Within these lymphoid tissues, immune activity is concentrated in regions called germinal centres, where the thread like tentacles of follicular dendritic cells (FDCs) form networks that trap invaders.

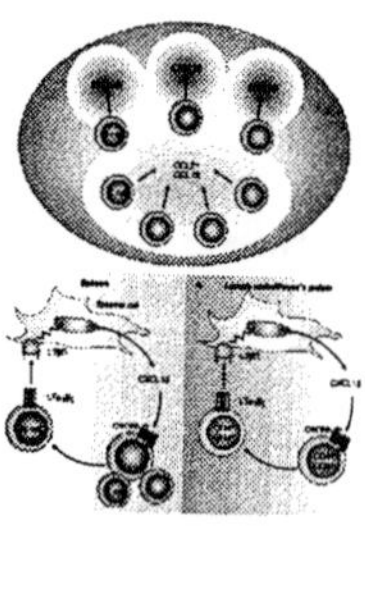

■ **lymphoid tissue**
tissue made up white blood cells and lymphatic vessels.

■ **lymphoid tissues and organs**
collections of lymphocytes and related cells involved in immune responses.

■ **lymphokines**
cytokines (chemical messengers) produced by lymphatic cells.

■ **lymphoma**
cancers of the lymphatic system, often of T or B lymphocytes. There are many categories of lymphoma, including lymphoblastic, cleaved, non-cleaved, burkitt's, and hodgkin's disease. Many lymphomas count as an aids diagnosis.

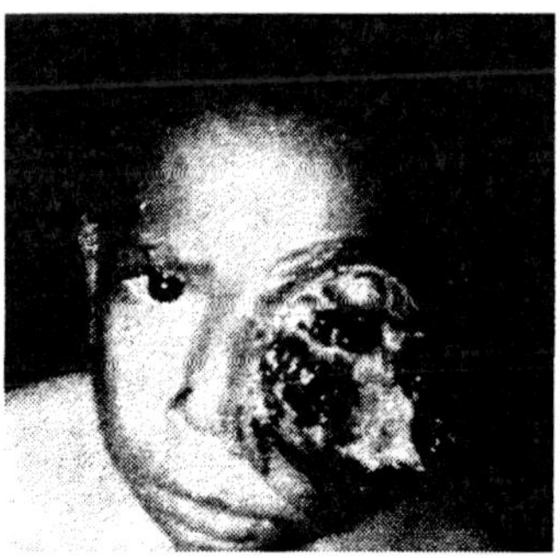

■ **lysate**
remains of cells and virions that are released after lysis of cells.

■ **lyse**
to burst.

■ **lysis**
rupture and destruction of a cell.

■ **lysogenic conversion**
change in the properties of bacteria as a result of carrying a prophage.

■ **lysogens**
bacteria that carry a prophage integrated into their chromosome.

■ **lysogeny**
an association where a prokaryote contains a prophage and the virus genome is replicated in synchrony with the host chromosome.

■ **lysosome**
cell organelle containing digestive enzymes.

■ **lysozyme**
enzyme that degrades the peptidoglycan layer of bacterial cell wall.

■ **m protein**
heat and acid resistant protein found in the cell walls of Group A streptococci.

■ **macconkey agar**
type of selective and differential bacteriological medium used to isolate gram negative rods that typically reside in the intestine

■ **macroenvironment**
overall environment in which an organism lives.

■ **macrofauna**
soil animals that are > 1000 micrometers in length (e.g., vertebrates, earthworms, and large arthropods).

■ **macrolides**
a family of antibiotics with wide spectrum activity, including clarithromycin, azithrom-ycin, and erythromycin. Some macrolides are sometimes used as parts of combination therapy for *mycobacterium avium.*

■ **macromolecule**
very large molecule composed of repeating subunits.

■ **macronutrient**
substance required in large amounts for growth, usually attaining a concentration of > 500 mg kg^{-1} in mature plants. Usually refers to N, P, K, Ca, Mg and S.

■ **macrophage**
large scavenger cell that ingests degenerated cells, blood tissue and foreign particles, and secretes messenger proteins (monokines) involved in inflammatory reactions, lymphocyte activation and acute systemic immune responses. Macrophages exist in large numbers throughout the body and are key to the development of immunity to a variety of organisms. Along with their precursor blood cell, the monocyte, macrophages are a major reservoir of HIV infection.

■ **macropore**
larger soil pores, generally having a minimum diameter between 30 and 100 micrometers, from which water drains readily by gravity.

■ **magnetic resonance imaging (MRI)**
medical imaging that uses radio frequency radiation as its source. MRI is a non-invasive diagnostic technique that can provide information on the

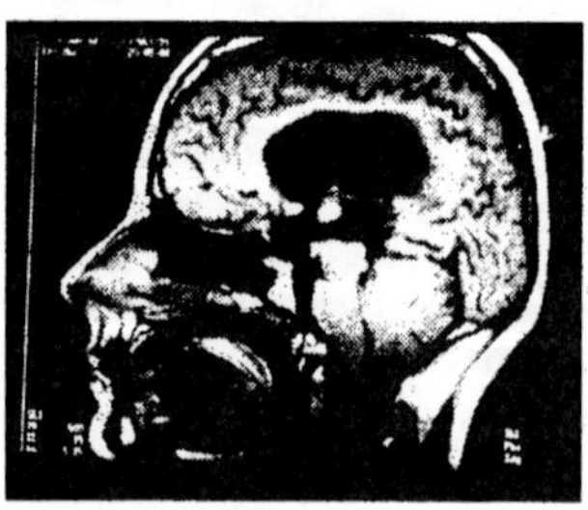

form and function of internal tissues and organs of the body.

- **magnetotaxis**
  movement by bacterial cells containing magnetite crystals in response to a magnetic field.

- **major histocompatibility complex (MHC)**
  two classes of molecules of the surfaces of antigen presenting cells. Antigen is complexed with MHC I or MHC II, and presented to an effecter cell. Antigen without MHC is ignored. Discordant MHC type is the source of graft versus host disease and other rejection phenomena. MHC class i is used for presentation to cd8 cells. Class ii is used to present antigen to cd4 cells.

- **malabsorption syndrome**
  decreased intestinal absorption resulting in loss of appetite, muscle pain and weight loss.

- **malaise**
  vague feeling of uneasiness or discomfort.

- **malignant**
  cells or tumours growing in an uncontrolled fashion.

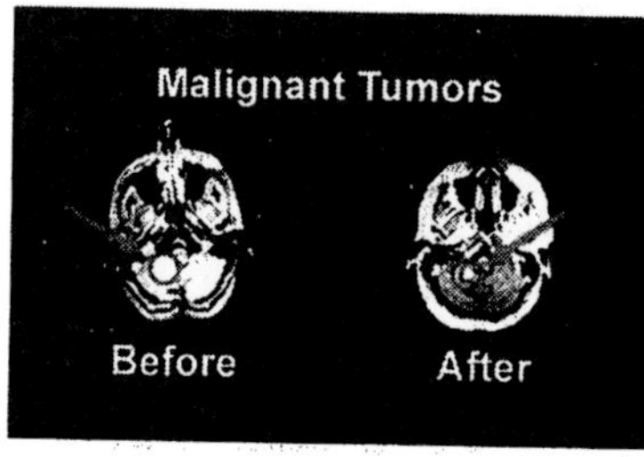

- **malignant tumour**
  abnormal growth of cells no longer under normal control which have the potential to spread to other parts of the body.

- **malnutrition**
  faulty nutrition resulting from poor diet, under eating or abnormal absorption of nutrients from the gastrointestinal tract.

- **MALT**
  abbreviation for mucosal associated lymphoid tissue

- **mammalian artificial chromosomes**
  vectors that can be used to clone large fragments of DNA into animal cells.

- **management trial**
  trial that is designed primarily to provide information on the value of a treatment in normal usage, typically analysed by intention to treat.

■ **manifestation**
signs or symptoms by which a disease state is known.

■ **manual of operations**
document or collection of documents that describes the procedures used in a centre or set of centres in a clinical trial (e.g., manual of operations for study clinics, coordinating centre manual of operations.)

■ **manure**
excreta of animals, with or without an admixture of bedding or litter, fresh or at various stages of decomposition or composting. In some countries the term may denote any fertilizer material.

■ **marinol**
brand name for dronabinol.

■ **mass flow (nutrient)**
movement of solutes associated with net movement of water.

■ **mast cell**
granulocyte found in tissue. The contents of the mast cells, along with those of basophils, are responsible for the symptoms of allergy.

■ **mast cells**
granule containing tissue cells similar in appearance and function to the basophils of the blood, with receptors for the FC portion of IGE, important in the inflammatory response and immediate allergic reactions.

■ **matching placebo**
pill (capsule or tablet) that is designed to resemble in shape, texture, size, taste, etc., a therapeutically active drug and that is used as the control treatment.

■ **matric potential**
portion of the total soil water potential due to the attractive forces between water and soil solids as represented through adsorption and capillarity.

■ **MBC**
abbreviation for minimum bactericidal concentration.

■ **mean**
commonly referred to as the 'average', the mean of a set of quantities is the sum of the quantities, divided by the number of quantities summed.

■ **mean corpuscular volume (MCV)**
the average volume of erythrocytes, conventionally expressed in per cubic micrometers.

■ **mechanical vector**
organism such as a fly that physically moves contaminated material from one location to another.

■ **median**
the value such that for a series of ranked quantities, one half are above the median, and one half are below. For example, the median for a set of cd4 counts is that value which half the counts are less than, and half more.

■ **medical device**
diagnostic or therapeutic contrivance that does not interact chemically with a person's body. Includes diagnostic tests, kits, pacemakers, arterial grafts, intra-ocular lens and orthopaedics pins.

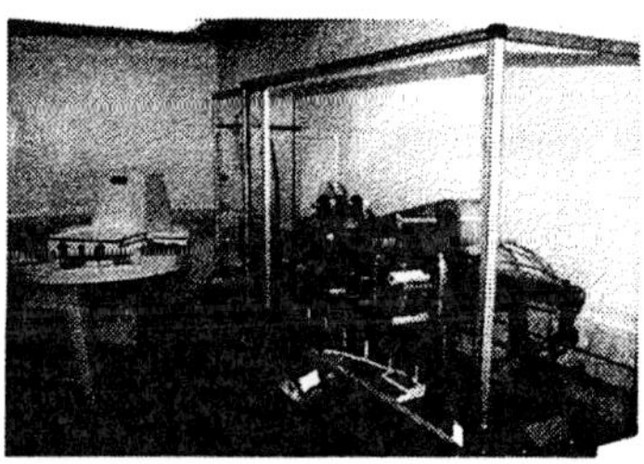

■ **medical officer**
staff member at the division of aids in charge of a particular protocol.

■ **medium (pl. media)**
any material used for growing organisms.

■ **medlars**
medical literature analysis retrieval system.

■ **medline**
medical literature analysis retrieval system on line. A computer searchable database of published medical literature.

■ **mega**
prefix meaning a million times, as in megagram, a million grams.

■ **megace**
brand name of megestrol acetate.

■ **megestrol acetate**
synthetic hormone used in patients to increase appetite and weight gain.

■ **meiosis**
in eukaryotes, reduction division, the process by which the change from diploid to haploid occurs.

■ **melting**
de-naturating of double stranded DNA.

■ **membrane**
thin sheet or layer of pliable tissue (or lipids in the case of cells)

that serves as a semi permeable covering.

■ **membrane attack complex (MAC)**
complex of the later components of complement that inserts through the cell membrane, resulting in lysis of the cell.

■ **membrane filtration**
method employing a membrane filter that is used to determine the number of bacteria in a liquid sample with a relatively low number of organisms.

■ **membrane proteins**
specialised proteins embedded in the membrane bi-layer; some function as receptors and others function as transport proteins.

■ **memory cells**
lymphocytes specific for an antigen that persist in the body after an immune response to that antigen, upon subsequent exposure to the same antigen they differentiate and usually proliferate to become effector cells.

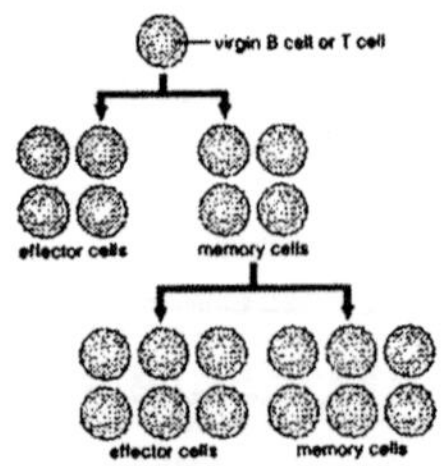

■ **memory response**
(anamnestic response) enhanced immunological response to a second or subsequent dose of antigen.

■ **memory T cell**
persistent t cells that bear a receptor for a specific antigen that was previously encountered in the course of illness or vaccination. Memory t cells allow a rapid response to pathogens that the body has been previously exposed to.

■ **meninges**
membranes surrounding the brain or spinal cord. Part of the so called 'blood brain barrier'.

■ **meninges**
membranes covering the brain and spinal cord.

■ **meningitis**
an inflammation of the meninges.

■ **mepron**
brand name of atovaquone.

■ **merozoite**
stage in the life cycle of certain protozoa, such as the malaria causing *plasmodium* species.

mesh
medical subject heading.

mesofauna
soil animals between 200 to 1000 micrometers in length, including nematodes, oligochaete worms, smaller insect larvae, and small arthropods.

mesophile
organism whose optimum temperature for growth falls in an intermediate range of approximately 15 to 40°c.

messenger RNA (m-RNA)
single stranded RNA synthesised during transcription from DNA that binds to ribosomes and directs the synthesis of protein.

meta analysis
a quantitative method for combining the results of many studies into one set of conclusions. Generally done from a literature review, a meta analysis is more a review than an analysis, properly speaking.

metabolism
sum total of all the chemical reactions in a cell.

metabolite
any product of metabolism.

metachromatic granules
polyphosphate granules found in the cytoplasm of some bacteria that appear as different colours when stained with a basic dye.

metastasis
transfer of a disease producing agent (e.g., cancer cells or bacteria) from an original site of disease to another part of the body with development of a similar lesion in the new location (e.g., spread of cancer from an original site to other sites in the body).

methanogenesis
biological production of methane.

methanogenic bacterium (methanogen)
methane producing prokaryote, member of the archaea.

methanogens
group of archaea that generate energy by oxidising hydrogen gas, using CO_2 as a terminal electron acceptor. This process generates methane (CH_4).

methanotroph
organism capable of oxidising methane.

■ **MHC**
abbreviation for major histocompatibility complex.

■ **MIC**
abbreviation for minimum inhibitory concentration.

■ **micro**
prefix mean small, or one millionth, as in microgram, a millionth of a gram.

■ **microaerophile**
organism that requires a low concentration of oxygen for growth. Sometimes indicates an organism that will carry out its metabolic activities under aerobic conditions but will grow much better under anaerobic conditions.

■ **microaerophiles**
organisms that require small amounts of oxygen (2% to 10%) for growth, but are inhibited by higher concentrations.

■ **microaerophillic bacteria**
bacteria that grow only in 2 to 10% of O_2.

■ **microaggregate**
clustering of clay packets stabilised by organic matter and precipitated inorganic materials.

■ **microbes**
microscopic living organisms, including bacteria, protozoa, and fungi.

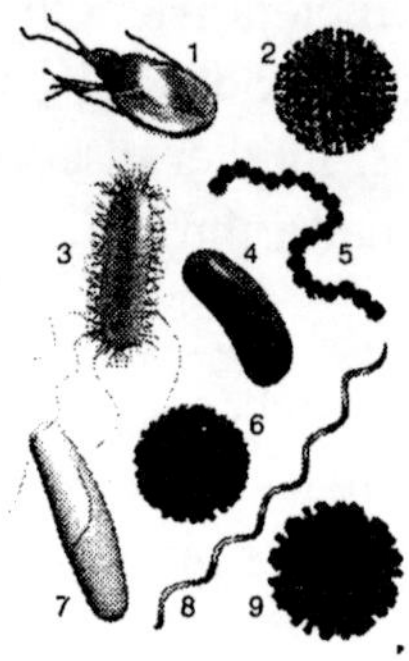

■ **microbial biomass**
total mass of micro-organism alive in a given volume or mass of soil.

■ **microbial population**
total number of living microorganisms in a given volume or mass of soil.

■ **microbicide**
agent (e.g., a chemical or antibiotic) that destroys microbes.

■ **microbiology**
study of micro-organisms.

■ **microcosm**
community or other unit that is representative of a larger unity.

■ **microencapsulated**
surrounded by a thin layer of

protection, a mean of protecting a drug or vaccine from rapid breakdown.

■ **microenvironment**
environment immediately surrounding an individual micro-organism.

■ **microfauna**
protozoa, nematodes and arthropods generally < 200 micrometers long.

■ **microfilaments**
cytoskeleton structures of eukaryotic cells that enable the cell cytoplasm to move.

■ **microflora**
bacteria (including actinomycetes), fungi, algae and viruses.

■ **microhabitat**
clusters of micro-aggregates with associated water within which microbes function. May be composed of several microsites (e.g., aerobic and anaerobic).

■ **micrometer**
one millionth of a meter, or 10^{-6} meter, the unit usually used for measuring micro-organisms.

■ **micronutrient**
a trace element; an organic compound like a vitamin that is essential but only in small amounts for physical health, growth and metabolism.

■ **micro-organism (microbe)**
living organism toc small to be seen with the naked eye (< 0.1 mm), includes bacteria, fungi, protozoans, microscopic algae, and viruses.

■ **micropore**
relatively small soil pore, generally found within structural aggregates and having a diameter < 30 micrometers.

■ **microsite**
small volume of soil where biological or chemical processes differ from those of the soil as a whole, such as an anaerobic micro-site of a soil aggregate or the surface of decaying organic residues.

■ **microsporidiosis**
disease resulting from infection with a protozoal pathogen from the *microsporidia* order, similar in symptoms (diarrhoea, cramps) and often misdiagnosed as cryptosporidiosis.

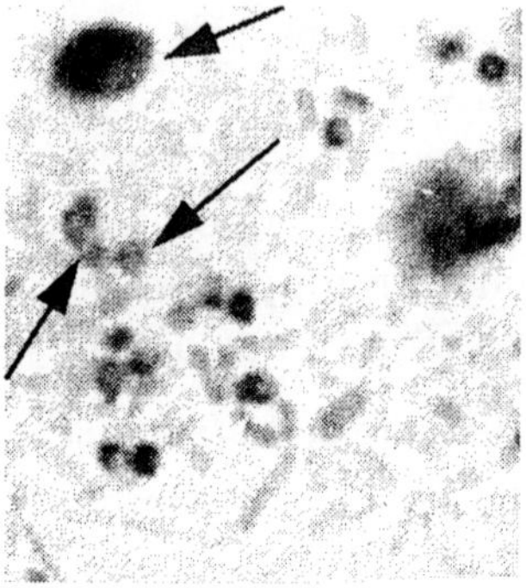

■ **microtubules**
cytoskeleton structures of a eukaryotic cell that form mitotic spindles, cilia and flagella; long hollow cylinders composed of tubulin.

■ **microvillus (pl. Microvilli)**
tiny cylindrical process from laminar surfaces of cells such as those lining the intestine, increases surface area of the cell.

■ **milli**
prefix meaning one thousandth, as in milligram, a thousandth of a gram.

■ **mineralisation**
conversion from organic to inorganic form, stabilisation.

■ **minimum bactericidal concentration (MBC)**
lowest concentration of a specific anti-microbial medication that kills 99.9% of a given strain of bacteria.

■ **minimum inhibitory concentation**
the smallest amount of a substance, when diluted, which kill pathogens or stop them from reproducing. Usually means concentration required to achieve ed90.

■ **minus ( ) strand (1)**
the DNA strand that is used as a template for RNA synthesis.

■ **miracidium**
first larval form of a fluke, hatching from the ovum as a ciliated organism.

■ **mismatch repair**
repair mechanism in which a repair enzyme recognises improperly hydrogen bonded bases and excises a short stretch of nucleotides containing these bases.

■ **mitochondria**
organelle in eukaryotic cells that releases ATP.

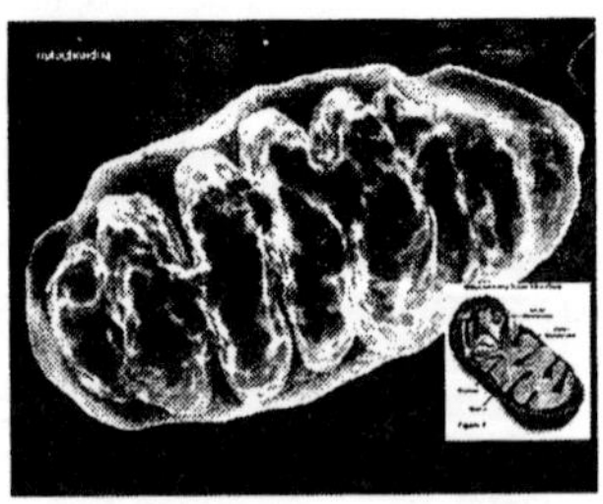

mitochondrion (pl. mitochondria)
eukaryotic organelle responsible for processes of respiration and oxidative phosphorylation.

mitogen
substance that induces cell division

mitosis
highly ordered process by which the nucleus divides in eukaryotes.

mixotroph
organism able to assimilate organic compounds as carbon sources while using inorganic compounds as electron donors. Compare with autotroph and heterotroph.

MMWR
abbreviation for morbidity and mortality weekly report, published by the centres for disease control (CDC).

mn
a strain of HIV used in vaccine development.

mold
filamentous fungus.

mole
amount of a chemical in grams equal to the atomic weights of all the atoms in a molecule of that chemical and contains 10^{23} molecules.

molecular postulates
group of criteria used to determine the cause of an infectious disease by using genetic and other molecular techniques.

molecular weight
relative weight of an atom or molecule based on a scale in which the h atom is assigned the weight of 1.0.

molecule
result of two or more atoms combining by chemical bonding.

molluscum contagiosum
infectious skin condition characterised by small whitish papules, generally on the face or the trunk.

monitoring boundaries
set of values formed by a line or set of lines (or curves), usually specified before or shortly after the start of patient recruitment, which, if exceeded, indicates the existence of a test control treatment difference that satisfies certain statistical properties (e.g., has a

p value of less than a certain size). The boundaries will be used as a basis for stopping the trial when developed in conjunction with a sequential design, but not necessarily when used in conjunction with a fixed sample size design. Z values larger in absolute values are declared statistically significant. Boundaries are designed to control the overall type i error.

■ **monobactams**
group of anti-microbial medications that interferes with peptidoglycan synthesis, very resistant to b lactamases.

■ **monocistronic**
RNA transcript that encodes one gene.

■ **monoclonal antibodies**
antibodies produced by a hybridoma or antibody producing cell source for a specific antigen. Monoclonal antibodies are useful as a tool for identifying specific protein molecules.

■ **monoclonal antibody**
antibody produced from a single clone of cells. This antibody has uniform structure and specificity.

■ **monocyte**
antigen presenting white blood cell, monocytes mature into macrophages.

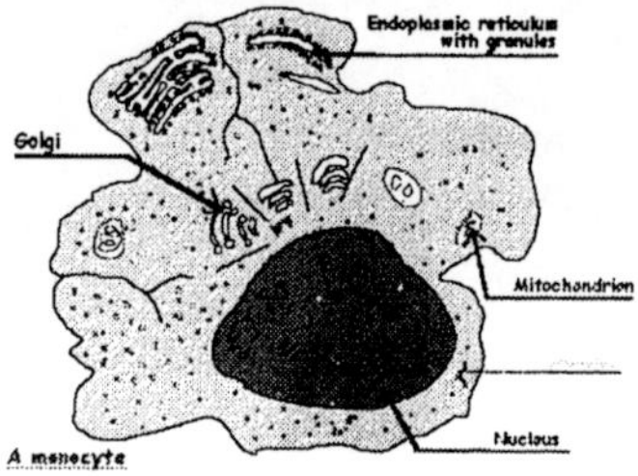

■ **monokaryon**
fungal hypha in which compartments contain one nucleus.

■ **monomer**
repeating subunit of a polymer.

■ **mononuclear phagocyte system (MPS)**
system of mononuclear cells (monocytes and macrophages) scattered throughout the body that are highly efficient at phagocytosis, formerly known as the reticuloendothelial system.

■ **monosaccharide**
sugar.

■ **monotherapy**
single drug, prescribed by itself.

■ **monovalent vaccine**
vaccine that is specific for only one antigen.

■ **morbidity**
condition of being diseased or sick.

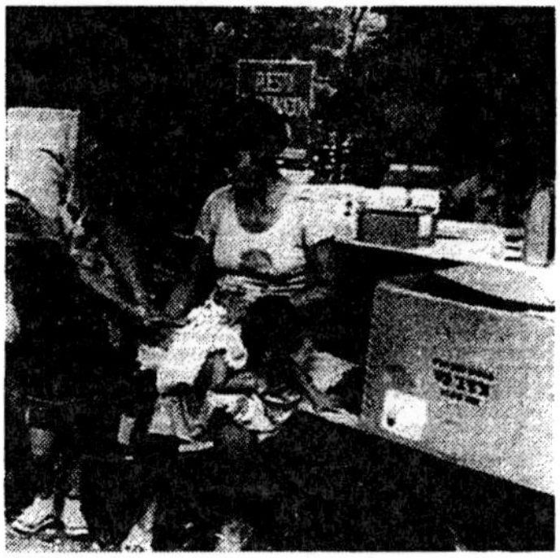

■ **morbidity illness**
most often expressed as the rate of illness in a given population at risk.

■ **morbidity rate**
number of cases of a specific disease per given population at risk.

■ **mordant**
substance that increases the affinity of cellular components for a dye.

■ **morphology**
form or shape of a particular organism or structure.

■ **mortality**
condition of being dead.

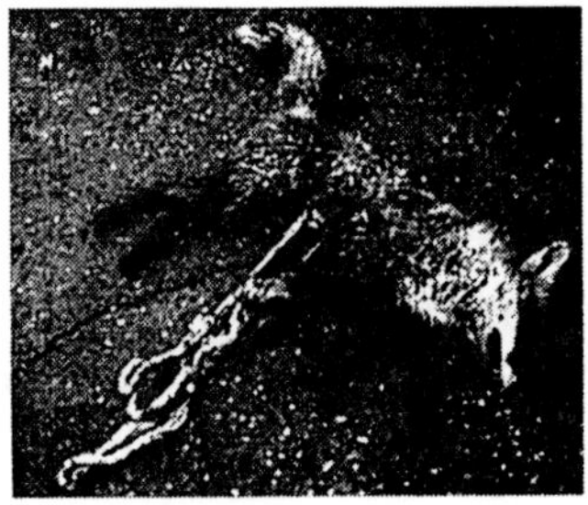

■ **mortality rate**
fraction of people who die from a given disease.

■ **most probable number (MPN)**
method for estimating microbial numbers in soil based on extinction dilutions.

■ **motility**
movement of a cell under its own power.

■ **m-RNA**
messenger RNA.

■ **mucigel**
gelatinous material at the surface of roots grown in normal nonsterile soil. It includes natural and modified plant mucilages, bacterial cells, and their metabolic products (e.g., capsules and slimes), and colloidal mineral and organic matter from the soil.

■ **mucilage**
gelatinous secretions and exu-

dates produced by plant roots and many micro-organisms.

■ **mucociliary escalator**
moving layer of mucus and cilia lining the respiratory tract that traps bacteria and other particles and moves them into the throat.

■ **mucocutaneous**
pertaining to the mucous membranes and the skin, e.g., mouth, vagina, lips, anal area.

Mucocutaneous Leishmaniasis

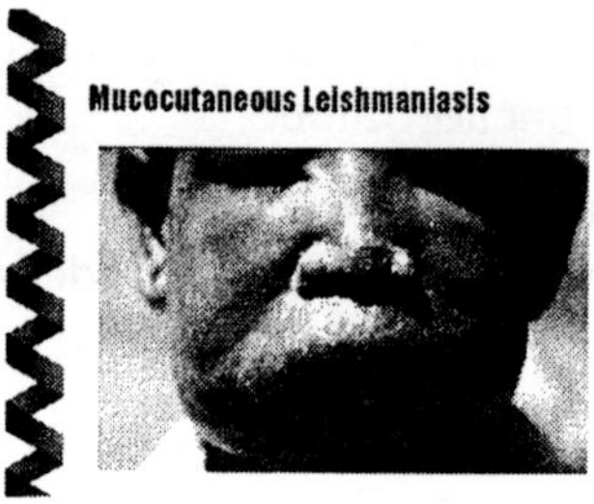

■ **mucosal**
pertaining specifically to the mucous membranes

■ **mucosal immunity**
resistance to infection across the mucous membranes. Dependent on immune cells and antibodies present in the lining of the urogenital tract, gastrointestinal tract and other parts of the body exposed to the outside world.

■ **mucosal associated lymphoid tissue (MALT)**
lymphoid tissue present in the mucosa of the respiratory, gastrointestinal and genitourinary tracts.

■ **mucous membrane**
a moist layer of tissue that lines body cavities or passages that have an opening to the external world (e.g., the lining of the mouth, nostrils or vagina).

■ **mulch**
any material such as straw, sawdust, leaves, plastic film, and loose soil, that is spread upon the surface of the soil to protect the soil and plant roots from the effects of raindrops, soil crusting, freezing, or evaporation.

■ **multicentre clinical trial**
clinical trial involving two or more clinical centres and a common study protocol.

■ **multiple cloning site**
small sequence of DNA that contains several unique restriction enzyme recognition sites into which foreign DNA can be cloned.

■ **multiple comparisons**
a term used to refer to the fact

that two or more treatment comparisons, each involving the same outcome measure, are made or are to be made at a designated time point in the course of the trial. The comparison may involve all members of the treatment groups or subsets (e.g., as in analyses involving subgroups of patients defined by the presence or absence of some baseline characteristic.). Also applies to comparisons among several subgroups and/ or use of several endpoints.

■ **multiple comparisons problem**
a term referring to the fact that significant findings will appear by chance alone if enough different comparisons are tested. For example, in an infinitely large data set, results with a significance level of 0.05 will occur on the average every twentieth time.

■ **multiple outcomes**
a term used to refer to the fact that a trial involves several different outcome measures, each of which is used or is to be used to make treatment comparisons.

■ **municipal solid waste**
combined consumer and commercial waste generated within a defined geographic area

■ **mushroom**
large, sometimes edible, fruiting body produced by some fungi.

■ **mutagen**
substance that causes the mutation of genes.

■ **mutant**
organism, population, gene, or chromosome that differs from the corresponding wild type by one or more base pairs.

■ **mutation**
heritable change in the base sequence of the DNA of an organism.

■ **mutualism**
association in which both partners benefit.

■ **myambutol**
a brand name of ethambutol.

■ **myasthenia**
gravis autoimmune disease characterised by muscle weakness, caused by autoantibodies.

■ **mycelex**
brand name of clotrimazole.

■ **mycelium (pl. Mycelia)**
tangled, matlike mass of fungal hyphae.

■ **mycobacterium avium complex (MAC)**
common opportunistic infection caused by two very similar mycobacterial organisms, *mycobacterium avium* and *m. Intracellulare*. It can spread through the bloodstream to infect lymph nodes, bone marrow, liver, spleen, spinal fluid, lungs and intestinal tract. Symptoms of MAC include prolonged wasting, fever, fatigue and enlarged spleen. Mac infection is one of the diseases making up the aids definition.

■ **mycobacterium kansasii**
another member of the mycobacteria family, sometime mistaken for MAC.

■ **mycobacterium**
any bacterium of the genus mycobacterium or a closely related genus.

■ **mycobutin**
brand name of rifabutin.

■ **mycology**
study of fungi.

■ **mycophagous**
organisms that consume fungi, such as mycophagous nematodes.

■ **mycoplasma**
group of bacteria without a cell walls that do not revert to walled forms. Phylogenetically related to clostridia.

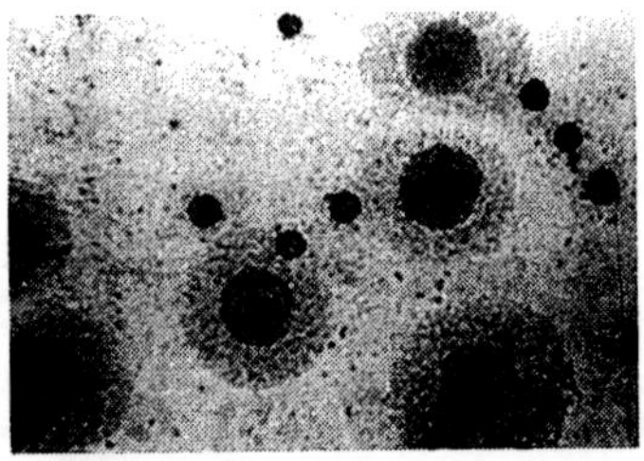

■ **mycorrhiza**
symbiotic relationship between certain fungi and the roots of plants.

■ **mycorrhizosphere**
unique microbial community that forms around a mycorrhiza.

■ **mycosis**
any disease caused by a fungus.

■ **mycovirus**
virus that infects fungi.

■ **myelin**
a substance that sheathes nerve cells, acting as an electric insulator that facilitates

the conduction of nerve impulses.

▸ Myelination of PNS and CNS Axons

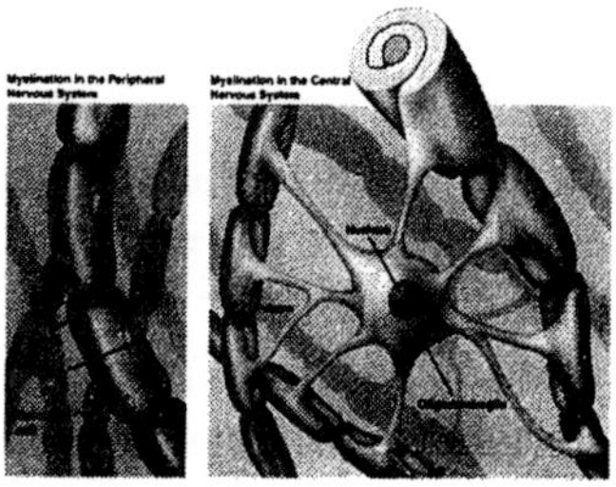

■ **myelitis**
inflammation of the spinal cord, or of the bone marrow.

■ **myelopathy**
degenerative process involving the spinal cord.

■ **myelosuppression**
impairment of the blood cell producing function of the bone marrow.

■ **myelotoxic**
toxic to the bone marrow.

■ **myopathy**
a degenerative condition of the muscles. Can be caused by both HIV and AZT.

■ **N acetylglucosamine**
(NAG) one of the two alternating subunits of the glycan chains that make up peptidoglycan.

■ **N acetylglucosamine and N acetylmuramic acid**
sugar derivatives in the peptidoglycan layer of bacterial cell walls.

■ **NAD**
abbreviation for nicotinamide adenine dinucleotide, a derivative of the vitamin niacin that is important in the transfer of hydrogen atoms in metabolic processes.

■ **NADH**
abbreviation for the reduced form of nicotinamide adenine dinucleotide, a diffusible electron carrier.

■ **NADPH**
abbreviation for the reduced form of nicotinamide adenine dinucleotide, a diffusible electron carrier.

■ **naive T cell**
a newly formed t cell that has not yet been exposed to antigen.

■ **nano**
prefix meaning one billionth, as in nanogram, a billionth of a gram.

■ **nanometer**
one millionth of a millimeter.

■ **nanopore**
soil pore having dimensions measured in nanometers. Materials encased in nanopores are beyond the reach of microorganisms and enzymes.

■ **narrow host range plasmid**
plasmid that only replicates in one or a few closely related species of bacteria.

■ **narrow spectrum antimicrobials**
antimicrobial medications that inhibit or kill a limited range of bacteria.

■ **natal**
relating to birth.

■ **natural history of disease**
the course of a disease when left untreated

■ **natural history study**
study of the natural development of something (such as an organism or a disease) over a period of time.

■ **natural killer (NK) cell**
a type of lymphocyte (white blood cell) that lyses infected or cancerous cells. NK response does not require antigen presentation to lymphocytes.

■ **natural selection**
selection by the environment of those cells best able to grow in that environment

■ **nebuliser**
device used to reduce liquid medication to extremely fine cloudlike particles, useful in delivering medication to deeper parts of the respiratory tract (e.g., into the lungs).

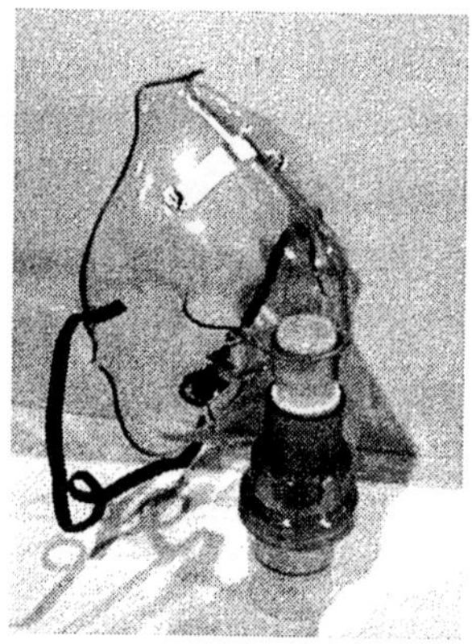

■ **nebupent**
brand name of pentamidine.

■ **necrolysis**
shedding of surface components of tissue, such as cells from internal body surfaces, due to death of a portion of tissue.

■ **necrosis**
cell death and decay.

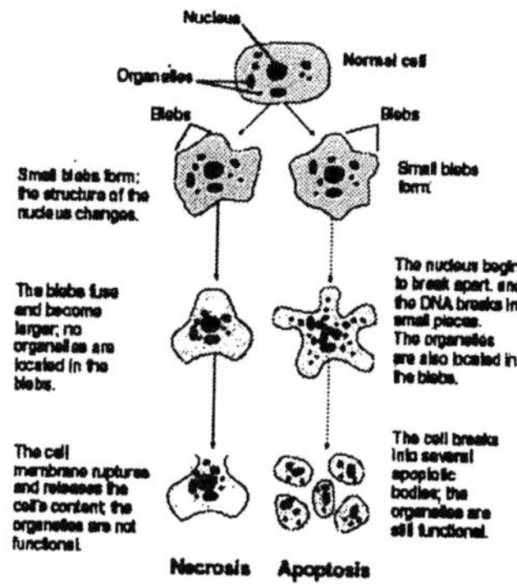

■ **necrotic**
dead, refers to dead cells or tissues in contact with living cells, as necrotic tissue in wounds.

■ **necrotising**
causing necrosis.

■ **necrotrophic**
nutritional mechanism by which an organism produces a battery of hydrolytic enzymes to kill and break down host cells and then absorb nutritional compounds from the dead organic matter.

■ **Nef**
one of the regulatory genes of the HIV virus. Three HIV regulatory genes Tat, Rev and Nef and three so called auxiliary genes Vif, Vpr and Vpu contain information necessary for the production of proteins that control the virus's ability to infect a cell, produce new copies of the virus or cause disease.

■ **negative ( ) sense strand of RNA**
that does not act as m-RNA, strand of DNA that is not transcribed into m-RNA.

■ **negative control**
inactive control treatment.

■ **negative staining**
staining technique that employs acidic dye to stain the background against which colourless cells can be seen.

■ **negri body**
viral inclusion body characteristic of rabies.

■ **nematode**
multicellular eukaryote defined as an unsegmented, usually microscopic roundworm. Various species feed on plants, animals, fungi, and bacteria.

■ **neonatal**
concerning the first four weeks of life after birth.

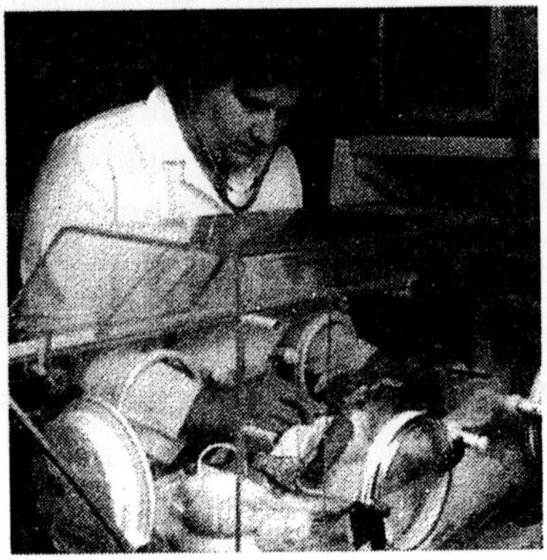

tremities, loss of deep tendon responses, and decrease in sensitivity to touch stimulation.

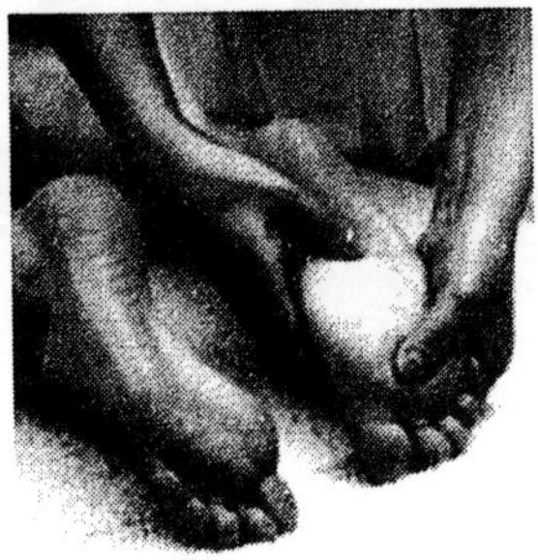

■ **neoplasm**
an abnormal and uncontrolled growth of tissue, a tumour.

■ **nephrotoxic**
poisonous to the kidneys.

■ **neupogen**
brand name of filgrastim

■ **neuralgia**
a sharp, shooting pain along a nerve pathway.

■ **neurologic**
pertaining to the brain or nervous system.

■ **neuropathy**
abnormal and degenerative state of the nervous system. HIV, some treatments, and other diseases can cause a peripheral neuropathy marked by burning tingling sensations in the ex-

■ **neurotransmitter**
any of a group of substances released from the terminations of nerve cells when they are stimulated, that cross to the adjacent cell and cause it to be excited or inhibited.

■ **neutralism**
lack of interaction between two organisms in the same habitat.

■ **neutralisation tests**
tests in which antibodies neutralise viruses by preventing them from infecting cells or neutralise toxins by binding to them and making them nontoxic.

■ **neutralisation**
process by which an antibody binds to specific antigens,

thereby 'neutralising' the micro-organism.

■ **neutralising antibody**
antibody that neutralises (renders harmless) the infectivity of micro-organisms, particularly viruses.

■ **neutralising domain**
section of the HIV envelope protein gp120 that elicits antibodies with neutralizing activities.

■ **neutrexin**
brand name of trimetrexate.

■ **neutron**
uncharged component of an atom found in the nucleus.

■ **neutropenia**
abnormally low number of neutrophils (white blood cells) in the circulating blood.

■ **neutrophil**
called polymorphonuclear neutrophil (pmn). It is a white blood cell that plays a central role in defence of a host against infection. Neutrophils engulf and kill foreign microorganisms.

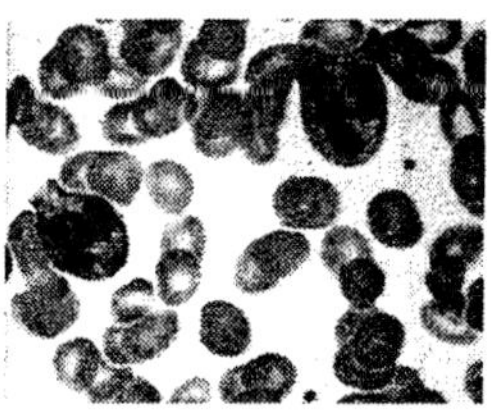

■ **neutrophiles**
organisms that can live and multiply within the range of ph 5 (acidic) to ph 8 (basic) and have a ph optimum near neutral (ph 7).

■ **neutrophils**
actively phagocytic leukocytes with granules containing antimicrobial and degradative substances that destroy engulfed organisms and materials, professional phagocytes.

■ **nevaripine**
an antiretroviral drug of the non nucleoside reverse transcription inhibitor family. These drugs target the same enzyme as AZT and the other nucleoside drugs, but are chemically different.

■ **niche**
functional role of a given organism within its habitat.

■ **nicotinamide adenine dinucleotide (NAD+)**
important coenzyme, functioning as a hydrogen and electron carrier in a wide range of redox reactions; the oxidized form of the coenzyme is written NAD^+, the reduced form as NADH.

■ **nicotinamide adenine dinucleotide phosphate (NADP+)**
important coenzyme, functioning as a hydrogen and electron carrier in a wide range of redox reactions; the oxidised form of the coenzyme is written $NADP^+$, the reduced form as NADPH.

■ **nitrate reduction (biological)**
process whereby nitrate is reduced by plants and micro-organisms to ammonium for cell synthesis (nitrate assimilation, assimilatory nitrate reduction) or to various lower oxidation states (N_2, N_2O, NO,) by bacteria using nitrate as the terminal electron acceptor in anaerobic respiration.

■ **nitrification**
conversion of NH_3 to nitrate (NO_3^-).

■ **nitrifying bacteria**
chemolithotrophs capable of carrying out the transformations from NH_3 to NO_2 or NO_2 to NO_3.

■ **nitrogen cycle**
sequence of biochemical changes wherein nitrogen is used by a living organism, transformed upon the death and decomposition of the organism, and converted ultimately to its original state of oxidation.

■ **nitrogen fixation**
conversion of nitrogen gas to ammonia.

■ **nitrogenase**
specific enzyme system required for biological N_2 fixation.

■ **NK cell**
large granular, non T, non B lymphocyte that can recognise and destroy certain cells that it senses as foreign in a non-specific fashion.

■ **nodule**
swelling on the root of a leguminous plant caused by rhizobium; the site of nitrogen fixation.

■ **nodulins**
unique proteins produced in root hairs or nodules in response to rhizobial infection.

■ **nomarski differential interference contrast microscope**
type of microscope that has a device for separating light into two beams that pass through the specimen and then recombine. Light waves are out of phase when they recombine, resulting in the three di-

mensional appearance of material in the specimen.

■ **nomenclature**
system of naming organisms.

■ **Non Nucleoside Reverse Transcriptase Inhibitor (NNRTI)**
class of drugs including nevaripine and delaviridine that targets the same reverse transcriptase enzyme of HIV as the nucleoside drugs like AZT, DDI, etc. NNRTI's have been characterised by strong antiviral activity, followed by extremely rapid acquisition of resistance by exposed virus.

■ **non communicable diseases**
disease that cannot be transmitted from one individual to another.

■ **non competitive inhibition**
type of enzyme inhibition that results from a molecule binding to the enzyme at a site other than the active site.

■ **noncompliance**
not in compliance with a designated procedure. Usually in reference to some treatment or data collection procedure

■ **noncompliant**
absence of a compliant state in relation to a designated procedure.

■ **non conjugative plasmid**
plasmid that lacks some of the genetic information required for its transfer to other bacteria by conjugation.

■ **non critical items**
medical instruments and surfaces such as stethoscopes and countertops that only come into contact with unbroken skin

■ **noncyclic photophosphorylation**
type of phosphorylation in which high energy electrons are drawn off to generate reducing power. Electrons must still be returned to chlorophyll, but they must come from a source such as water.

■ **non polar**
possessing hydrophobic (water repelling) characteristics and not easily dissolved in water.

■ **non polar covalent bond**
bond formed by sharing electrons between atoms that have

equal attraction for the electrons.

■ **non required follow up visit**
any visit by the patient to the clinic after the randomisation visit that is not required for data collection purposes. The visit may be initiated by the patient or by study personnel, and includes interim follow up visits, monitoring for toxicities, and post trial follow up visits. Event driven data such as adverse experiences and overtly clinical events may be collected, otherwise data generated at such visits are not generally used to satisfy data collection needs for required follow up visits, unless they take place within the time windows for those visits and all necessary procedures are carried out during the visits.

■ **non specific immunity**
immune responses that are non-specific with respect to the infectious agent or other material involved, and that are not affected by prior exposures.

■ **normal microbial flora**
that group of micro-organisms that colonises the body surfaces but does not usually cause disease. Also called normal flora.

■ **northern blot**
procedure that is similar in principle to a southern blot, except that it uses a nucleic acid probe to detect sequences of RNA.

■ **nosocomial**
a term for an infection or illness that was acquired in a hospital, or other health care facility.

■ **nosocomial infection**
infection acquired during hospitalisation.

■ **notifiable diseases**
group of diseases that are reported to the CDC by individual states; typically these diseases are of relatively high incidence or otherwise a potential danger to public health.

■ **NSAID**
non-steroidal anti inflammatory (i.e., counteracting inflammation) drug.

■ **nuclear membrane**
membrane that separates the nucleus from the cytoplasm in eukaryotic cells.

■ **nucleic acid hybridisation**
technique in which single strands of DNA are mixed to-

gether and allowed to re-associate. The degree to which the single strands re-associate indicates how complementary the strands are to one another.

■ **nucleic acid**

organic substance, found in all living cells, in which the hereditary information is stored and from which it can be transferred. Nucleic acid molecules are long chains that generally occur in combination with proteins. The two chief types are DNA (deoxyribonucleic acid), found mainly in cell nuclei, and RNA (ribonucleic acid), found mostly in cytoplasm. Each nucleic acid chain is composed of subunits called nucleotides, each containing a sugar, a phosphate group, and one of four bases adenine (symbolised a), guanine (g), cytosine (c) and thymine (t). RNA contains the sugar ribose instead of deoxyribose and the base uracil (u) instead of thymine. The specific sequences of nucleotides constitute the cell's genetic information each three nucleotide DNA sequence specifies one particular amino acid. The long sequences of DNA nucleotides thus correspond to the sequences of amino acids in the cell's proteins. In order to be expressed as protein, the genetic information is carried to the protein synthesising machinery of the cell, usually in the cell cytoplasm. Forms of RNA mediate this process. DNA not only provides information, but also specifies its own exact replication. The cell replicates its DNA by making a complementary copy of its exact nucleotide sequence t for every a, c for every g, g for every c, a for every t. Although the triplet nucleotide code seems to be universal, the actual sequences of the nucleotides vary according to the species and individual. See also gene; genetic engineering; mutation.

■ **nucleic acids**

ribonucleic acid (RNA) and deoxyribonucleic acid (DNA).

■ **nucleocapsid**

viral nucleic acid and its protein coat.

■ **nucleoid**

region of a prokaryotic cell containing the DNA.

■ **nucleoli**

bodies in the nucleus that become enlarged during protein synthesis and contain the DNA template for ribosomal RNA.

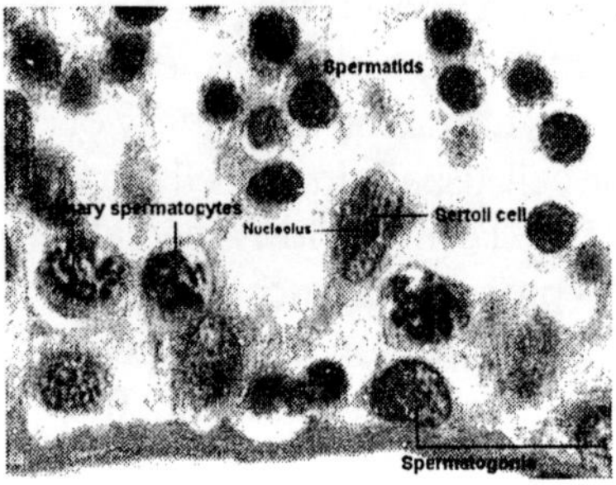

■ **nucleolus**
region within the nucleus where ribosomal RNA's are synthesised.

■ **nucleophilic compound**
chemical that attracts or is drawn to electron deficient regions in other chemicals; reducing agents act as nucleophilic compounds.

■ **nucleoside**
nucleotide without the phosphate group.

■ **nucleoside analog**
nucleosides are related to nucleotides, the subunits of nucleic acids; however, they do not carry the phosphate groups of, the nucleotides. Nucleoside analogs generally are synthetic compounds similar to one of the components of DNA or RNA; a general type of antiviral drug (e.g., acyclovir and AZT).

■ **nucleoside analogue reverse transcriptase inhibitors**
family of antiviral compounds including AZT, DDI, DDC, D4T, 3TC, FLT, PMEA, and others. These compounds are phosphorylated into nucleotide analogues, and interfere with the activity of the viral enzyme reverse transcriptase.

■ **nucleosome**
unit of the chromatin of eukaryotic cells that consists of a complex of histones around which the linear DNA wraps twice.

■ **nucleotide**
monomeric unit of nucleic acid, consisting of a sugar (pentose), a phosphate, and a nitrogenous base.

■ **nucleotide array technology**
use of a solid support to which a two dimensional arrangement of numerous different single stranded DNA fragments of known sequences has been attached.

■ **nucleus**
membrane enclosed structure containing the genetic material (DNA) organised in chromo-

somes.

nuisance bloom
Odiferous scum caused when buoyant cyanobacteria cells float to the surface of a body of stagnant water, and then lyse and decay.

null cell
lymphocyte that develops in the bone marrow and lacks the characteristic surface markers of the b and t lymphocytes. Null cells represent a small proportion of the lymphocyte population. Stimulated by the presence of antibody, null cells can attack certain cellular targets directly and are known as 'natural killer' or NK cells.

null hypothesis (statistics)
hypothesis that postulates no underlying difference in the populations or groups being compared with regard to the factor, trait, characteristic, or condition of interest.

null treatment hypothesis
hypothesis that states that the true underlying effect of the test treatment, as expressed by a specified outcome measure, is no more or less than for the control treatment.

numerical taxonomy
method of classification based on the phenotypes of prokaryotes; determines the relatedness of different organisms based on the percentage of characteristics that two groups have in common.

nutrient
substance taken by a cell from its environment and used in catabolic or anabolic reactions.

nutrition
processes involved in the taking in and metabolism of food material by living plants and animals.

nystatin
a brand name of clotrimazole.

O antigen
antigenic polysaccharide portion of lipopolysaccharide, the molecule that makes up the outer leaflet of the outer membrane of Gram negative bacteria.

objective lens
lens of a compound microscope that is closest to the specimen.

obligate
adjective referring to an environmental factor (for example,

oxygen) that is always required for growth.

- **obligate aerobes**
  organisms with an absolute requirement for oxygen.

- **obligate anaerobes**
  organisms that cannot multiply if O_2 is present; they are often killed by traces of O_2 because of its toxic derivatives.

- **obligate fermenters**
  organisms that can grow in the presence of O_2 but never use it as a terminal electron acceptor; also called aerotolerant anaerobes.

- **obligate intracellular parasites**
  organisms that grow only inside living cells

- **O'brien fleming monitoring boundary**
  set of criteria used to determine how data can be looked at during interim reviews, and how much potential error may be caused through looking. Used in constructing the stopping rules for a trial

- **observational study**
  follow up study where clinical interventions are not specified by protocol. Ideally, data collection activities are similar to an intervention study.

- **observed treatment difference**
  actual treatment difference observed either at the end of the trial or at some designated time point during the trial.

- **occlusion bodies**
  masses of viruses inside or outside cells

- **ocular**
  pertaining to the eye.

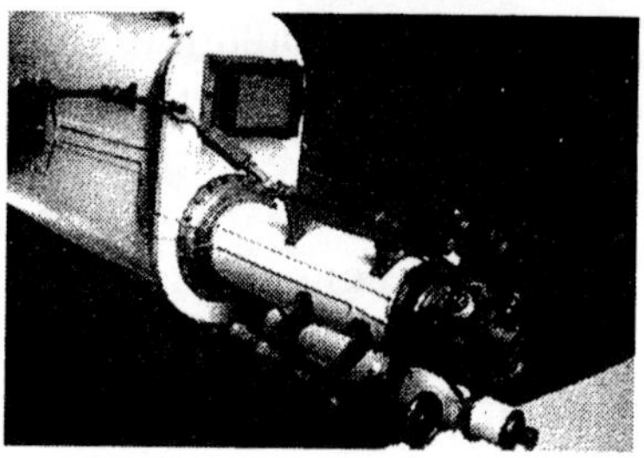

- **ocular lens**
  lens of a compound microscope that is closest to the eye.

- **off label**
  usage of a medication for other purposes than the specific ones appearing in the labelling

- **okazaki fragment**
  nucleic acid fragment synthesised as a result of the discontinuous replication of the lag-

ging strand of DNA.

- **oligonucleotide**
short chain of nucleotides.

- **oligosaccharide**
short chains of monosaccharide subunits joined together by covalent bonds. Shorter than a polysaccharide.

- **oligotroph**
micro-organism specifically adapted to grow under low nutrient supply. Thought to subsist on the more resistant soil organic matter and be little affected by the addition of fresh organic materials. Sometimes a synonym for autochthonous.

- **oligotrophic environment**
an environment that is deficient in nutrients.

- **oncogene**
gene whose activity is involved in turning a normal cell into a cancer cell

- **one tailed alternative hypothesis**
alternative to the null hypothesis that specifies a range of permissible values of all which lie to one side of the null value (e.g., all favouring one treatment).

- **one tailed test (statistics)**
a statistical test of significance based on the null value of no difference versus the set of all alternative values that are either to the right or to the left of the null value (e.g., the set indicating a positive treatment effect in a clinical trial).

- **oogonium**
specialised sexual structure formed as a female gametangium by fungus like organisms in the phylum oomycota.

- **oospore**
thick walled spore formed within an oogonium by fungus like organisms in the phylum oomycota.

- **open label trial**
clinical trial in which a study physician or study patient decides on the treatment to be administered. Non random clinical trial.

- **open reading frames (ORFS)**
stretches of DNA, generally longer than 300 bp, that begin with a start codon and end with a stop codon, they suggest that the region encodes a protein.

- **open system**
method used to maintain cells in a state of continuous growth by

continuously adding nutrients and removing waste products; also called a continuous culture

- **open label trial**
clinical trial in which doctors and participants know which drug or vaccine is being administered.

- **operator**
region located immediately downstream of a promoter to which a repressor can bind. Binding of the repressor to the operator effectively prevents RNA polymerase from progressing past that region and blocks transcription.

- **operon**
group of linked genes that are controlled as a single unit.

- **opine**
unusual amino acid derivative; the portion of the ti plasmid of *agrobacterium tumefaciens* that is transferred to plant cells directs the recipient cells to synthesise this compound.

- **opportunist**
organism that causes disease only in hosts with impaired defence mechanisms, also called opportunistic pathogens.

- **opportunistic infection**
illness caused by an organism that usually does not cause disease in a person with a normal immune system. People with advanced HIV infection suffer opportunistic infections of the lungs, brain, eyes and other organs.

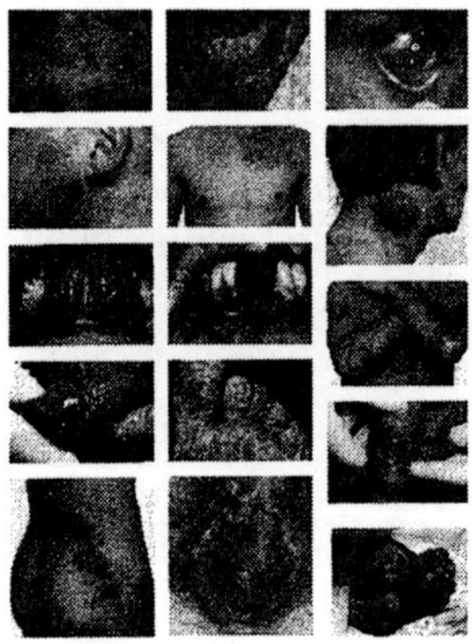

- **opportunistic infections**
infection in an immune compromised person caused by an organism that does not usually cause disease in healthy people. Many of these organisms are carried in a latent state by virtually everyone, and only cause disease when given the opportunity of a damaged immune system.

- **opsonization**
enhanced phagocytosis, usu-

ally caused by coating of the particle to be ingested with either antibody or complement components.

- **opthalmia neonatorum**
eye infection of newborns caused by *neisseria gonorrhoeae*, which is acquired from infected mothers during the birth process.

- **optical (or stereoisomer)**
isomer mirror image of a compound.

- **optimum growth temperature**
temperature at which a microorganism multiplies most rapidly.

- **order**
taxonomic classification between class and family.

- **organ**
structure composed of different tissues coordinated to perform a specific function.

- **organelle**
structure within a cell that performs a specific function.

- **organic chemical**
any chemical based on carbon. Frequently including oxygen, hydrogen and nitrogen.

- **organic matter**
material that contains carbon atoms bonded to other carbon atoms.

- **organic soil**
soil that contains a high percentage ($>200\ g\ kg^{-1}$, or >120 180 $g\ kg^{-1}$ if saturated with water) of organic carbon.

- **organotroph**
organism that obtains reducing equivalents (stored electrons) from organic substrates.

- **origin**
location where the process of replication in a nucleic acid begins.

- **origin of replication**
distinct region of a DNA molecule at which replication is initiated.

- **origin of transfer**
short stretch of nucleotides, a part of which is transferred first when a plasmid is transferred to a recipient cell; necessary for plasmid transfer.

- **oropharyngeal**
relating to that division of the pharynx between the soft palate and the epiglottis. Pharynx is a tube that connects the mouth and nasal passages with

the esophagus, the connection to the stomach. Epiglottis is a thin, valve like structure that covers the glottis, the opening of the upper part of the larynx (the part of the throat containing the vocal cords), during swallowing.

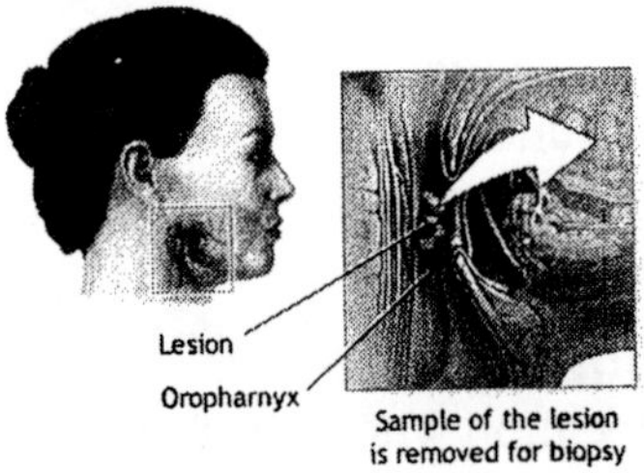

■ **orphan drug**

category for medications used to treat diseases that occur rarely, so there is little financial incentive for industry to develop them. Orphan drug status gives the manufacturer specific financial incentives to provide the drug.

■ **osmosis**

movement of water across a membrane from a dilute solution to a more concentrated solution.

■ **osmotic potential**

portion of total soil water potential due to the presence of solutes in soil water.

■ **osmotic pressure**

pressure exerted by water on the cytoplasmic membrane due to a difference in the concentration of molecules on each side of the membrane.

■ **osmotolerant**

organisms that can tolerate relatively high salt concentrations, up to approximately 10% Nacl.

■ **O specific polysaccharide side chain**

the portion of LPS that is directed away from the membrane, at the end opposite of Lipid A, because its composition varies, it can be used to identify species or strains.

■ **outbreak**

cluster of cases occurring during a brief time interval and affecting a specific population; may herald the onset of an epidemic.

■ **outcome variable**

an observation recorded for patients in the trial at one or more time points after enrollment for the purpose of assessing the effects of the study treatments.

outer membrane
in prokaryotic cells, the unique lipid bi-layer of gram negative cells that surrounds the peptidoglycan layer.

outlier
any value, reading, or measurement that is far outside established limits or the central range of the data and, for this reason, is questioned or considered to be in error.

ovary
part of the female reproductive system. One of a pair of female gonads (a gamete producing gland) found on each side of the lower abdomen, beside the uterus, in a fold of the broad ligament. At ovulation, an egg is extruded from a follicle on the surface of the ovary under the stimulation of certain hormones.

oven dry soil
soil that has been dried at 105°c until it reaches constant mass.

oxazolidinones
group of anti-microbial drugs that interferes with protein synthesis.

oxic
containing oxygen, aerobic. Usually used in reference to a microbial habitat.

oxidase test
rapid biochemical test used to detect cytochrome c.

oxidation
removal of an electron.

oxidation state
number of electrons to be added (or subtracted) from an atom in a combined state to convert it to the elemental form.

oxidation reduction (redox) reaction
coupled pair of reactions, in which one compound becomes oxidised, while another becomes reduced and takes up the electrons released in the oxidation reaction.

oxidative phosphorylation
synthesis of ATP involving a membrane associated electron transport chain and the creation of a proton motive force. Also called electron transport chain phosphorylation.

oxidative stress
physiological effects of increased levels of free radicals and oxidating molecules, associated with disease and aging; effects include cell membrane

damage and cell death.

- **oxygenic photosynthesis**

photosynthetic reaction that synthesises carbohydrate from CO_2 and H_2O with the release of oxygen.

- **p value**

probability of obtaining a given outcome due to chance alone. For example, a study result with a significance level of $p<0.05$ implies that 5 times out of 100 the result could have occurred by chance.

- **P24 antigen**

a core protein making up the nucleocapsid of the HIV virus, p24 was thought at one time to be a surrogate marker for disease progression. Now it is recognised that some long term asymptomatics have relatively high elevations of p24, while others die never having been positive (anything less than 10 picograms/mole is effectively negative)

- **p24**

within the envelope of the HIV virus is a bullet shaped core made of another protein, p24, that surrounds the viral RNA.

- **package insert**

document furnished by the manufacturer of a drug for use when dispensing the drug, which indicates approved uses, contraindications, and potential side effects.

- **PAHO**

pan Americans health organisation.

- **palindrome**

two stretches of DNA on opposite strands that are identical when oriented in the same direction, i.e. 5' to 3' or 3' to 5'.

- **palliative**

treatment which provides symptomatic relief, but not a cure.

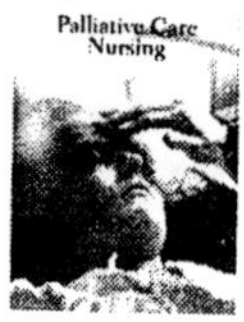

- **pancreas**

gland situated near the stomach that secretes a digestive fluid into the intestine through one or more ducts and also secretes the hormone insulin.

- **pancreatitis**

inflammation of the pancreas that can produce severe pain

and debilitating illness. See also pancreas.

- **pancytopenia**
  deficiency of all cell elements of the blood.

- **pandemic**
  worldwide epidemic.

- **pap smear**
  method for the early detection of cancer and other abnormalities of the female genital tract, especially of the cervix and uterus, employing exfoliated cells (cells that have been shed into vaginal fluid) and a special staining technique for microscopic examination that differentiates diseased tissue. Also known as papanicolaou smear after George Papanicolaou, the American cytologist who developed this method and published it in 1943.

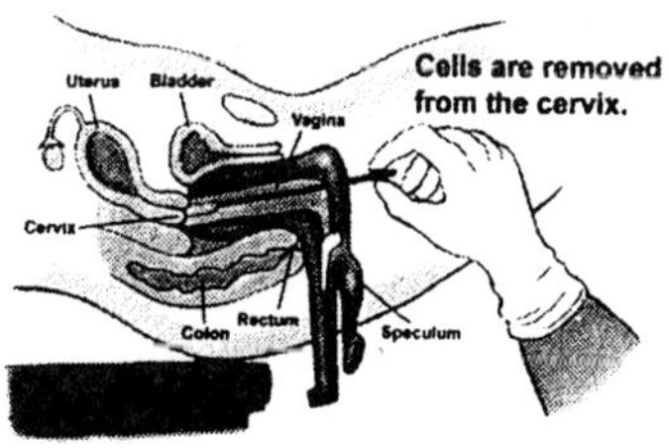

- **papilloma**
  benign tumour (as a wart or condyloma) resulting from an overgrowth of epithelial tissue on papillae of vascularised connective tissue (as of the skin).

- **papillomavirus**
  family of papova viruses associated with sexually transmitted diseases, including condylomata. Certain papillomavirus variants have also been associated with cervical cancer, particularly in HIV infected women.

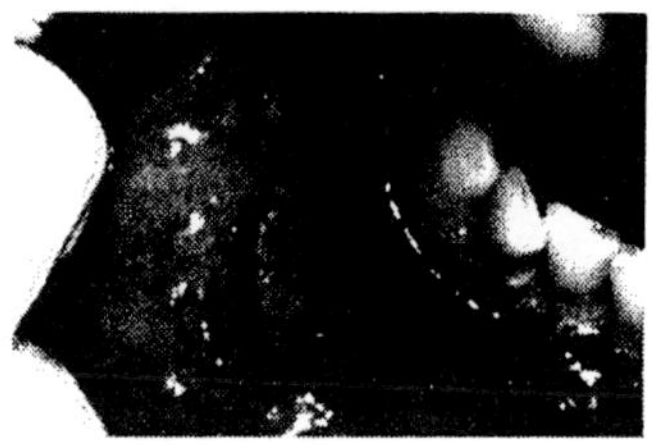

- **papule**
  small raised bump or protrusion on the skin

- **para aminobenzoic acid (PABA)**
  intermediate in the pathway for folic acid synthesis in bacteria, sulpha drugs have a similar structure to PABA.

- **parallel track**
  system of distributing experimental drugs to patients who are unable to participate in ongoing clinical efficacy trials and have no other treatment options.

■ **parasexual cycle**
nuclear cycle in which genes of haploid nuclei recombine without meiosis.

■ **parasite**
plant or organism that lives on or in the host, deriving nourishment from it. Some cause inflammation, but others cause infection and destroy tissue. Human parasites include fungi, yeast, bacteria, protozoa, worms and viruses.

■ **parasitism**
association in which one organism, the parasite, benefits at the expense of the other organism, the host.

■ **parenchyma**
the tissue of an organ (as distinguished from supporting or connective tissue).

■ **parent strain**
refers to the original strain of a bacterium, often used in place of wild type strain.

■ **parenteral**
not in or through the digestive system. For example, parenteral can pertain to blood being drawn from a vein in the arm or introduced into that vein via a transfusion (intravenous), or to injection of medications or vaccines through the skin (subcutaneous) or into the muscle (intra-muscular).

■ **paresthesia**
abnormal sensations, numbness, tingling, burning.

■ **paromomycin (humatin)**
antibiotic used for treating intestinal infections.

■ **partially blinded clinical trial**
clinical trial in which some, but not all, of the study treatments are administered in a single or double blinded fashion.

■ **participant**
study participant.

■ **particle density**
density of the soil particles, the dry mass of the particles being divided by the solid (not bulk) volume of the particles, in contrast with bulk density.

■ **particle size**
effective diameter of a particle measured by sedimentation, sieving or micrometric methods.

■ **passive diffusion**
process in which molecules flow freely into and out of a cell so that the concentration of any

particular molecule is the same on the inside as it is on the outside of the cell.

- **passive immunity**
  protective immunity resulting from the transfer of immune serum or immune cells produced by other individuals or animals.

- **passive immunotherapy/ passive immunisation**
  infusion of antibodies from another individual. As distinguished from actively stimulating an immune response in the recipient

- **pasteurisation**
  process using mild heat to reduce microbial numbers in heat sensitive materials.

- **pathogen**
  organism or virus that can cause disease.

- **pathogenesis**
  process by which disease develops.

- **pathogenicity**
  ability of a parasite to inflict damage on the host.

- **pathogenicity islands**
  short fragments of DNA in bacteria that code for factors that cause disease and have been transferred from disease causing organisms.

- **pathogen suppressive soil**
  soil where a pathogen does not establish or persist, a pathogen establishes but causes little or no damage, or a pathogen causes disease for a while, but the disease becomes less important even though the pathogen persists in soil.

- **patient close out**
  process of separating patients from a clinical trial at the end of treatment and follow up.

- **patient close out stage**
  stage of a trial in which patients leave a trial. The end of treatment and follow up.

- **patient follow up**
  process involving periodic contact with patients enrolled in a clinical trial for the purpose of administering the assigned treatment(s), observing the effects of treat-ment(s), modifying the course of treatment(s), or for collecting required data.

- **patient identification number**
  a unique sequence of numbers, or numbers and letters, that are

used to identify a patient.

- **patient population**
  study population.

- **patient recruitment**
  process of identifying suitable patients for enrolment into a clinical trial.

- **patient recruitment goal**
  number of patients scheduled to be enrolled into the trial. Usually set before the trial starts, or shortly thereafter, via a sample size calculation or via practical considerations.

- **PCR (polymerase chain reaction)**
  highly sensitive test that can detect and/or DNA fragments of viruses or other organisms in blood or tissue. PCR works by repeatedly copying genetic material using heat cycling, and enzymes similar to those used by cells.

- **peat**
  unconsolidated soil material consisting largely of un-decomposed, or only slightly decomposed, organic matter accumulated under conditions of excessive moisture.

- **pectin**
  important component of the plant cell walls containing chains of galacturonic acid that is often esterified with a methyl group.

- **pediatric**
  relating to the medical specialty concerned with the development, care and treatment of children from birth through adolescence.

- **peer review**
  process by which new scientific or medical findings, announced by one researcher, are reviewed by other scientists or physicians before these findings are published.

- **peliosis hepatis**
  serious condition characterised by formation of blood filled cysts in the liver, caused by *bartonella henselae*, usually a complication of aids or other severe immunodeficiency.

- **pellicle**
  relatively rigid layer of proteinaceous elements just beneath the cell membrane in many protozoa and algae.

- **Pelvic Inflammatory Disease (PID)**
  a painful gynaecological condition usually caused by infec-

tion, where disease spreads upward from the vagina into the pelvic cavity.

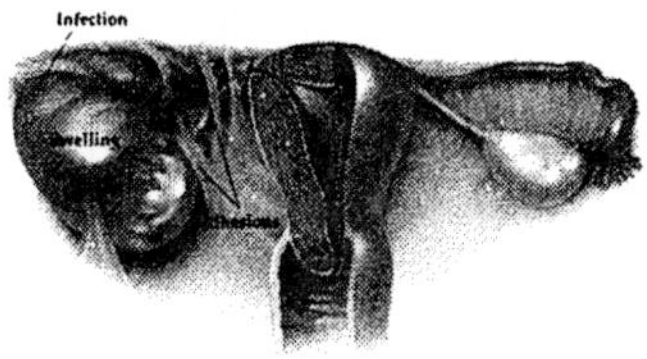

■ **penicillin**

antibiotic that interferes with the synthesis of the peptidoglycan portion of bacterial cell walls.

■ **penicillin enrichment**

method for increasing the relative proportion of auxotrophic mutants in a population by killing off the growing prototrophic cells with penicillin.

■ **penicillin binding proteins (PBPS)**

target of b lactam antimicrobial drugs; their role in bacteria is peptidoglycan synthesis.

■ **pentam**

brand name of pentamidine.

■ **pentamer**

polymer composed of five monomeric structural units.

■ **pentamidine**

antibiotic effective in an IV formulation against PCP. An aerosolised form is used to prevent PCP.

■ **pentamidine**

approved anti-protozoal drug used for the treatment and prevention of pneumocystis carinii pneumonia (PCP) infection. It can be delivered intravenously or intramuscularly or inhaled as an aerosol. Aerosolised pentamidine is approved for the prophylaxis of PCP in HIV positive individuals with cd4+ counts below 200 per cubic millimeter or for those with prior episodes of PCP. The drug is also known under the names pentam and nebupent.

■ **pentose phosphate pathway**

metabolic pathway that converts glucose to pyruvate, generating reducing power in the form of NADPH, and two precursor metabolites.

■ **peptide**

short string of amino acids. Peptides are small proteins.

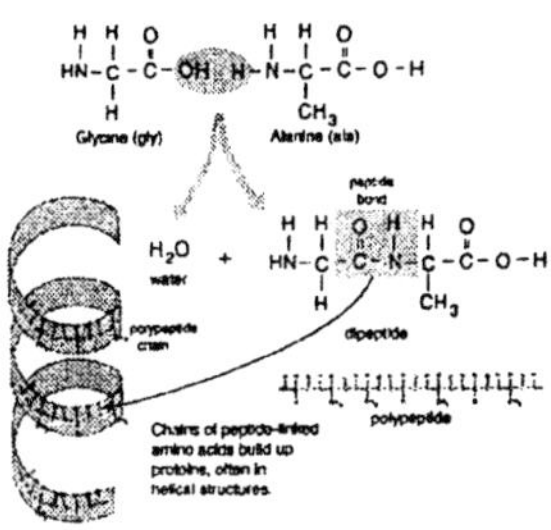

- **peptide bond**
  covalent bond formed between the –COOH group of one amino acid and the $-NH_2$ group of another amino acid; characteristic of proteins.

- **peptide interbridge**
  component of the peptidoglycan layer of gram positive bacteria; the short chain of amino acids that links the peptide side chains of adjacent n acetylmuramic acid molecules.

- **peptide or p site**
  first site on the ribosome to which the t RNA binds to begin translation.

- **peptidoglycan**
  macromolecule found only in bacteria that provides rigidity to the bacterial cell wall. The basic structure of peptidoglycan is an alternating series of two major subunits n acetylmuramic acid (NAM) and n acetylglucosamine (NAG). These chains are cross linked by peptide chains.

- **peptidoglycan layer**
  rigid backbone of the bacterial cell wall, composed of repeating subunits of n acetylmuramic acid and n acetylglucosamine and a number of amino acids.

- **peptone**
  common component of bacteriological media, consists of proteins originating from any of a variety of sources that have been hydrolysed to amino acids and short peptides by treatment with enzymes, acids or alkali.

- **perforin**
  molecule produced by t cytotoxic cells and nk cells, functions in killing target cells by forming a pore through the target cell membrane.

- **perianal**
  around the anus.

- **peribacteroid membrane**
  plant derived membrane surrounding one to several rhizobia within host cells of legume nodules

- **perinatal**
  relating to the period around the time of birth.

- **peripheral**
  toward the outside, or at the extremities.

- **peripheral blood mononuclear cell (PBMC)**
  cells in the bloodstream with one nucleus.

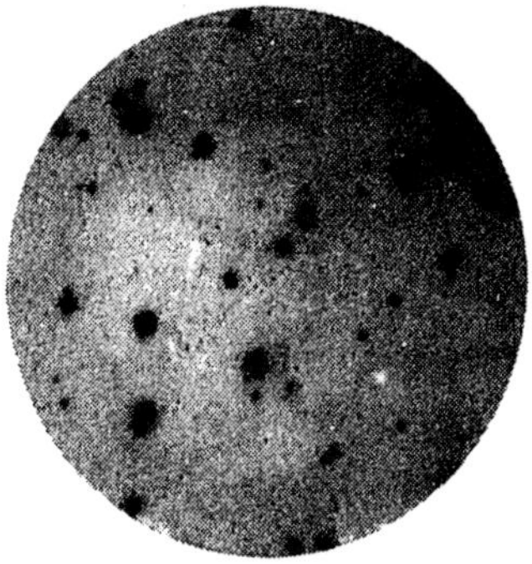

■ **peripheral neuropathy**
a disorder of the nerves that usually involves the feet or hands and sometimes the legs, arms and face. Symptoms may include numbness, a tingling or burning sensation, sharp pain, weakness and abnormal reflexes.

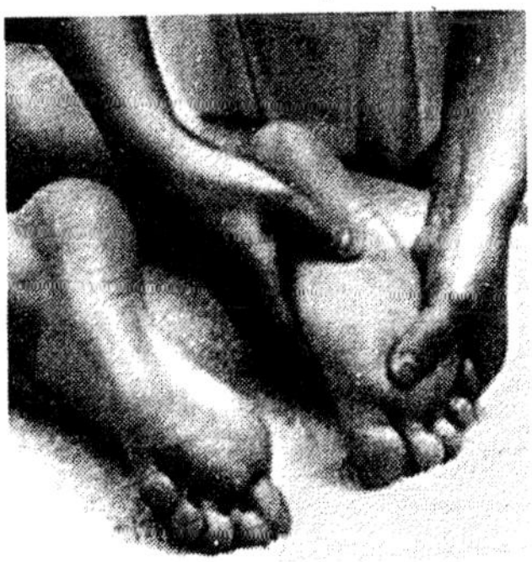

■ **periplasm**
periplasmic gel Very narrow gel that lies between the cell wall and the cytoplasmic membrane in Gram negative bacteria.

■ **periplasmic space**
area between the cell membrane and the cell wall in gram negative bacteria, containing certain enzymes involved in nutrition.

■ **perithecium**
flask shaped ascocarp open at the tip, containing asci of fungi in the phylum ascomycota.

■ **peritrichous flagella**
distribution of flagella over the entire surface of a cell.

■ **peritrichous flagellation**
having flagella attached to many places on the cell surface.

■ **permanent wilting point**
greatest water content of a soil at which indicator plants, growing in that soil wilt and fail to recover when placed in a humid chamber. Often estimated by the water content at 1.5 mpa soil matric potential.

■ **peroxidase enzymes**
enzymes found in neutrophil granules, saliva, and milk that together with hydrogen perox-

ide and halide ions make up an effective anti-microbial system.

- **persistent**
  refers to infection in which the causative agent remains in the body for long periods of time often without causing symptoms of disease.

- **persistent generalised lymphadenopathy (PGL)**
  chronic, diffuse, non-cancerous lymph node enlargement. Typically it has been found in those with immune system disturbances who develop frequent and persistent bacterial, viral and fungal infections.

- **petechia (pl. petechiae)**
  small purplish spot on the skin or mucous membrane caused by hemorrhage.

- **petri dish**
  two part dish of glass or plastic often used to contain medium solidified with agar, on which bacteria are grown.

- **peyer's patch**
  lymphatic tissue lining the intestines. One of the largest areas of lymphatic tissue in the body. May take over some of the role of the thymus in adults

- **ph**
  scale of 0 to 14 that expresses the acidity or alkalinity of a solution.

- **phage**
  abbreviation for bacteriophage.

- **phage induction**
  process by which phage DNA is excised from bacterial DNA

- **phagocystosis**
  the consumption and destruction of foreign materials by white blood cells like macrophages

- **phagocyte**
  a cell that is able to ingest and destroy foreign matter, including bacteria.

- **phagotrophic**
  form of feeding where animals, such as protozoans, engulf particulate nutrients, such as bacterial cells or detritus.

- **pharmacokinetic**
  concerning the study of how a drug is processed by the body, with emphasis on the time required for absorption, duration of action, distribution in the body and method of excretion.

- **phase contrast microscope**
  type of light microscope that employs special optical devices

to amplify the difference in the refractive indexes of cells and the surrounding medium, increasing the contrast of the image.

- **phase I trial**
first stage in testing a new drug in humans. The studies are usually done to generate preliminary information on the chemical action and safety of the drug using normal healthy volunteers. Usually done without a comparison group.

- **phase II trial**
second stage in testing a new drug in humans. Generally carried out on patients with the disease or condition of interest. The main purpose is to evaluate activity, and possibly provide preliminary information on treatment efficacy and to supplement information on safety obtained from phase i trials. Usually, but not always, designed to include a control treatment and random allocation of patients to treatment.

- **phase II/III**
special classification arising from the aids context where greater testing of efficacy occurs earlier.

- **phase III trial**
third and usually final stage in testing a new drug in humans. Concerned primarily with assessment of dosage effects and efficacy and safety. Usually designed to include a control treatment and random allocation to treatment. Once this phase is completed the drug manufacturers may request permission to market the drug, assuming the results of the phase i, ii and iii trials are consistent with such a request.

- **phase IV trial**
generally, a randomised controlled trial that is designed to evaluate the long term safety and efficacy of a drug for a given indication .Usually carried out after licensure of the drug for that indication.

- **phase variation**
reversible change in antigenicity of a structure, such as the flagella of salmonella species.

- **phenotype**
observable properties of an organism.

- **phenotypic mixing or transcapsidation**
exchange of protein coats by

two viruses when two virions infect the same cell

- **phosphobacterium**
bacterium that is especially good at solubilizing the insoluble inorganic phosphate in soil.

- **phosphodiester bond**
type of covalent bond linking nucleotides together in a polynucleotide.

- **phospholipid**
lipid that has a phosphate molecule as part of its structure.

- **phosphorus cycle**
sequence of transformations undergone by phosphorus where it is transformed between soluble and insoluble, and organic and inorganic forms.

- **phosphorylation**
process of adding phosphorus to a compound. Often done within the body by enzymes named 'kinases'. The nucleoside drugs, like AZT, Ddi, ddc, etc. All need to be phosphorylated in the body before they become active.

- **phosphotransferase system**
type of group translocation in which the transported molecule is phosphorylated as it passes through the cytoplasmic membrane.

- **photic zone**
uppermost layer of a body of water or soil that receives enough sunlight to permit the occurrence of photosynthesis.

- **photoautotroph**
organism able to use light as its sole source of energy and carbon dioxide as sole carbon source.

- **photoheterotroph**
organism able to use light as a source of energy and organic materials as carbon source.

- **photooxidation**
chemical reaction occurring as a result of absorption of light energy in the presence of oxygen.

- **photophosphorylation**
processes that utilise light as an energy source to drive the synthesis of ATP.

- **photoreactivation (or light repair)**
breakage of the covalent bonds joining thymine dimers in the

light thereby restoring the DNA to its original state.

- **photosynthesis**
process of using light energy to synthesise carbohydrates from carbon dioxide.

- **photosystems**
protein complexes within which chlorophyll and other light gathering pigments are organised; located in special photosynthetic membranes.

- **phototaxis**
movement toward light.

- **phototroph**
organism that uses light as the energy source to drive the electron flow from the electron donors, such as water, hydrogen, or sulphide.

- **phycobilin**
water soluble pigment that occurs in cyanobacteria and functions as the light harvesting pigments for photosystem II.

- **phycobiliproteins**
light harvesting pigments of cyanobacteria, they absorb energy from wavelengths of light that are not well absorbed by chlorophyll.

- **phylogenetic tree**
type of diagram that depicts the evolutionary heritage of organisms.

- **phylogeny**
evolutionary relatedness of organisms.

- **phylum**
collection of similar classes. A collection of similar phyla comprises a kingdom. A phylum may also be called a division.

- **phytohemagglutinin (pha)**
a plant chemical used to stimulate the multiplication of white blood cells.

- **phytoplankton**
floating and swimming algae and photosynthetic prokaryotic organisms of lakes and oceans.

- **pico**
prefix meaning a one trillionth, as in picogram, a trillionth of a gram.

- **PID**
patient identification number. A unique identifier that refers to a particular patient, yet preserves

confidentiality for record keeping

■ **pilot study**
preliminary study designed to indicate whether a larger study is practical.

■ **pilus (pl. pili)**
hairlike appendages on many gram negative bacteria that function in conjugation and for attachment.

■ **pinocytosis**
process by which eukaryotic cells take in liquid and small particles from the surrounding environment by internalising and pinching off small pieces of their own membrane, bringing along a small volume of liquid and any material attached to the membrane.

■ **pituitary gland**
small, oval endocrine gland that lies at the base of the brain. It is called the master gland because the other endocrine glands depend on its secretions for stimulation. The pituitary has two distinct lobes, anterior and posterior. The anterior lobe secretes at least six hormones human growth hormone, which stimulates overall body growth; ACTH (adrenocorticotropic hormone), which controls steroid hormone secretion by the adrenal cortex, thyrotropic hormone, which stimulates the activity of the thyroid gland, and three gonadotropic hormones, which control growth and reproductive activity of the gonads (ovaries and testes). The posterior lobe secretes antidiuretic hormone, which causes water retention by the kidneys, and oxytocin, which stimulates the mammary glands to release milk and also causes uterine contractions. An overactive pituitary during childhood can cause gigantism; during adulthood, it can cause acromegaly. Dwarfism results from pituitary deficiency in childhood.

■ **placebo**
an inactive substance against which investigational treatments are compared for efficacy.

Pituitary Gland

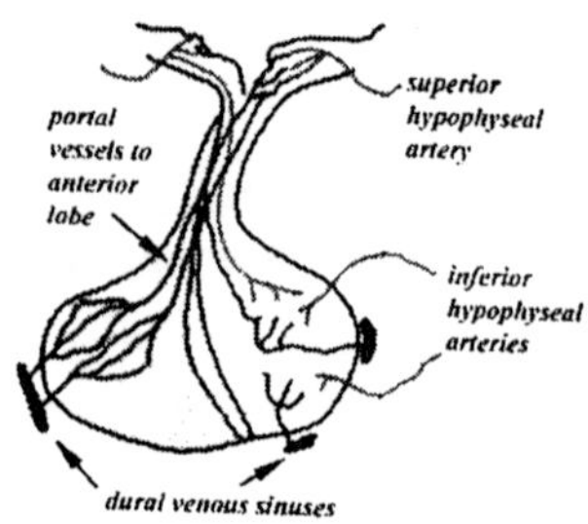

■ **placebo controlled study**
method of investigation of drugs in which an inactive substance (the placebo) is given to one group of patients, while the drug being tested is given to another group. The results obtained in the two groups are then compared.

■ **placebo effect**
physical or emotional change occurring after a substance is taken or administered that is not the result of any special property of the substance. The change may be beneficial, reflecting the expectations of the patient and, often, the expectations of the person giving the substance.

■ **placebo controlled clinical trial**
clinical trial in which patients assigned to the control treatment receive a placebo.

■ **placenta**
combination of foetal and maternal cells that serves as the organ of exchange for nutrients and other chemicals between mother and foetus during pregnancy.

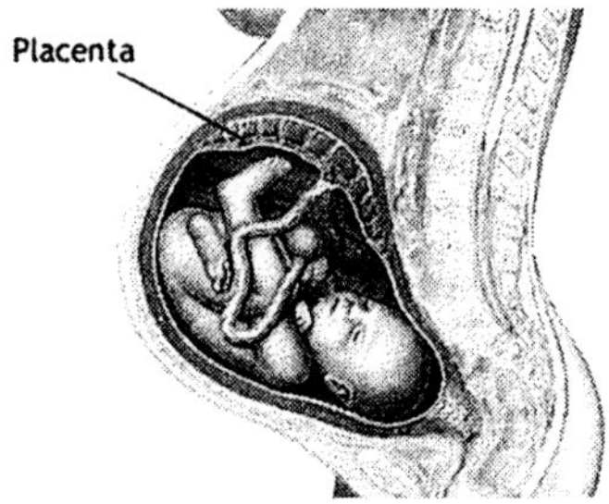

■ **plankton**
primarily microscopic organisms floating freely in most waters.

■ **plant growth promoting rhizobacteria (PGPR)**
broad group of soil bacteria that exert beneficial effects on plant growth usually as root colonizers. Many members of the genus *Pseudomonas*.

■ **plaque**
localised area of lysis or cell inhibition caused by virus infection on a lawn of cells.

■ **plasma**
fluid portion of non-clotted blood.

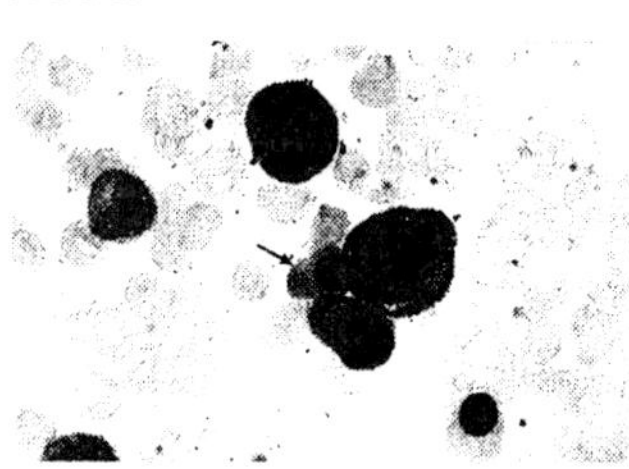

■ **plasma cell**
end cell of the b cell series, fully differentiated to produce and secrete large amounts of antibody.

■ **plasma membrane**
semipermeable membrane that surrounds the cytoplasm in a cell, cytoplasmic membrane.

■ **plasma**
that 10 percent of the blood that contains nutrients, electrolytes (dissolved salts), gases, albumin, clotting factors, wastes and hormones.

■ **plasmapheresis**
selective removal of certain proteins or antibodies from the blood (followed by reinjection of the blood). This process is sometimes used in the treatment of some peripheral neuropathies and is an integral part of passive immunotherapies for HIV.

■ **plasmid**
covalently closed, circular piece of DNA which, as an extrachromosomal genetic element, is not essential for growth.

■ **plasmogamy**
fusion of the contents of two cells, including cytoplasm and nuclei.

■ **plasmolysis**
process in which water diffuses out of a cell, causing the cytoplasm to dehydrate and shrink from the cell wall.

■ **plastid**
specialised cell organelles containing pigments or protein materials.

■ **plate count**
method used to determine the number of viable cells in a specimen by determining the number of colonies that arise when the specimen is added to an agar medium.

■ **platelets**
active agents of inflammation when damage occurs to a blood vessel. They are not actually cells, but fragments released by megakaryocyte cells. Megakaryocyte is a large cell in the bone marrow whose function is to produce platelets. When vascular damage (i.e., damage to blood vessels) occurs, the platelets stick to the vascular walls, forming clots to prevent the loss of blood. Thus, it is important to have adequate numbers of normally functioning platelets to

maintain effective coagulation of the blood. There are drugs that can potentially alter the platelet count, making it necessary to monitor the count. Also, some people with HIV infection develop thrombocytopenia (a condition characterised by a platelet count of less than 100,000 platelets per cubic millimetre of blood). The normal value for men is 154,000 354,000 platelets per cubic millimetre of blood. For women, it is 162,000 380,000 platelets per cubic millimetre of blood.

- **pleomorphic**
bacteria that characteristically vary in shape.

- **pleurisy**
inflammation of the pleura, membranes that line the lung and chest cavity; often marked by a sharp pain associated with breathing.

- **plus (+) strand (1)**
the DNA strand that is complementary to the strand used as a template for RNA synthesis. (2) of the two RNA molecules that can theoretically be transcribed from double stranded DNA, the one that can be translated to make a protein; also called the sense strand.

- **PMN**
abbreviation for polymorphonuclear neutrophils.

- **pneumocystis carinii pneumonia**
opportunistic pneumonitis often seen in HIV infected patients. PCP generally produces a dry, hacking cough. Although previously thought to be a protozoa, and responsive to anti protozoal treatment, recent genetic analysis suggest that *p carinii* is closer to the funguses.

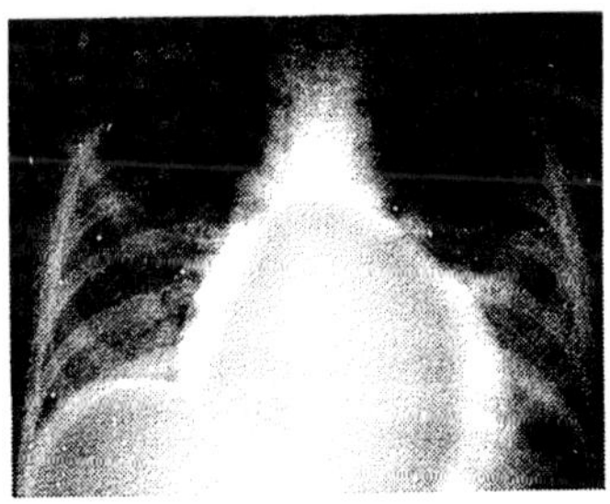

- **pneumocystis carinii pneumonia (PCP)**
protozoal infection of the lungs.

- **pneumonia**
inflammation of the lungs accompanied filling of the air sacs with fluids such as pus and

blood

■ **pneumonic plague**
disease that develops when *yersinia pestis* infects the lungs.

■ **PO**
abbreviation for 'by mouth' (as opposed to intravenous, intramuscular, etc.).

■ **point mutation**
mutation in which only a single base pair is involved.

■ **polar**
possessing hydrophilic characteristics and generally water soluble.

■ **polar covalent bond**
bond formed by sharing electrons between atoms that have unequal attraction for the electrons.

■ **polar flagellation**
condition of having flagella attached at one end or both ends of the cell.

■ **polarity (1)**
the degree of affinity that an atom has for electrons. This results in positive or negative charges on atoms in a molecule.

■ **poly**
a tail series of approximately 200 adenine derivatives that are added to the 3' end of a MRNA transcript in eukaryotic cells; thought to stabilise the transcript and enhance translation.

■ **poly beta hydroxybutyrate (PHB)**
common storage material of prokaryotic cells consisting of beta hydroxybutyrate or other beta alkanoic acids.

■ **polycistronic (polygenic)**
refers to m-RNA containing transcripts of many genes in a single molecule.

■ **polyclonal antiserum**
mixture of antibodies to a variety of antigens or to a variety of determinants on a single antigen.

■ **polymer**
large molecule formed by polymerisation of monomeric units.

■ **polymerase chain reaction**
method used to create millions of copies of a given region of DNA in only a matter of hours.

■ **polymerase**
any of several enzymes that catalyse the formation of DNA or RNA from precursor substances in the presence of preexisting DNA or RNA acting as templates (i.e., patterns).

■ **polymorphic**
having different distinct forms at various stages of the life cycle.

■ **polymorphonuclear neutrophil (PMN)**
phagocytic cells that together with the macrophages are known as 'professional phagocytes.'

■ **polyneuritis**
inflammation of many nerves at once.

■ **polyneuropathy**
neuropathy involving a number of different nerves

■ **polysaccharide**
long chain of monosaccharides (sugars) linked by glycosidic bonds.

■ **polysome**
strings of ribosomes attached by strands of m-RNA.

■ **polyvalent vaccine**
vaccine that is active against multiple viral strains.

■ **pore space**
portion of soil bulk volume occupied by soil pores.

■ **porin**
protein channel in the lipopolysaccharide layer of gram negative bacteria.

■ **porosity**
volume of pores in a soil sample (nonsolid volume) divided by the bulk volume of the sample.

■ **portal of entry**
place of entry of micro-organisms into the host.

■ **portal of exit**
place where infectious agents leave the host to find a new host.

■ **positive (+) sense strand strand of RNA**
a which acts as m-RNA. The strand of DNA that gives rise to m-RNA.

■ **post hoc analyses**
analyses conducted after the results are available that were not defined before the start of the trial. Such analyses are particularly prone to false positive claims or type i error.

■ **posterior**
rear side or behind.

■ **post herpetic neuralgia (PHN)**
literally 'pain following herpes' the term is usually applied to the severe pain that sometimes follows the healing of herpes zoster lesions.

■ **posthumous**
after death.

■ **post marketing surveillance**
term used to characterise any procedure, implemented after licensure of a drug for a given indication, that is designed to provide information on the actual use of the drug for that indication and on the occurrence of related side effects. The surveillance usually involves survey techniques rather than controlled trials.

■ **post mortem**
after death or after the event.

■ **post partum**
after giving birth.

■ **post stratification**
the process of classifying patients into strata after they have been enrolled in the study usually for data analysis purposes.

■ **potential energy**
stored energy, it can exist in a variety of forms including chemical bonds, a rock on the top of a hill, and water behind a dam.

■ **pour plate**
method for performing a plate count of micro-organisms. A known amount of a serial dilution is placed in a sterile petri dish and then a melted agar medium is added and the inoculum mixed well by gently swirling. After growth the number of colony forming units is counted.

■ **pour plate method**
method of inoculating an agar medium with bacteria while the agar is liquid and then pouring it into a petri dish where the agar hardens. The colonies grow both on the surface and within the medium.

■ **power**
probability of finding a treatment effect that actually exists, or of rejecting the null hypothesis when the alternative hypothesis is in fact true. In clinical trials, the power of the study design is the ability of the study to detect a postulated difference between treatment groups if it in fact exists. For example, if there is 'something going on' in the study, does the study design have the power to demonstrate it?

■ **precipitation reaction**
reaction of an antibody with a

soluble antigen to form an insoluble substance.

- **preclinical**
  generally refers to research that has been done before a compound is tried on humans, i.e. in vitro and animal studies

- **precursor cells**
  cells from which other cells are formed by natural processes.

- **precursor metabolites**
  metabolic intermediates that are produced in catabolic pathways but can be siphoned off for use in anabolic pathways.

- **predation**
  relationship between two organisms whereby one organism (predator) engulfs or captures and digests the second organism (prey).

- **premature termination**
  early termination of a trial before data are sufficiently strong to be convincing.

- **prenatal**
  relating to the period before birth.

- **prerandomisation examination**
  any examination that is part of the evaluation process of a patient for enrolment into a trial and that is carried out before the randomisation examination.

- **prerandomisation visit**
  any visit made to the clinic by a potential study patient for the purpose of evaluation for enrolment into the trial and that takes place prior to the randomisation visit.

- **presumptive**
  presumed. In the context of diagnosis, one that is not definitely made, but where signs and symptoms make it exceedingly likely to be the proper one, even without confirmatory evidence. Diagnosis of cmv retinitis by characteristic appearance, without using a biopsy is an example if a presumptive diagnosis.

- **prevalence**
  total number cases, both old and new, in a given population at risk at a point in time.

- **primary culture**
  cells taken and grown directly from the tissues of an animal.

- **primary drug resistance (PDR)**
  resistance of bacteria or other pathogens to drugs which exists prior to the beginning of treatment.

- **primary immune response**
  immune response that occurs upon first exposure to an antigen.

- **primary infection**
  infection in a previously healthy individual, such as measles in a child who has not had measles before.

- **primary lymphoid organs**
  organs in which lymphoid stem cells mature, including the thymus and bone marrow.

- **primary metabolites**
  compounds synthesised by a cell during the log phase.

- **primary outcome**
  the event or condition the trial is designed to ameliorate, delay, or prevent.

- **primary outcome variable**
  the outcome variable that is designated or regarded as key in the design or analysis of the results of a trial. Generally, the variable used for sample size calculations in the design of the trial or, when no sample size calculation is made, for the main avenue of data analyses. The primary outcome monitored in interim analyses.

- **primary producer**
  organism that adds biomass to the ecosystem by synthesising organic molecules from carbon dioxide and simple inorganic nutrients.

- **primary stain**
  first dye applied in a multi step differential staining procedures, generally stains all cells.

- **primary structure**
  refers to the sequence of amino acids in a protein.

- **primase**
  enzyme that synthesises small fragments of RNA to serve as primers for DNA synthesis during DNA replication.

- **primer**
  RNA molecule that initiates the synthesis of DNA.

- **principal investigator**
  designation used to denote the individual named on a grant who is responsible for directing the proposed research

- **prion**
  infectious crystallising protein, which affects the brain.

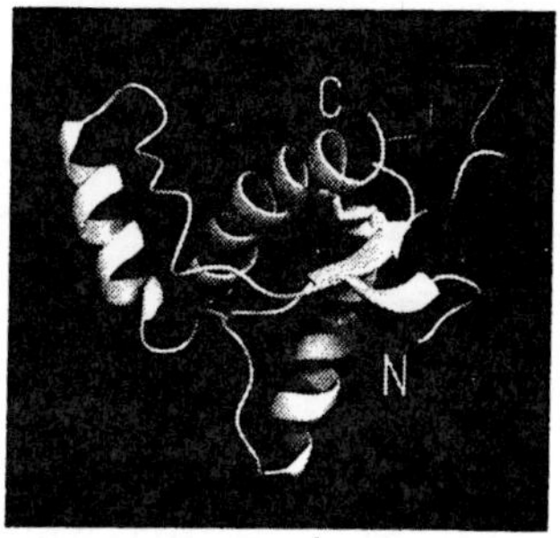

■ **Prn**
abbreviation meaning 'take as needed', usually applied to prescription drugs.

■ **procrit**
brand name of erythropoietin

■ **proctitis**
inflammation of the rectum.

■ **prodromal**
pertaining to symptoms indicating the onset of a disease. May include symptoms prior to those adequate for accurate diagnosis.

■ **prodrome**
symptom that indicates the onset of a disease.

■ **prodrug**
chemical precursor of a drug that is converted into the desired substance in the body.

■ **production**
stage of biogeochemical recycling in which producer organisms convert carbon dioxide or other inorganic compounds into organic materials.

■ **productive infection**
virus infection in which more virions are produced.

■ **progenitor**
parent or ancestor.

■ **proglottid**
one of the segments that make up most of the body of a tapeworm.

■ **prognosis**
the probable future course of a disease.

■ **progression of disease**
common endpoint used in aids clinical trials. The entity 'progression of disease' usually consists of new occurrences of non recurrent aids defining illnesses or death.

■ **progressive multicocal leukoencephalopathy (PML)**
opportunistic infection resulting from reactivation or new infection with the jc virus.

■ **project officer**
individual in the sponsoring agency who is responsible for dealing with technical, scientific, and programmatic aspects of a grant or contract funded project.

■ **prokaryote**
prokaryotic cell characterised by lack of a nuclear membrane and the absence membrane bound organelles.

■ **prokine**
brand name of sargramostim

■ **promoter**
site on DNA where the RNA polymerase binds and begins transcription.

■ **propagated epidemic**
outbreak of contagious disease in which the infectious agent is transmitted to others, resulting in steadily increasing numbers of people becoming ill.

■ **propagule**
cell unit capable of developing into a complete organism.

■ **prophage**
latent form of a temperate phage whose DNA has been inserted into the host's DNA.

■ **prophage**
state of the genome of a temperate virus when it is replicating in synchrony with that of the host, typically integrated into the host genome.

■ **prophylactic trial**
trial that is designed to assess the efficacy of a treatment procedure aimed at preventing the development or progression of a specific disease or condition.

■ **prophylaxis**
prevention of disease.

■ **prospective follow up study**
study in which people with a specific attribute or characteristic are identified and then observed for some period of time thereafter for the occurrence of the outcome or condition of interest, usually disease or death. The study may or may not involve a comparison group. Clinical trials represent a special subset of prospective follow up studies.

■ **prospective study**
study that looks ahead to see if the risk factors identified by a retrospective study predict a tendency to develop the disease.

■ **prosthetic group**
tightly bound, non-protein portion of an enzyme, not the same as coenzyme.

■ **protease**
enzyme that degrades protein, encoded by HIV and the target of several anti HIV medications.

protease inhibitor

new class of experimental antiretroviral drugs that work by inhibiting the HIV protease. Some examples include saquinavir, indinavir and ritonavir.

protease inhibitors

HIV protease is an aspartyl enzyme essential to the replicative life cycle of HIV. The three dimensional molecular structure of the HIV protease has been fully determined. Pharmaceutical developers are therefore able to rationally design compounds to inhibit it and thus interfere with replication of the virus.

protein A

Protein produced by *Staphylococcus aureus* that inhibits phagocytosis of the organism by binding to the FC portion of antibodies.

proteins

any of the group of highly complex organic compounds found in all living cells. Protein is the most abundant class of all biological molecules, comprising about 50 percent of cellular dry weight. Classified by biological function, proteins include the enzymes, which catalyse cellular reactions; collagen, keratin and elastin, which are structural, or support, proteins; haemoglobin and other transport proteins, casein, ovalbumin and other nutrient proteins; antibodies, which are necessary for immunity; protein hormones, which regulate metabolism; and proteins such as actin and myosin, the contractile muscle proteins that perform mechanical work. Structurally, proteins are large molecules composed of one or more chains of varying amounts of the same 22 amino acids, which are linked by peptide bonds. Each protein is characterised by a unique and invariant amino acid sequence. Protein chains may contain hundreds of amino acids; some proteins also incorporate phosphorus or such metals as iron, zinc and copper. The amino acid sequence also determines the molecule's three dimensional structure; this so called native state is required for proper bio logical function. The information for the syntheses of the specific amino acid sequences from free amino acids is carried by the cell's nucleic acid.

protist
designation for eukaryotic organisms other than plants, animals and fungi, may be unicellular or multi-cellular.

protista
old taxonomic term referring to algae, fungi, and protozoa (collectively, the eukaryotic protists), and the prokaryotes.

protocol
detailed plan for a clinical trial that states the trial's rationale, purpose, drug or vaccine dosages, length of study, routes of administration, who may participate and other aspects of trial design.

proton
positively charged component of an atom found in the nucleus.

proton motive force
form of energy generated by the electron transport chain, which expels protons to create a chemiosmotic gradient.

protooncogene
genes in the bodies of animals that code for proteins that activate transcription.

protoplasm
complete cellular contents, cytoplasmic membrane, cytoplasm, and nucleus; usually considered the living portion of the cell, thus excluding those layers peripheral to the cell membrane.

protoplast
cell from which the wall has been removed.

prototroph
organism that has no organic growth requirements other than a source of carbon and energy.

protozoa
family of unicellular organisms including amoebas, that are the simplest form of animal life. Protozoa can be a cause of parasitic disease. In aids, toxoplasmosis, pneumocystis carinii, giardia, and cryptosporidium belii are among the most harmful protozoa.

protozoan (pl. protozoa)
unicellular eukaryotic microorganisms that move by either protoplasmic flow (amoebae), flagella (flagellates) or cilia (ciliates). Most species feed on bacteria, fungi or detrital particles

■ **provirus**
latent form of a virus in which the viral DNA is incorporated into the chromosome of the host.

■ **pruritic**
causing itching.

■ **pruritus**
itching rash.

■ **pseudomonad**
member of the genus *pseudomonas*, a large group of gram negative, obligatory respiratory (never fermentative) bacteria.

■ **pseudopodium (pl. pseudopodia)**
protrusion of an amoeboid cell formed by the extrusion or streaming of the cytoplasm (but still enclosed in the membrane) for the purpose of movement or feeding.

■ **pseudopods**
transient arm like extensions formed by phagocytes and protozoa, they surround and enclose extracellular material, including bacteria, during the process of phagocytosis.

■ **pseudovirion**
virus like particle.

■ **p site (peptidyl site)**
site on the ribosome where the t-RNA that temporarily carries the elongating amino acid chain resides.

■ **psychrophile**
micro-organism that grows best between –5° and 15°c.

■ **psychrotroph**
organism that can grow well at low temperatures but has an optimum temperature above 15°c.

■ **pulmonary**
pertaining to the lungs.

■ **pulsed field gel electrophoresis**
type of gel electrophoresis that is used to separate very large fragments of DNA.

■ **pulsenet**
surveillance network to facilitate the tracking of food borne disease outbreaks, catalogues the rflps of certain pathogenic organisms..

■ **pure culture**
culture that contains only a single strain of an organism.

■ **purified protein derivative (PPD)**
the most common test for exposure to *m. Tuberculosis*, the bacteria that causes TB. In the ppd

test, a small amount of protein from TB is injected under the skin. If the patient has been previously infected, they will mount a delayed type hypersensitivity reaction, characterised by a hard red bump called an induration.

- **purine**
  component of RNA and DNA. The two major purines are adenine and guanine.

- **purulent**
  infected and producing pus.

- **pus**
  thick, opaque, often yellowish material that forms at the site of infection, made up of dead neutrphils and tissue debris.

- **putrefaction**
  digestion of proteins by enzymes to yield foul smelling products.

- **pyoderma**
  any skin disease characterised by production of pus.

- **pyogenic**
  pus producing.

- **pyrimethamine (daraprim)**
  antibiotic used in treating toxoplasmosis, and rarely for the treatment or prophylaxis of PCP

- **pyrimidine**
  component of RNA and DNA. The three major pyrimidines are thymidine, cytosine and uracil.

- **pyrogens**
  fever inducing substances.

- **pyruvate**
  end product of glycolysis, a precursor metabolite used in the synthesis of amino acids.

- **Q10**
  relative increase in a reaction rate with temperature. It is expressed as the increase over a 10°c interval.

- **Q4H**
  common abbreviation for 'every four hours'. Also, q5h, would be every five hours, q6h would be every six, etc.

- **Qapacc**
  see 'quality assurance, performance assessment, and capacity committee'

- **QID**
  common abbreviation for 'four times a day'.

- **quadrant**
  one section of something that has been divided into four equal parts

■ **qualitative**
of, relating to, or expressed in relative or subjective terms impossible to precisely quantify.

■ **quality assurance**
any procedure, method or philosophy for collecting, processing, or analysing data that is aimed at maintaining or improving the reliability or validity of the data and the associated procedures used to generate them.

■ **quantitative**
of, relating to or expressed in terms of quantity.

■ **quartenary structure**
level of structure of a protein molecule resulting from the interaction of one or more protein chains.

■ **quaternary ammonium compounds**
cationic (positively charged) detergents that are non toxic enough to be used to disinfect food preparation surfaces. Also called quats.

■ **quorum sensing**
communication between bacteria by means of small molecules, permitting the bacteria to sense when there is an adequate quorum or number of organisms present to activate virulence genes.

■ **R plasmids**
plasmids that encode resistance to one or more anti-microbial medications.

■ **radial immunodiffusion test**
quantitative antigen antibody precipitation in gel test in which one reactant is distributed throughout the gel and the other reactant diffuses into the gel producing a ring of precipitation.

■ **radiculopathy**
infection or other damage of the peripheral nerves and spinal roots, accompanied by weakness, numbness, and eventual paralysis. Radiculopathy is distinguished from peripheral neuropathy frequently by its asymmetric presentation

■ **radioallergosorbent test (RAST)**
radioimmunoassay that measures the ige antibody reacting with a specific antigen, used in the diagnosis of immediate allergies.

■ **radiography**
use of x rays in diagnosis

- **radioimmunoassay (RIA)**
competitive inhibition assay using a radioactively labelled reactant to measure antigens or antibodies.

- **radiology**
science of diagnosis and/or treatment using radiant energy. Includes x rays, MRI, destruction of tumours by radiation, etc.

- **rales**
sounds in the lungs, often indicative of disease.

- **random (general)**
having no specific pattern or objective. Of or designating a chance process in which the occurrence of previous events is of no value in predicting future events. From old french, *random*, meaning force, violence, impetuosity.

- **random allocation**
method for assigning patients to treatment using a random process.

- **random number**
number generated or drawn via some defined random process.

- **random process**
any method or procedure whose output is random (i.e., cannot be predicted by any means).

- **random variable**
variable that may assume any one of a number of different values, where the set of possible values is determined by a probability distribution, such as binomial or normal.

- **randomisation**
process of assigning patients to treatment using a random process, such as via use of a table of random numbers.

- **randomisation visit**
visit where the participant is randomly assigned to treatment.

- **randomised**
having been assigned to a treatment via a random process. Normally considered to have occurred when the randomisation schedule is sent to the unit pharmacist, so they can then dispense the appropriate drug.

- **randomised controlled clinical trial**
clinical trial that involves at least one test treatment and one control treatment, concurrent enrolment and follow up of the test and control treated groups, and in which

the treatments to be administered are selected by a random process, such that neither the patients nor the persons responsible for their selection or treatment can influence the assignments, and where the assignments remain unknown to the patients and clinic staff until the patients have been determined to be eligible for enrolment into the trial (and then in blinded trials may be revealed to patients and clinic personnel only by letter or number codes).

■ **randomised trial**
study in which participants are randomly assigned to either a treatment arm or placebo arm of a clinical trial.

■ **raw data**
measurements and observations recorded on study data forms.

■ **reactogenicity**
capacity to produce adverse reactions.

■ **reading frames**
grouping of a stretch of nucleotides into sequential triplets. A MRNA molecule has three reading frames, but only one is typically used in translation.

■ **reannealing**
process where two complementary single strands of DNA automatically hybridise back into a single, double stranded molecule upon cooling.

■ **recalcitrant**
resistant to microbial attack.

■ **receptor**
structure on a cell which joins with proteins to produce changes in cellular function.

■ **receptor mediated endocytosis**
type of pinocytosis that allows cells to internalise extracellular ligands that bind to the cell's receptors.

■ **recombinant**
produced by genetic engineering in the laboratory.

■ **recombinant DNA**
DNA molecule containing DNA originating from two or more sources.

■ **recombinant vaccines**
subunit vaccines produced by genetic engineering.

■ **recombinant**
organism whose genome contains integrated genetic mate-

rial from a different organism.

■ **recombination**
process by which genetic elements in two separate genomes are brought together in one unit.

■ **record**
paper or electronic document that contains or is designed to contain a set of facts related to some occurrence, transaction, or the like

■ **rectum**
very bottom most portion of the lower intestine, including the anus.

■ **recurrence**
return or flare up of a condition thought cured or in remission

■ **redox reactions**
transfer of electrons from one compound to another; one compound becomes reduced and the other becomes oxidised.

■ **reducing agents**
compounds that readily donate electrons to another compound, thereby reducing the other compound.

■ **reducing equivalent (power)**
electrons stored in reduced electron carriers such as NADH, NADPH and $FADH_2$.

■ **reduction**
process by which a compound accepts electrons.

■ **reduction potential**
inherent tendency of a compound to act as an electron donor or an electron acceptor. Measured in millivolts.

■ **reductive dechlorination**
removal of Cl as Cl from an organic compound by reducing the carbon atom from CCl to CH.

■ **refraction**
bending of light rays that occurs when light passes from one medium to another.

■ **refractory**
resistant to treatment, as of a disease.

■ **regimen**
any particular treatment plan specifying which drugs are used, in what doses, according to what schedule, and for how long.

■ **regression**
any of several statistical techniques concerned with predicting some variables by knowing others. Regression is used to answers such questions as 'how well can I predict the values of

one variable, (such as survival) by knowing the value of another variable' (such as treatment assignment)

- **regression analysis**

methods of explaining or predicting the variability of a dependent variable using information about one or more independent variables, or techniques for establishing a regression equation. The equation indicates the nature and closeness of the relationship between two or more variables, specifically the extent to which you can predict some by knowing other, the extent to which some are associated with others. The equation is often represented by a regression line, which is the straight line that comes closest to approximating a distribution of points in a scatter diagram.

- **regression to the mean**

phenomenon that occurs when a second determination or measurement is made only on those individuals with an extreme initial determination or measurement.

On average, the second determination or measurement tends to be less extreme than the initial one. Term originally coined by Sir Francis Galton (1886) to characterise the tendency for tall parents to produce shorter offspring and vice versa. Another example might be an imaginary trial that only enrolled people with fevers. Since the normal state ('mean') of humans is to be a febrile, even a placebo would appear effective. Regression to the mean is a particular concern with measures that are highly variable. Imagine a trial that required one low cd4 count for entry, say below 100. Chances are many eligible participants regularly have cd4 counts greater than 100, yet due to random error and variability were low that day. A measurement of the whole group two weeks later might show raised cd4 count averages, although there was no true gain. Perhaps best phrased as 'everything is better by morning'.

- **regular follow up visit**

required follow up visit, the main purpose of which is to enable clinic personnel to carry out treatment assessment and data collection procedures, as specified in the study protocol. Called regular because such visits are normally required at fixed periods over the course of follow up. Does not include visits done simply for treatment application or treatment adjustment.

- **regulatory genes**
as related to HIV three regulatory HIV genes tat, rev and nef and three so called auxiliary genes vif, vpr and vpu contain information for the production of proteins that control (i.e., regulate) the virus's ability to infect a cell, produce new copies of the virus or cause disease.

- **regulatory protein**
protein that binds to DNA, either blocking or enhancing the function of RNA polymerase.

- **regulatory T cells**
T cells that direct other immune cells to perform special functions. The chief regulatory cell, the cd4+ T cell or T helper cell, is HIV's chief target.

- **regulon**
set of related genes that are transcribed as separate units but are controlled by the same regulatory protein.

- **remission**
reduction of the severity or duration of a condition, or the abatement of symptoms altogether over a period of time.

- **renal**
of, or pertaining to the kidney

- **replica plating**
technique for the simultaneous transfer of organisms in separated colonies from one medium to another medium.

- **replication**
the action or process of reproducing exact copies of one's self.

- **replication fork**
in DNA synthesis, the site at which double helix is being unwound to expose the single strands that can function as templates.

- **replicon**
piece of DNA that is capable of replicating, contains an origin of replication.

- **reporter gene**
gene that has a detectable phenotype and can be fused to a gene of interest, providing a mechanism by which to moni-

tor the expression of the gene of interest.

- **repressible pathway**
  pathway in which the enzymes are not synthesised when the end product of the pathway is present.

- **repression**
  process by which the synthesis of an enzyme is inhibited by the presence of an external substance (the repressor).

- **repressor**
  protein that binds to the operator site and prevents transcription.

- **reservoir**
  source of a disease producing organism.

- **resistance (bacterial, fungal or viral)**
  refers to the ability of some pathogens to grow and multiply even in the presence of certain drugs which normally kill them. (Such strains are referred to as 'drug resistant strains.')

- **resistance factor (r factor)**
  plasmid that carries genetic information for resistance to one or more chemotherapeutic agents.

- **resistance plasmid (r plasmid)**
  plasmid that carries genetic information for resistance to one or more antibiotics and heavy metals.

- **resolve**
  to clearly separate.

- **respiration**
  sum total of metabolic steps in the degradation of foodstuffs when the electron acceptor is an inorganic compound.

- **respiration**
  catabolic reactions producing ATP in which either organic or inorganic compounds are primary electron donors and exogenous compounds are the ultimate electron acceptors.

- **respire**
  to use the processes of respiration.

- **response regulator**
  regulatory protein of a two component regulatory system; receives a phosphoryl group from the membrane spanning sensor.

- **response variable**
  outcome variable.

■ **restriction endonuclease**
enzyme that recognises and cuts DNA at specific purine and pyrimidine sites.

■ **restriction enzyme**
type of enzyme that recognises and cleaves a specific sequence of DNA.

■ **restriction fragment length polymorphism (RFLP)**
pattern of fragment sizes obtained by digesting DNA with one or more restriction enzymes.

■ **reticulate body**
fragile, replicating, non infectious intracellular form of *chlamydia* species.

■ **reticuloendothelial cells**
system of interstitial cells that includes all the phagocytic cells, which trap and consume foreign agents, except the leukocytes circulating in the bloodstream. This system forms a network throughout the body and is another of the body's defence systems against invading organisms in the connective tissues of the body.

■ **retina**
back part of the eye that senses light and forms images.

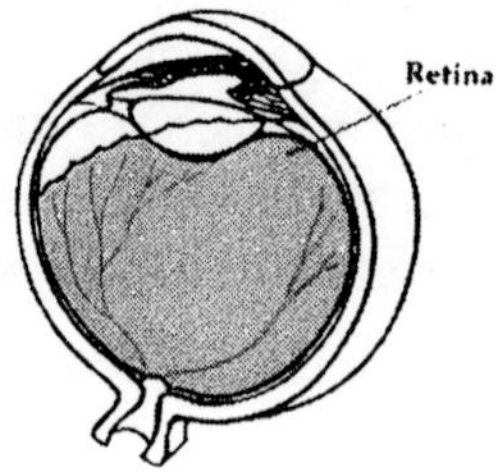

■ **retinitis**
inflammation of the retina, linked in AIDS to CMV infection. Untreated, it can lead to blindness.

■ **retrospective study**
type of study done following a disease outbreak; compares the actions and events surrounding clinical cases with those of controls.

■ **retrovirus**
a class of viruses, which copy genetic material using RNA as a template for making DNA (HIV is a retrovirus).

■ **retroviruses**
group of viruses that carry their genetic information as single stranded RNA. They have the enzyme reverse transcriptase, which forms a copy of DNA that is then integrated into the host

cell chromosome.

■ **rev**
one of the regulatory genes of the HIV virus. Three HIV regulatory genes tat, rev and nef and three so called auxiliary genes vif, vpr and vpu contain information necessary for the production of proteins that control the virus's ability to infect a cell, produce new copies of the virus or cause disease.

■ **reverse transcriptase**
enzyme that synthesises double stranded DNA complementary to an RNA template.

■ **reversion**
process by which a second mutation corrects a defect caused by an earlier mutation.

■ **review group**
group of individuals, normally recruited by the sponsoring agency or its representative, charged with the review of a specific research proposal or set of research proposals for scientific merit. Study section.

■ **reye's syndrome**
often fatal condition characterised by vomiting, coma, brain and liver damage, mostly occurring in children treated with aspirin for influenza or chickenpox.

■ **RFLP**
restriction fragment length polymorphism pattern of fragment sizes obtained by digesting DNA with one or more restriction enzymes.

■ **rheumatoid arthritis**
severe crippling autoimmune disease of the joints, caused by cytokines from inflammatory th1 cells and immune complexes.

■ **rhizobacteria**
bacteria that aggressively colonise roots.

■ **rhizobia**
bacteria capable of living symbiotically in roots of leguminous plants, from which they receive energy and often fix molecular dinitrogen. Collective common name for *rhizobium* and closely related genera.

■ **rhizoid**
rootlike structure that helps to hold an organism to a substrate.

■ **rhizomorph**
mass of fungal hyphae organised

into long, thick strands usually with a darkly pigmented outer rind and containing specialised tissues for absorption and water transport.

- **rhizoplane**
plant root surfaces and usually strongly adhering soil particles.

- **rhizosphere**
zone around plant roots containing organic materials exuded by the roots.

- **rhizosphere**
zone of soil immediately adjacent to plant roots in which the kinds, numbers or activities of micro-organisms differ from that of the bulk soil.

- **rhizosphere competence**
ability of an organism to colonise the rhizosphere.

- **rhodamine**
fluorescent dye that binds to a compound found only in the cells wall of members of the genus *mycobacterium.*

- **rhumab (recombinant human monoclonal antibody)**
hybrid recombinant anti ige molecule being tested in the treatment of asthma.

- **RIA**
abbreviation for radioimmunoassay

- **ribavirin**
antiviral drug, used for treatment of respiratory syncytial virus infection. May have some activity against HIV.

- **ribonucleic acid (RNA)**
macromolecules in a cell that play a role in converting the information coded by the DNA into amino acid sequences in protein.

- **ribose**
5 carbon sugar found in rna.

- **ribosomal rna (RRNA)**
types of RNA found in the ribosome, some participate actively in the process of protein synthesis.

- **ribosome**
spherical structure that assembles proteins after being fed the genetic instructions by MRNA.

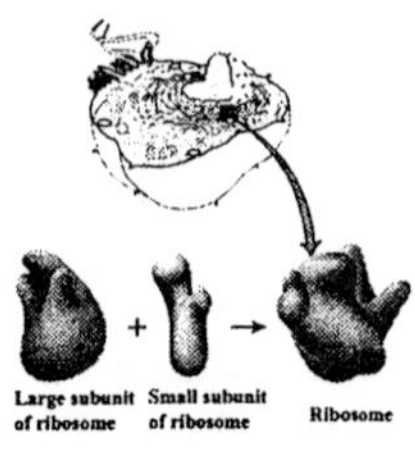

■ **ribosome binding site**
sequence of nucleotides on MRNA to which a ribosome binds. The first time the codon for methionine (aug) appears after that site, translation generally starts.

■ **ribotyping**
technique used to distinguish among related strains, detects rflps in ribosomal RNA genes.

■ **ribozymes**
RNA molecules that have a catalytic function.

■ **rifabutin (mycobutin)**
antibiotic used as a component in the combination treatment of *mycobacterium avium* complex. Rifabutin is also the only drug currently approved for the prevention of mac.

■ **rifadin**
brand name of rifampin.

■ **rifamate**
combination of rifampin and isoniazid in one pill.

■ **rifampin (rifadin, rimactane)**
antibiotic used alone, or as a component in the combination treatment of tuberculosis.

■ **rifamyc[illegible]s**
group of antimicrobial medications that block transcription.

■ **rimactane**
brand name of rifampin

■ **risk factor**
anything in the environment, personal characteristics, or events that make it more or less likely one might develop a given disease or experience a change in health status.

■ **risk factor analysis**
any analysis, usually involving regression or subgroup analyses, that is aimed at identifying risk factors for a given disease or condition.

■ **risk factors**
specific conditions associated with high frequencies of disease.

■ **RNA**
abbreviation for ribonucleic acid.

■ **RNA polymerase**
enzyme that catalyses the synthesis of RNA using a DNA template.

■ **rod**
cylindrical shaped bacterium, also called a bacillus.

■ **rolling circle replication**
mechanism of DNA replication

in which a single strand of DNA is synthesised.

- **root nodule**
specialised structure occurring on roots, especially of leguminous plants, in which bacteria fix dinitrogen and make it available for the plant.

- **rough endoplasmic reticulum**
organelle where proteins that are not located in the cytoplasm are synthesised

- **round worm (or nematode)**
helminth that is often parasitic and causes disease.

- **R RNA**
ribosomal RNA

- **R strategy**
ecological strategy where organisms rely on high reproductive rates for continued survival within the community. Populations of r strategists are subject to extreme fluctuations.

- **RTF**
abbreviation for resistance transfer factor.

- **Rubisco**
enzyme that initiates the calvin cycle by joining CO_2 to the 5 carbon compound ribulose 1, 5 bisphosphate.

- **Rx**
common abbreviation for 'prescription'.

- **saline**
salt water.

- **saline soil**
soil containing sufficient soluble salt to adversely affect the growth of most crop plants.

- **salinity**
amount of salt in a solution.

- **salmonella**
ubiquitous family of bacteria, salmonella can cause serious disseminated disease in HIV positive patients.

- **salt**
skin associated lymphoid tissues.

- **salvage therapy**
treatment used when the usual treatment(s) have failed. A last ditch option.

- **sample size**
number of patients required for a trial. In planning an interventional trial, a sample size is calculated , taking into account the frequency of the condition to be prevented or delayed, the anticipated effec-

tiveness of the treatment thought to be clinically significant, and variables such as predicted drop outs and crossover. The sample size is a calculated value that takes all of the above into account, and makes a statistically significant result likely within the prescribed amount of time.

- **sand**
  soil particle between 0.05 and 2.0 mm in diameter.

- **sanitisation**
  elimination of pathogenic or deleterious organisms, insect larvae, intestinal parasites and weed seeds.

- **sanitise**
  process of substantially reducing the microbial populations on objects to acceptably safe public health levels.

- **saprophyte**
  nonparasitic nutritional mechanism by which an organism obtains its food exclusively from the degradation of nonliving organic material.

- **saquinavir (invirase)**
  protease inhibitor drug made by Hoffman laroche.

- **sarcoma**
  malignant tumour of the skin or soft tissues.

- **sargramostim (granulocyte macrophage colony stimulating factor, GM CSF)**
  recombinant version of an endogenous cytokine that stimulates the production of white blood cells. Can be used for treatment of neutropenia attendant upon chemotherapy, or treatment with AZT, but filgrastim is usually used instead, because of concerns that sargramostim may increase HIV replication.

- **SAS**
  statistical analysis system (a package of data analysis programs).

- **saturated**
  refers to a fatty acid that contains no double bonds

- **scanning electron microscope (SEM)**
  type of electron microscope that scans a beam of electrons scans back and forth over the surface of a specimen, used for observing surface details, but not internal structures of cells.

- **scanning probe microscopes**
microscope that make it possible to view images at an atomic scale, produces a map showing the bumps and valleys of atoms on a surface.

- **scanning tunnelling microscope**
type of scanning probe microscope with a sharp metallic probe that causes electrons to tunnel between the probe and a conductive surface.

- **schizogony**
process of multiple fission in which the nucleus divides a number of times before individual daughter cells are produced.

- **schizont**
multinucleate stage in the development of certain protozoa, such as the ones that cause malaria.

- **sclerotium**
modified fungal hyphae that form a compact, hard vegetative resting structure with a thick pigmented outer rind.

- **scolex**
attachment organ of a tapeworm, the head end.

- **scrapie**
common name for a neurological disease of sheep thought to be caused by a prion.

- **seborrheic dermatitis**
chronic inflammatory disease of the skin of unknown etiology (i.e., cause or origin), characterised by moderate erythema, dry, moist or greasy scaling, and yellow crusted patches on various areas,

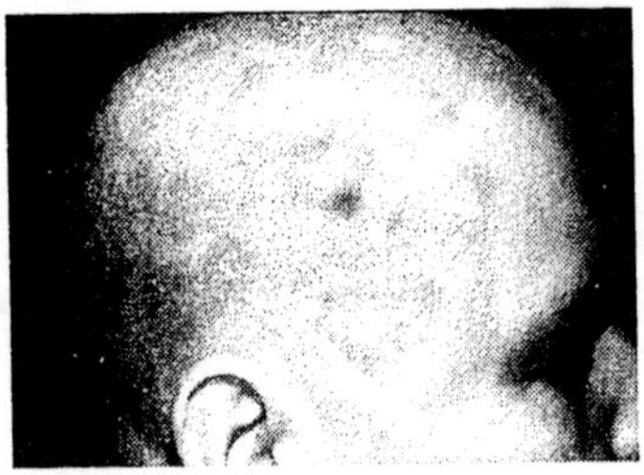

including the mid parts of the face, ears, supraorbital regions (above the orbit of the eye), umbilicus (the navel), genitalia, and especially the scalp

- **sebum**
oily secretion of the sebaceous glands of the skin.

- **secondary (memory) response**
enhanced immune response that occurs upon second or subsequent exposure to specific antigen, caused by the rapid activation of long lived memory cells.

- **secondary infection**
infection that occurs along with

or immediately following another infection, usually as a result of the first infection

- **secondary lymphoid organs**
  peripheral lymphoid organs throughout the body where mature lymphocytes function in immune responses, including the adenoids, tonsils, spleen, appendix, and lymph nodes, among others.

- **secondary metabolite**
  product of intermediary metabolism released from a cell, such as an antibiotic.

- **secondary metabolites**
  metabolic products synthesised during late log and stationary phase.

- **secondary outcome variable or secondary endpoint**
  outcome variable that is known or believed to be related to the primary outcome variable and that is used, in addition to the primary outcome variable, for evaluation of treatments in the trial (e.g. the use of CD4 as a secondary endpoint in a antiretroviral trial with mortality as it's primary endpoint, where CD4 trends are presumed to be associated with survival)

- **secondary structure**
  refers to the arrangement of amino acids in a protein. The two major arrangements are helices and sheets.

- **secretion system**
  mechanism by which bacterial pathogens transfer gene products into host cells to cause endocytosis or other effects.

- **segmented virus**
  virus more than one RNA molecule enclosed in the capsid.

- **selectable marker**
  gene that encodes a selectable phenotype such as antibiotic resistance.

- **selective enrichment**
  method of increasing the relative proportion of one particular organism in a mixed population by providing conditions in a broth that enhance the growth of the desired organism and including a selective agent that inhibits the growth of other organisms.

- **selective medium**
  medium that allows the growth of certain types of micro-organisms in preference to others. For example, an antibiotic containing medium

allows the growth of only those micro-organisms resistant to the antibiotic.

■ **selective toxicity**
causing greater harm to a pathogen than to the host.

■ **selectively permeable membrane**
membrane that allows some but not other molecules to pass through freely.

■ **self assembly**
spontaneous formation of a complex structure from its component molecules without the aid of enzymes.

■ **self transmissible plasmid**
plasmid that codes for all of the information necessary for its own transfer.

■ **semiconservative replication**
type of nucleic acid replication that results in each of the two double stranded molecules containing one of the original strands (the template strand) and one newly synthesised strand.

■ **semi critical items**
medical instruments such as endoscopes that come into contact with mucous membranes, but do not penetrate body tissue.

■ **semipermeable**
material that allows the passage of some but not other molecules.

■ **sense strand of the two RN**
molecules that can theoretically be transcribed from double stranded DNA, the one that can be translated to make a protein, also called the plus (+) strand.

■ **sensitisation**
prior immunisation. Allergic reactions to an antigen occur only in sensitised individuals who have been exposed to that particular antigen.

■ **sepsis**
bloodstream infection.

■ **septic tank method**
method of treating sewage in which wastes are collected in a large tank and degraded by anaerobic organisms, with the resulting fluid stabilised in a drainage field by aerobic organisms.

■ **septicemia**
disease due to sepsis

■ **septra**
brand name of trimethoprim sulphamethoxazole

■ **septum (pl. septa)**
crosswall (partition) dividing a parent cell into two daughter cells during binary fission or occurring between adjacent cells in hyphae.

■ **serial dilutions**
series of dilutions, usually two-fold or tenfold, used to determine the concentration of a substance in solution.

■ **seroconversion**
change from negative serum without specific antibodies to serum positive for specific antibodies.

■ **serogroup**
micro-organisms within a species that are the same antigenically as determined by specific antisera.

■ **serologic test**
any of a number of tests that are performed on the clear, liquid portion of blood (serum). Often refers to a test which determines the presence of antibodies to antigens such as viruses.

■ **serology**
study of antigen antibody reactions *in vitro*.

■ **seroprevalence**
as related to HIV infection the proportion of persons who have serologic (i.e., pertaining to serum) evidence of HIV infection at any given time.

■ **serostatus**
refers to the presence or absence of antibodies in the serum portion of blood.

■ **serotonin**
basic amine, stored in mast cell granules, that upon release can cause contraction of some smooth muscles and increased vascular permeability, a mediator of inflammation.

■ **serotype**
strain that has a characteristic antigenic structure that differs from other strains, also called a serovar.

■ **serum**
clear, non cellular, fluid portion of the blood.

■ **sex pilus**
thin protein appendage required for attachment of one bacterium to another prior to DNA transfer by conjugation.

■ **sexually transmitted disease (STD)**
also called venereal disease. A contagious disease usually acquired by sexual intercourse or

genital contact. Historically, the five venereal diseases were gonorrhea, syphilis, chancroid, granuloma inguinale and lymphogranuloma venereum. To these have been added scabies, herpes genitalis and anorectal herpes and warts, pediculosis, trichomoniasis, genital candidiasis, molluscum contagiosum, nonspecific urethritis, chlamydial infections, cytomegalovirus and aids.

■ **SF2**
a strain of HIV used in vaccine development.

■ **shake tube**
tube of agar medium that has been uniformly inoculated with a bacterial culture in order to determine the oxygen requirement of that organism.

■ **sham**
something false presented to be genuine, a spurious imitation. Derived from the word shame, meaning trick or fraud.

■ **sham procedure**
a procedure designed to resemble the real one and that is performed on a patient for the purpose of masking the patient or the patient's study physician as to whether the patient has received the real procedure. A placebo procedure.

■ **sheath**
tubular structure formed around a chain of cells or around a bundle of filaments.

■ **SHIV**
genetically engineered hybrid virus having an HIV envelope and an SIV core

■ **shock**
condition with multiple causes characterised by low blood pressure and circulation of the blood inadequate to sustain normal function of vital organs. Septic shock results from growth of microorganisms in the body. Toxic shock results from a circulating exotoxin.

■ **side effects**
the action or effect of a drug beyond what it is supposed to do. The term usually refers to undesired or negative effects, such as headache, skin irritation, or liver damage(although side effects can be expected or unexpected, desired or undesired. Experimental drugs must be evaluated for both immediate and long term side effects.

■ **siderophore**
nonporphyrin metabolite secreted by certain micro-organisms that forms a highly stable coordination compound (chelate) with iron, a high affinity iron binding compound. There are two major types catecholates and hydroxamates.

■ **sigma (s) factor component of RN**
polymerase that is recognises the promoter.

■ **signal sequence**
characteristic series of hydrophobic amino acids at the amino terminal end of proteins that are destined for secretion; functions as a tag, directing transport of the protein through the membrane.

■ **signal transduction**
process that transmits information from outside of a cell to the inside, allowing that cell to respond to changing environmental conditions.

■ **signature sequences**
characteristic sequences in the genes that encode ribosomal RNA that can be used to classify or identify certain organisms.

■ **significance level (statistics)**
the permissible type I error level for a test of the null hypothesis with a specified test statistic. The null hypothesis not rejected if the test statistic yields a p value which is larger than the specified level and is rejected if it is equal to or less than this value.

■ **significance test**
test of significance.

■ **significance testing (statistics)**
the act of carrying out a test of significance.

■ **significance (clinical)**
statistical significance does not necessarily imply that the results have practical implications or are clinically significant from the clinician's point of view, and vice versa.

■ **significance (statistical)**
infers that an observation was unlikely to have occurred by chance alone. Statistical significance is often based on a p value <0.05. Below this level, the smaller the p value, the greater the statistical significance.

■ **signs**
effects of a disease observed by examining the patient.

■ **silt**
soil particle with a diameter between 0.002 and0.05 mm.

■ **simian immunodeficiency virus (SIV)**
retrovirus closely related to HIV, which causes disease in monkeys

■ **similarity coefficient**
numerical value that can be used to classify prokaryotes based on their phenotypic characteristics.

■ **simple diffusion**
movement of molecules or ions from a region of high concentration to a region of low concentration, does not involve transport proteins.

■ **simple randomisation**
unrestricted randomisation.

■ **simple staining**
staining technique that employs a basic dye to impart colour to cells.

■ **single blind**
where certain persons (e.g., study physicians) are informed of some fact or condition whereas other persons (e.g., patients) are purposefully denied information regarding that fact or condition. Used to minimize the placebo effect or different reporting of symptoms based on patient attitude toward the treatment they believe they are taking.

■ **single blinded clinical trial**
clinical trial in which treatments are administered in such a manner that patients in the trial are not informed of whether they have been assigned to the test or control treatment, but clinic staff are.

■ **single cell protein (SCP)**
use of micro-organisms such as yeast and bacteria as a protein source.

■ **sinusitis**
infection of the sinus cavities in the head, often bacterial.

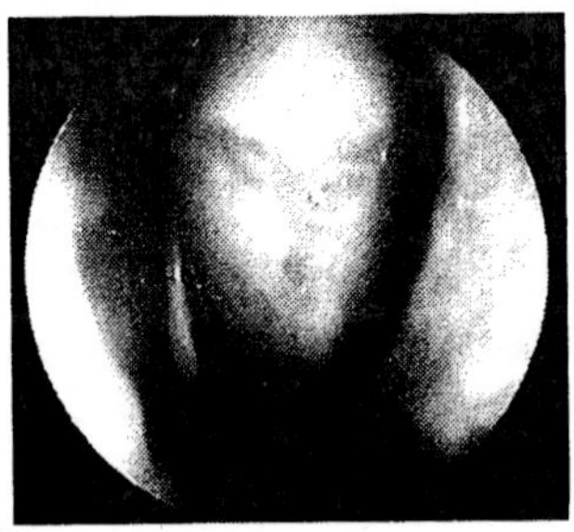

■ **site**
in ecology, area described or defined by its biotic, climatic, and soil conditions as related to its capacity to produce vegetation.

- **site specific recombination**
  mechanism by which a piece of DNA becomes part of a larger piece of DNA, involves identical sequences on each piece of DNA.

- **site visit**
  visit to a centre or prospective centre in a trial by personnel from outside that centre for the purpose of assessing its performance or performance potential in the trial.

- **site directed mutagenesis**
  insertion of a different nucleotide at a specific site in a molecule using recombinant DNA methodology.

- **skin associated lymphoid tissue (SALT)**
  secondary lymphoid tissue consisting of collections of lymphoid cells under the skin.

- **slime layer**
  type of glycocalyx that is diffuse and irregular.

- **slime mould**
  terrestrial organism that is similar to the fungi but not related genetically.

- **smear**
  in a staining procedure, the film obtained by placing a drop of a liquid containing a microbe on a glass microscope slide and allowing it to air dry.

- **smooth endoplasmic reticulum**
  organelle of eukaryotic cells that is the site of lipid synthesis and degradation and calcium ion storage.

- **soft endpoint**
  soft outcome.

- **soft outcome**
  any outcome measure that is subject to major errors of interpretation or measurement. Usually, a measurement or assessment that depends on clinical judgment, or is founded in symptom.

- **soil**
  unconsolidated mineral or material on the immediate surface of the earth that serves as a natural medium for the growth of land plants.

- **soil aggregate**
  unit of soil structure generally < 10 mm in diameter and formed by natural forces and substances derived from root exudates and microbial products which cement smaller particles into larger units.

■ **soil atmosphere**
gases occupying the pore space in soil. Generally characterised as having a greater percentage of carbon dioxide and a lesser percentage of oxygen than the overlying air.

■ **soil biochemistry**
branch of soil science concerned with enzymes and the reactions, activities, and products of soil micro-organisms.

■ **soil extract**
solution separated from a soil suspension or from a soil by filtration, centrifugation, suction or pressure.

■ **soil horizon**
layer of soil or soil material approximately parallel to the land surface and differing from adjacent genetically related layers in physical, chemical, and biological properties or characteristics such as colour, structure, texture, consistency, kinds and number of organisms present, and degree of acidity or alkalinity.

■ **soil microbiology**
branch of soil science concerned with soil inhabiting micro-organisms and their functions and activities.

■ **soil organic matter (SOM)**
organic fraction of the soil exclusive of un-decayed plant and animal residues. Often synonymous with humus.

■ **soil population**
all the organisms living in the soil, including plants and animals

■ **soil pore**
that part of the bulk volume of soil not occupied by soil particles. Soil pores have also been referred to as interstices or voids.

■ **soil quality**
continued capacity of soil to function as a vital living system to sustain biological productivity, maintain the quality of the environment, and promote plant, animal, and human health.

■ **soil salinity**
amount of soluble salts in a soil. The conventional measure of soil salinity is the electrical conductivity of a saturation extract.

■ **soil science**
science dealing with soils as a natural resource on the surface of the earth including soil for-

mation, classification and mapping, and physical, chemical, biological, and fertility properties of soils per se and these properties in relation to their use and management.

- **soil series**
  conceptualised class of soil bodies (polypedons) that have limits and ranges more restrictive than all higher taxa. The soil series serve as a major vehicle to transfer soil information and research knowledge from one soil area to another.

- **soil solution**
  aqueous liquid phase of the soil and its solutes.

- **soil structure**
  combination or arrangement of primary soil particles into secondary particles, units, or peds. The secondary units are characterised and classified on the basis of size, shape, and degree of distinctness into classes, types, and grades, respectively.

- **soil texture**
  relative proportions of the various soil separates in a soil. The major textural classes are sand, silt, and clay.

- **soil water potential (total)**
  amount of work that must be done per unit quantity of pure water in order to transport reversibly and isothermically an infinitesimal quantity of water from a pool of pure water, at a specified elevation and at atmospheric pressure, to the soil water (at the point under consideration). Informally, the amount of energy that must be expended to extract water from soil. The total potential (of soil water) consists of the following gravitational potential, matric potential, and osmotic potential.

- **solarisation**
  method to control pathogens and weeds where moistened soil in hot climates is covered with transparent polyethylene plastic sheets, thereby trapping incoming radiation.

- **solute**
  dissolved molecules.

- **Sos repair**
  complex, inducible repair process used to repair highly damaged DNA.

■ **southern blot**
hybridisation of single stranded nucleic acid (DNA or RNA) to DNA fragments immobilised on a filter.

■ **sparfloxacin**
an-experimental flouroquinolone antibiotic active against *mycobacterium avium* complex.

■ **spatial variability**
variation in soil properties, laterally across the landscape, at a given depth, or with a given horizon.

■ **specialised transduction**
transfer of only specific bacterial genes by phage from one bacterium to another.

■ **species**
in microbiology, a collection of closely related strains sufficiently different from all other strains to be recognised as a distinct unit.

■ **specific activity**
amount of enzyme activity units per mass of protein. Often expressed as micromoles of product formed per unit time per milligram of protein. Also used in radiochemistry to express the radioactivity per mass of material (radioactive and non-radioactive).

■ **specific epithet**
designation of a particular organism in the binomial nomenclature system. For example, *coli* is the specific epithet of *escherichia coli*.

■ **specific immunity**
immune response that depends on the recognition and elimination of foreign antigens by specialised lymphocytes.

■ **spermosphere**
area of increased microbial activity around a germinating seed.

■ **spheroplast**
gram negative cell from which the cell wall has been removed, retains some portions of the outer membrane.

■ **spikes or attachment proteins**
structures on the outside of the virion that bind to host cell receptors.

■ **spirillum (plural spirilla)**
curved rod long enough to form spirals.

■ **spirochete**
type of long helical cell with a flexible cell wall that is characterised by an axial filament.

■ **spleen**
lymphoid organ in the abdominal cavity that is an important centre for immune system activities.

■ **splenomegaly**
enlarged spleen.

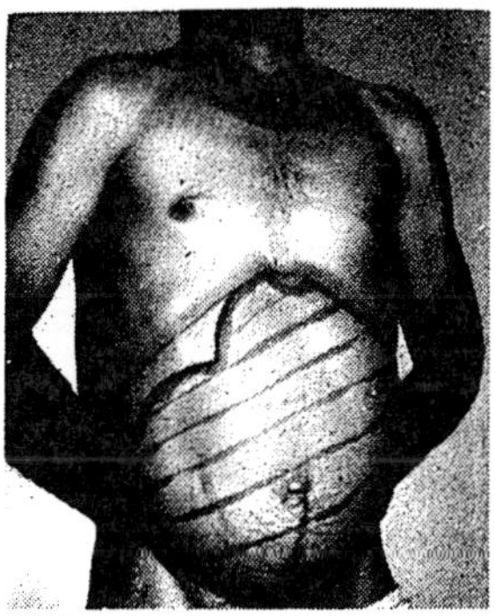

■ **splicing**
process that removes introns from eukaryotic precursor RNA to generate m-RNA.

■ **spoilage**
biochemical changes in foods that are perceived as undesirable.

■ **spontaneous generation**
discredited theory that organisms can arise from nonliving matter.

■ **spontaneous mutation**
mutation that occurs naturally without the addition of mutagenic agents.

■ **sporadic**
occurring in a population widely spaced in time and place.

■ **sporangiospore**
spore formed within a sporangium by fungi in the phylum zygomycota.

■ **sporangium**
fungal structure which converts its cytoplasm into a variable number of sporangiospores, formed by fungi in the phylum zygomycota.

■ **spores**
specialised reproductive cell. Asexual spores germinate without uniting with other cells, whereas sexual spores of opposite mating types unite to form a zygote before germination occurs.

■ **sporogenesis**
in bacteria, a complex, highly ordered sequence of morphological changes during which a

bacterial vegetative cell produces a specialized cell greatly resistant to environmental adversity. Eukaryotes can also experience sporogenesis.

■ **sporozoite**
elongated infectious form of certain protozoa, for example, in malaria, the form entering the body from a mosquito bite, infectious for liver cells.

■ **spread plate**
technique used to cultivate bacteria by uniformly spreading a suspension of cells onto the surface of an agar plate.

■ **sputum**
material coughed from the lungs.

■ **stabilisation**
conversion of organic to inorganic matter.

■ **standard deviation**
a statistic that shows the spread or dispersion of scores in a distribution of scores. In other words, a measure of dispersion. The more widely the scores are spread out, the greater the standard deviation. The standard deviation is the square root of the variance. For example imagine trued groups of patients. In one cd4 cell counts range from 310 650, in the other they range from 43 700. The standard deviation would be much greater for the second group.

■ **standard error**
short for 'standard error of the mean', or 'standard error of the estimate'. A statistic indicating how greatly the mean score of a single sample is likely to differ from the mean score of the population. It is the standard deviation of a sampling distribution of the means. The standard error of the mean indicates how much the sample mean differs from the expected value. The standard error of estimate is how much you are off when using a regression line to predict particular scores. In either case, the smaller the standard error, the better the sample statistic is an estimate of the population parameter. The standard error is a measure of sampling error, due to random fluctuations in the samples.

■ **standard treatment**
accepted mode of treatment for a given disease or condition.

Equivalent to the control treatment in clinical trials when chosen to mimic standard medical practice.

- **standards of care**

treatment regimen or medical management based on state of the art patient care.

- **start codon**

codon at which translation is initiated, in prokaryotes, typically the first aug after a ribosome binding site.

- **starter cultures**

strains of micro-organisms added to a food to initiate the fermentation process.

- **stationary phase**

period during the growth cycle of a population in which growth rate equals the death rate.

- **statistical significance**

term based on statistical tests that is used to denote the probability that the observed association could have occurred by chance alone. Does not refer to medical or biological significance of an association. For example, a statistical significance at the 1 percent level indicates a 1 in 100 chance that a result can be ascribed to chance.

- **statistical test, analysis of variance (ANOVA)**

statistical technique used to test the difference among the means of two groups or more regarding continuous data. The purpose of ANOVA is to test whether the observed differences among the means of these groups is significant or due to chance.

- **statistical test (chi square)**

statistical technique used to test the difference between groups regarding discrete (categorical) data. The purpose of chi square is to test whether differences between observed and expected frequencies are significant or due to chance.

- **statistical test (multiple regression)**

statistical technique used to assess the relationship between one dependent variable and two or more input variables. The purpose of multiple regression analysis is to measure the degree of association between variables or predict the dependent variable as a function of the input variables.

■ **statistical test (T test)**
statistical technique used to test whether the means of two groups differ significantly regarding continuous data. The purpose of the t test is to infer whether the difference between the means of two groups on one variable is statistically significant or due to chance.

■ **statistics (descriptive)**
intent of descriptive statistics is to summarise and present data, e.g., measures of central tendency (mean, mode, median) and measures of variability (standard deviation, variance, standard error of the mean).

■ **statistics (inferential)**
inference refers to making generalisations about a population on the basis of a sample from that population. The intent of inferential statistics is to determine whether differences between groups are real or due to chance.

■ **stavudine**
nucleoside antiretroviral drug recently approved for treatment of advanced HIV disease.

■ **steering committee (SC)**
committee responsible for directing the activities of a designated project

■ **stem cells**
cells from which all blood cells derive. Bone marrow is rich in stem cells.

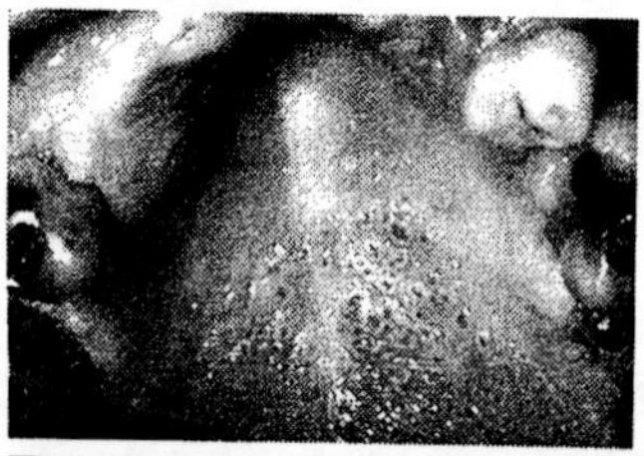

■ **stereoisomer (or optical isomer)**
mirror image of a compound.

■ **sterile**
completely free of all micro-organisms and viruses, an absolute term.

■ **sterilisation**
rendering an object or substance free of viable microbes.

■ **sterilising immunity**
immune response that completely eliminates an infection.

■ **steroids**
a large family of structurally similar chemicals. Various steroids have sex determining, anti inflammatory, and growth regulatory roles.

■ **sterol**
type of lipid that has a characteristic structure. Cholesterol is a common sterol.

■ **Steven Johnson Reaction**
severe allergic drug reaction. Steven Johnson is characterised by high fevers and desquamating rash, and is frequently fatal.

■ **Stevens Johnson Syndrome**
a severe and sometimes fatal form of erythema multiforme that is characterised by conjunctivitis (eye inflammation) and often results in blindness, Vincent's angina (trench mouth) and ulceration of the genitals and anus.

■ **sticky ends**
single stranded overhangs generated when DNA is digested with a restriction enzyme that cuts asymmetrically within the recognition sequence. Also called cohesive ends.

■ **stock culture**
culture stored for use as an inoculum in later procedures.

■ **stomatitis**
inflammation of the upper gastric tract, including the mouth.

■ **stop codon**
codon that does not code for an amino acid and is not recognised by a TRNA; signals the end of the protein.

■ **stop condition**
condition encountered when carrying out a procedure (e.g., completing a data form, performing a patient examination) that requires the person performing the procedure to terminate the procedure until or unless the condition can be removed

■ **stopping rule**
rule, usually set before or shortly after the start of patient recruitment, that specifies a limit for the observed test control treatment difference for the primary outcome, which, if exceeded, automatically leads to termination of the test or control treatment, depending on the direction of the observed difference.

■ **storage polysaccharide**
energy reserve deposited in the cell when there is an excess of carbon available. These are usually deposited as large granules in the cell. The most common example of a storage polysaccharide in plants is starch. Its counterpart in animal cells is glycogen.

■ **strain**
specific type, quality or disposition of a material.

■ **strata (pl. of stratum)**
a series of distinct levels or layers. In this book, generally subgroups of patients formed by classification on some variable or set of variables, usually baseline variables.

■ **stratification**
process of classifying observation units into strata.

■ **stratification variable**
variable used to classify the experimental or observational units into strata.

■ **stratified allocation**
method of treatment assignment in which patients are first classified into defined subgroups based on one or more baseline variables and then assigned to treatment within the defined subgroups.

■ **stratified randomisation**
treatment assignment process using stratified random allocation. Attempts to ensure balance by the stratification variable.

■ **stratum (sing. of strata)**
a layer, level, or defined subgroup.

■ **streak plate**
simplest and most commonly used technique for isolating bacteria. A series of successive streak patterns is used to sequentially dilute an inoculum on the surface of an agar plate.

■ **streptococcal pyrogenic exotoxins (SPES)**
family of genetically related poisonous proteins produced by certain strains of *Streptococcus pyogenes*, responsible for scarlet fever, toxic shock and 'flesh eating' necrotising fasciitis.

■ **stromatolite**
coral like mat of filamentous micro-organisms.

■ **structural isomers**
molecules that contain the same elements but in different arrangements and not mirror images. Structural isomers have different names.

■ **structural polysaccharide**
polysaccharide that serves primarily as a structural element in cell walls and coats and intercellular spaces, and connective tissue where they give shape, elasticity, or rigidity to plant or ani-

mal tissues and protection and support to unicellular organisms. Cellulose is the predominant structural polysaccharide in plant cell walls and chitin is abundant in fungal cell walls and insect exoskeletons.

■ **study**
general term used to refer to any one of a variety of research activities involving the collection, analysis, or interpretation of data.

■ **study manual of operations**
document or collection of documents that describes the procedures used in a centre or set of centres in a clinical trial (e.g., manual of operations for study clinics, coordinating centre manual of operations, protocol centre manual of operations).

■ **study participant**
term sometimes used in place of study patient when there is a desire to avoid the connotation of illness, as in trials involving well people.

■ **study patient**
term used to characterise an individual considered for enrolment or actually enrolled into a trial regardless of whether or not there is a perceived need for medical care.

■ **study physician**
physician associated with a study clinic who is responsible for administering the study treatments to patients in the trial or who is responsible for patient care, as dictated by the study protocol.

■ **study population**
set of patients enrolled in a trial.

■ **study protocol**
narrative document that describes the general design and operating features of a trial. Distinguished from the study manual of operations by its generality and absence of specific details needed for day to day execution of the trial.

■ **study section**
any review group, especially one that is chartered to carry out reviews of research applications in a general area of research and that meets at regular intervals during the calendar year to perform those reviews

- **subarachnoid space**
  space through which the spinal fluid circulates.

- **subclinical infection**
  an infection, or phase of infection, without readily apparent symptoms or signs of disease.

- **subcutaneous**
  beneath or introduced beneath the skin (e.g., subcutaneous injections).

- **subgroup**
  subpart of the study population distinguished by a particular characteristic or set of characteristics (e.g., males under age 45 at entry).

- **subgroup analysis**
  any data analysis that focuses on a selected subgroup or patients. Generally , any analysis that is aimed at elucidating treatment differences within a defined subgroup of patients.

- **subgrouping variable**
  a variable, such as age, used to classify patients (treatment units) into subgroups. Usually a baseline characteristic for most subgroup analyses in clinical trials.

- **substrate**
  substance on which an enzyme acts to form

- **substrate level phosphorylation**
  transfer of the high energy phosphate from a phosphorylated compound to ADP to form ATP.

- **subtype**
  genetic variant.

- **subunit HIV vaccine**
  genetically engineered vaccine that is based on only part of the HIV molecule.

- **subunit vaccines**
  vaccines made of products or portions of an agent, bacteria or viruses.

- **succession**
  gradual process brought about by the change in the number of individuals of each species of a community and by the establishment of new species that gradually replace the original inhabitants.

- **sucrose**
  disaccharide consisting of a molecule of glucose bonded to fructose, common table sugar

- **sugar phosphate backbone**
  series of alternating sugar and phosphates moieties of a DNA molecule.

■ **sulpha drug**
any of a class of synthetic chemical substances derived from sulphanilamide and used to treat bacterial infections. These drugs inhibit the action of para aminobenzoic acid, a substance bacteria needed in order to reproduce. Sulpha drugs are used primarily in the treatment of urinary tract infections and ulcerative colitis. Antibiotics have largely replaced them in the treatment of other bacterial infections.

■ **sulphadiazine**
sulpha antibiotic, sometimes used in the treatment of toxoplasmosis, especially in combination with pyrimethamine

■ **sulphadoxine**
sulpha antibiotic, only occasionally used in aids

■ **sulphanilamide**
antimicrobial drug that inhibits folic acid synthesis; one of the sulpha drugs.

■ **sulfate reducers**
group of obligate anaerobes that use sulfate (so_4^{2}) as a terminal electron acceptor, producing hydrogen sulfide as an end product.

■ **sulphur cycle**
sequence of transformations undergone by sulphur where it is taken up by living organisms, transformed upon death and decomposition of the organism, and converted ultimately to its original state of oxidation.

■ **sulphamethoxazole**
sulfa antibiotic, and half of the combination 'trimethoprim sulphamethoxazole', it is rarely used alone.

■ **sunit (for svedberg)**
unit of measurement that expresses the sedimentation rate of a compound; reflects the mass and density of the compound.

■ **superantigen**
investigators have proposed that a molecule known as a superantigen, either made by HIV or an unrelated agent, may stimulate massive quantities of cd4+ T cells at once, rendering them highly susceptible to HIV infection and subsequent cell death.

■ **superantigens**
molecules that stimulate T lymphocytes by binding to MHC

class II molecules and to part of the T cell receptor distinct from the antigen binding site, resulting in activation of many t cells, overproduction of cytokines, severe reactions, and sometimes fatal shock.

- **superficial mycoses**
fungal infections that affect the hair, skin or nails.

- **superoxide**
(O_2^-) toxic derivative of O_2.

- **superoxide dismutase**
enzyme that degrades superoxide to produce hydrogen peroxide.

- **suppressor t cells (t_8, Cd_8)**
subset of t cells that halt antibody production and other immune responses.

- **surface area**
area of the solid particles in a given quantity of soil or porous medium.

- **surface soil**
uppermost part of the soil, ordinarily moved in tillage, or its equivalent in uncultivated soils ranging in depth from 7 to 20 cm. Frequently designated as the surface layer, the ap layer, or the ap horizon.

- **surrogate marker**
a substitute, a person or thing that replaces another. In HIV disease, the number of cd4+ t cells and cd8+ cells is a surrogate immunological marker of disease progression.

- **surrogate outcome variable**
also called surrogate marker a test, measurement, score, or some other similar variable that is used in place of a clinical event (e.g., use of blood pressure change in place of clinical hypertension) in the design of a trial, or in summarising results from it. Used because the variable is believed to be correlated with the clinical event of interest and because of its perceived utility in yielding detectable treatment differences. CD4 was once believed to be a surrogate marker for death from AIDS.

- **surveillance**
close or continuous observation or testing (e.g., serosurveill-ance), used, among others, in epidemiology. Immunological surveillance, or immunosurvei-llance, is a monitoring process of the immune system that detects and destroys neoplastic (e.g., cancerous) cells and that tends to break

down in immunosuppressed individuals.

■ **survival analysis**
any method of data analysis that focuses on the length of survival.

■ **susceptible**
vulnerable or predisposed to a disease.

■ **swarmer cells**
motile cells of sheathed bacteria that disperse to new locations.

■ **sx**
common abbreviation for 'symptoms'.

■ **symbiosis**
living together in intimate association of two dissimilar organisms. The interactions between the organisms can be commensal or mutualistic.

■ **symmetric**
equally divided, and identical on both sides of a middle line; mirror image

■ **symporters**
transport systems in which the passage of one type of molecule or ion facilitates the transport of another.

■ **symptomatic**
showing clinical pathology or changes indicative of disease, such as HIV disease. Often symptomatic HIV disease means clinical evidence of HIV infection in absence of an aids diagnosis, indicative of, relating to or constituting the aggregate of symptoms of a disease.

■ **symptoms**
effects of a disease experienced by the patient.

■ **syncytia**
mass of cells which fuse together to form one 'giant cell.' in HIV infection this condition leads to direct cell to cell infection and continued HIV replication.

■ **syncytium (pl. syncytia)**
multinucleate body formed by the fusion of cells.

■ **syndrome**
group of symptoms and diseases that together are characteristic of a specific condition.

■ **synergism**
association between organisms that is mutually beneficial. Both populations are capable of surviving in their natural environment on their own although, when formed,

the association offers mutual advantages.

■ **synergistic**
acting together of agents to produce an effect greater than the sum of the effects of each agent

■ **synthesis**
in chemistry, the formation of a compound from simpler compounds or elements.

■ **synthetic medium**
medium in which the chemical composition and quantity of every component is known

■ **syntrophy**
interaction of two or more populations that supply each other's nutritional needs.

■ **syphilis**
disease (usually sexually transmitted) resulting from infection with the spirochete (a bacterium) treponema pallidum.

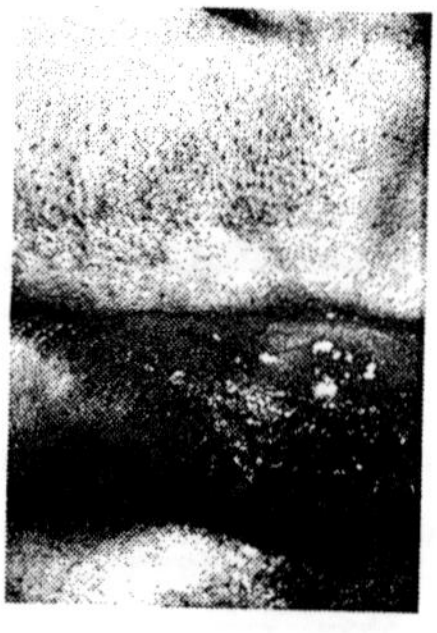

■ **systemic**
throughout the body. Sometimes applies to medications that are taken orally or parenterally that saturate the entire body.

■ **systemic infection**
infection in which the infectious agent spreads throughout the body

■ **systemic mycoses**
fungal infections that affect the tissues deep in the body.

■ **T cells**
lymphocytes that mature in the thymus; they originate from stem cells in bone marrow, differentiate in the thymus, and move through the blood stream to secondary lymphoid organs where they are responsible for cellular immune responses and function as helper cells in the antibody response.

■ **T cytotoxic cells**
CD8+ lymphocytes that recognise antigen on the surface of target cells and kill the target cells.

■ **t helper (th) cells**
CD4+ T lymphocytes that produce cytokines, influencing and helping the specific immune re-

sponse; two subgroups are Th1 and Th2.

- **T killer cells**

major component of cytotoxic lymphocyte response (ctl), responsible for lysing infected or cancerous cells. t killer cells (not to be confused by natural killer cells) are a subset of cd8+ lymphocytes.

- **T lymphocyte cells**

thymus dependent cells, coordinate the cell mediated immune system.

T-Cell Development in the Thymus

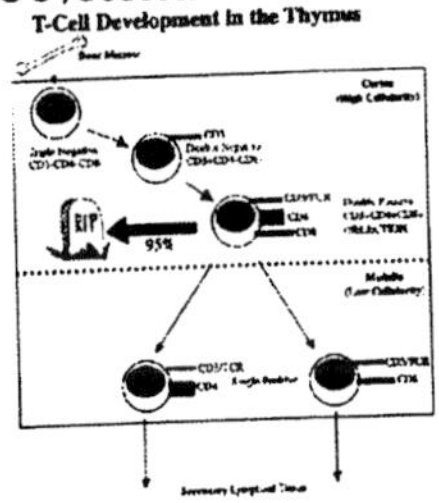

- **T lymphocyte proliferation assay**

measures the strength of response of t memory cells (a subgroup of T lymphocytes) to HIV..

- **t suppressor (ts) cells**

T lymphocytes that specifically suppress immune responses, often CD8+ T lymphocytes.

- **tandem repeat**

repetitive core sequence located in regions between human genes; probes that bind to tandem repeats are used in DNA fingerprinting.

- **tape worm**

(or cestode) helminth that is often parasitic and causes disease.

- **taq polymerase**

heat stable DNA polymerase of the thermophilic bacterium, *Thermus aquaticus*.

- **target DNA**

in the PCR procedure, the region to be amplified.

- **tat**

one of the regulatory genes of the HIV virus. Three HIV regulatory genes tat, rev and nef and three so called auxiliary genes vif, vpr and vpu contain information necessary for the production of proteins that control the virus's ability to infect a cell, produce new copies of the virus or cause disease. The tat gene is thought to enhance virus replication.

- **tautomeric shift**

movement of H atoms from one site on a nitrogenous base to another on DNA, alters the hydrogen bonding properties and therefore, may result in mutations.

■ **taxa**
groups into which organisms are classified.

■ **taxon (pl. taxa)**
a group into which related organisms are classified.

■ **taxonomy**
study of scientific classification and nomenclature.

■ **T cell dependent antigens**
proteins and other antigens that require the cooperation of CD4 Th2 and B cells for the production of antibodies.

■ **T cell independent antigens**
antigens that can stimulate the production of igm antibody without the aid of Th cells

■ **T DNA**
portion of the ti plasmid of *agrobacterium tumefaciens* that is typically transferred into a plant cell.

■ **teichoic acids**
all wall, membrane, or capsular polymers containing glycerophosphate or ribitol phosphate residues.

■ **teleomorph**
sexual stage in reproduction in which cells are formed by the process of meiosis and genetic recombination.

■ **temperate phage**
bacteriophage that can either become integrated into the host cell DNA as a prophage or replicate outside the host chromosome leading to cell lysis.

■ **temperate virus**
virus which upon infection of a host does not necessarily cause lysis but whose genome may replicate in synchrony with that of the host.

■ **template**
a gauge, pattern or mould used as a guide to the form of the piece being made. In biology, a molecule (such as DNA) that serves as a pattern for the generation of another macromolecule (e.g., messenger RNA).

■ **teratogenicity**
the production of physical defects in offspring in utero (i.e., causing birth defects).

■ **terminal electron acceptor**
chemical that is ultimately reduced as a consequence of chemotrophic metabolism.

■ **tertiary structure**
level of structure of a protein

described by its three dimensional nature. Two major shapes exist, globular and fibrous.

■ **test**
hard external covering or shell.

■ **test of significance**
the evaluation of observed data by calculating a specified test statistic and then deriving the associated p value

■ **test treatment**
the drug, device, or procedure to be evaluated in a particular trial.

■ **tetracyclines**
group of antimicrobial medications that interfere with protein synthesis.

■ **th1 cells**
CD4 T lymphocytes called inflammatory T cells because they produce cytokines that drive the development of cytotoxic T cells and that activate macrophages.

■ **TH1/TH2 cells**
subsets of T helper lymphocytes, involved in cell mediated immune responses. Th1 cells secrete il 1 and gamma interferon, which enhance cell mediated responses and inhibit both TH2 subset cell activity and the humeral immune responses. TH2 cells, the other subset of T helper cells, are also involved in cell mediated immune responses. TH2 cell activity and secretions are thought to inhibit cell mediated responses and to enhance the humeral response. TH2 cells secrete IL 4 and IL 10.

■ **TH2 cells**
CS4T lymphocytes that produce cytokines that stimulate B cells to produce antibodies.

■ **thallus**
vegetative body that is not differentiated into tissue systems or organs.

■ **therapeutic HIV vaccine**
vaccine designed to boost the immune response to HIV in persons already infected with the virus.

■ **therapeutic index**
ratio of minimum toxic dose to minimum effective dose of a medication.

■ **therapeutic trial**
trial designed to test the safety and efficacy of a particular drug, device, or procedure that is considered to have therapeutic value.

■ **thermal death time**
shortest period of time needed to kill all the organisms in a microbial population at a specific temperature and under defined conditions.

■ **thermophile**
organism whose optimum temperature for growth is between 45 and 85°c.

■ **thrombocytopenia**
decreased number of blood platelets (cells important for blood clotting).

■ **thrush**
infection of the mouth by *candida albicans.*

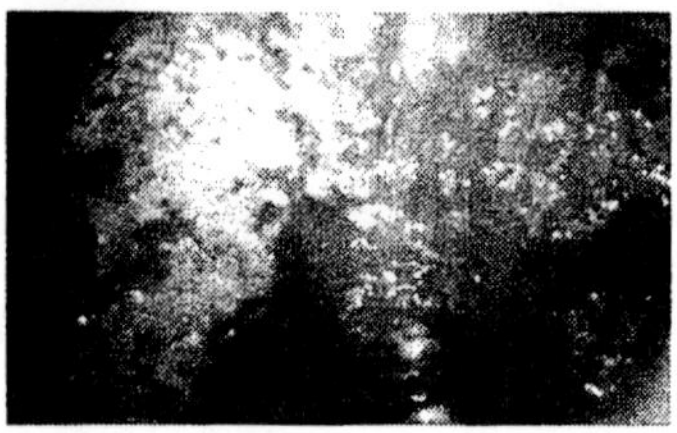

■ **thylakoids**
membrane bound disc like structures within the stroma of chloroplasts, they contain chlorophyll.

■ **thymine dimer**
two adjacent thymine molecules on the same strand of DNA joined together through covalent bonds.

■ **thymosin**
polypeptide hormone of the thymus that influences the maturation of t cells destined for an active role in cell mediated immunity.

■ **thymus**
primary lymphoid organ located in the upper chest in which t lymphocytes mature.

■ **TI plasmid**
conjugative tumour inducing plasmid present in the bacterium *Agrobacterium tunefaciens* which can transfer genes into plants.

■ **TID**
common abbreviation for 'three times a day'.

■ **time of enrolment**
time point at which a patient (treatment unit) is regarded as having officially entered the trial and after which is regarded as a part of the study population. Operationally, the time point at which the treatment assignment is revealed to clinic staff, or when treatment is initiated when assignments are known in advance of en-

rolment.

■ **time to event**
common manner of evaluating endpoints in clinical trials, time to event not only counts how many participants got a specified event, but how long it took to get it. Time to event allows patients to enrol non simultaneously, and still derive valid conclusions

■ **time window**
permissible time interval for performing a specified baseline or follow up examination.

■ **tissue culture**
culture of plant or animal cells that grows in an enriched medium outside the plant or animal.

■ **tissue**
collection of similar cells acting together to perform a particular function. There are four basic tissues in the body epithelial, connective, muscle and nerve.

■ **titer ('titre')**
laboratory measurement of the amount (or concentration) of a given component in solution.

■ **topical**
applied to the skin or other external area.

■ **topsoil**
layer of soil moved in cultivation.

■ **torulopsis glabrata**
fungal infection similar to *candida albicans*, but less susceptible to many of the treatments used for candida

■ **total parental nutrition (TPN)**
type of nutritional feeding that delivers all nutrients in liquid form through a plastic tube into a vein.

■ **toxemia**
circulation of toxins in the blood stream.

■ **toxicity**
the extent, quality or degree of being poisonous or harmful to the body.

■ **toxin**
harmful or poisonous agent.

■ **toxoid**
modified form of a toxin that is no longer toxic but is able to stimulate the production of antibodies that will neutralise the toxin.

■ **toxoplasmosis**
life threatening opportunistic

infection caused by a microscopic parasite (*toxoplasma gondii*) found in raw or undercooked meat and cat faeces. Symptoms may be so mild as to be barely noticeable or may be more severe with headache, lymphadenopathy, malaise, muscle pain, fever and dementia. Toxoplasmosis may lead to brain swelling, coma and death in people with suppressed immune systems.

■ **trace elements**

elements that are required in very minute amounts by all cells, they include cobalt, zinc, copper, molybdenum and manganese.

■ **trace gas**

gas other than nitrogen and oxygen in the atmosphere, particularly those gases that are active in the chemistry or radiation balance of the atmosphere.

■ **trachoma**

potentially serious chronic eye disease caused by certain strains of *chlamydia trachomatis*.

■ **transaminase**

liver enzyme. A laboratory test that measures transaminase levels is used to assess the health of the liver.

■ **transamination**

transfer of an amino group from an amino acid to another organic compound; converts the recipient compound to an amino acid.

■ **transcapsidation or phenotypic mixing**

exchange of protein coats in viral assembly when two virions infect the same cell.

■ **transcript**

fragment of RNA, synthesised using one of the two strands of DNA as a template.

■ **transcription**

process of transferring genetic information coded in DNA into messenger RNA (MRNA).

■ **transcutaneous**

the passage of substances through unbroken skin, as in absorption.

■ **transduction**

transfer of host genetic information via a virus or bacteriophage particle.

■ **transfer factor**

a fraction of white blood cells

that apparently 'transfers' capability to mount an immune response to a specific antigen.

■ **transfer RNA (TRNA)**
type of RNA that delivers the appropriate amino acid to the ribosome during translation.

■ **transformation**
transfer of genetic information into living cells as free DNA.

■ **transformed cells**
containing inheritable changes in bacterial or animal cells.

■ **transfusion reaction**
reaction characterised by fever, low blood pressure, pain, nausea, and vomiting, resulting from the transfusion of immunologically incompatible blood.

■ **transfusion**
process of transfusing fluid (such as blood) into a vein.

■ **transgenic**
plants and animals into which new DNA has been introduced.

■ **transient**
short lived, passing, not permanent.

■ **transition step**
step in metabolism that links glycolysis to the TCA cycle, converts pyruvate to acetyl COA.

■ **translation**
process by which genetic information in the messenger RNA directs the order of amino acids in protein.

■ **translocation**
advancement of a ribosome a distance of one codon during translation.

■ **transmissible spongiform encephalopathies**
group of fatal neuro-degenerative diseases of humans and animals in which brain tissue develops sponge like holes.

■ **transmission electron microscope (TEM)**
type of microscope that directs a beam of electrons at a specimen, used to observe fine details of cell structure.

■ **transmission**
in the context of HIV disease HIV is spread most commonly by sexual contact with an infected partner. The virus can enter the body through the mucosal lining of the vagina, vulva, penis, rectum or, very rarely, the mouth during sex. The likelihood of transmission is increased by factors that may

damage these linings, especially other sexually transmitted diseases that cause ulcers or inflammation. Studies of SIV infection of the genital membranes of nonhuman primates suggest that the sentinel cells known as mucosal dendritic cells may be the first cells infected. Infected dendritic cells may migrate to lymph nodes and infect other cells. HIV also is spread through contact with infected blood, most often by the sharing of drug needles or syringes contaminated with minute quantities of blood containing the virus. Children can contract HIV from their infected mothers either during pregnancy or birth, or postnatally, via breastfeeding. Current research indicates that the AIDS virus may be 100 to 1000 times more contagious during the first two months of infection, when routine aids tests are unable to tell whether people are infected.

■ **transport protein**
type of protein found in cell membranes that functions in the transport of certain compounds across the membrane, may be called a permease or a carrier.

■ **transposable element**
genetic element that can to move (transpose) from one site on a chromosome to another.

■ **transposition**
movement of a piece of DNA from one site in a molecule to another site in the same cell.

■ **transposon**
transposable element of which, in addition to genes involved in transposition, carries other genes; often confers selectable phenotypes such as antibiotic resistance.

■ **transposon mutagenesis**
insertion of a transposon into a gene, this inactivates the host gene leading to a mutant phenotype and also confers the phenotype associated with the transposon gene.

■ **treatment**
act of treating, as in caring for a patient.

■ **treatment allocation**
process of assigning patients to treatment

■ **treatment allocation design**
plan for assigning patients to treatment.

treatment arm
term sometimes used in place of study treatment, or study group, especially in aids and cancer trials.

treatment assignment
treatment to be administered to a patient, but may also mean treatment assigned to some other larger unit such as all members of a family or members of a hospital ward as indicated in the treatment allocation schedule.

treatment assignment probability
probability associated with a specified treatment assignment. The value is fixed over the course of patient enrolment in trials with fixed allocation designs. It changes in trials using adaptive allocation designs.

treatment block
block consisting of a pre-specified number of patients, all enrolled in reasonably close proximity to one another and assigned to the various study treatments in such a way so as to satisfy a preset allocation ratio.

treatment block size
number of allocations required for a specified treatment block. For example, a random allocation schedule for a trial involving two treatments constructed using blocks of size 8 and an allocation ratio of 1:1, would require constraints on the assignment process such that the specified allocation ratio is satisfied after every eighth assignment.

treatment comparison
any comparison involving two or more of the study treatment groups for a designated outcome or follow up variable.

treatment compliance
degree to which a patient follows his assigned treatment regimen.

treatment crossover
change of treatment for a patient in a clinical trial involving a switch of study treatments. The switch may be planned, as in a crossover trial, or may be unplanned, as in the case of a noncrossover trial in which a patient assigned to one treatment is exposed to one of the other study treatments sometime dur-

ing the trial. Unplanned cross-overs are called 'drop out' and 'drop in'.

■ **treatment difference**
difference observed between the test and control treated groups of patients for some specified outcome measure.

■ **treatment effect**
effect attributed to the test treatment. Usually in clinical trials inferred from a comparison of the test and control treated groups of patients using observed results for a specified outcome measure

■ **treatment failure**
refers to individuals who fail to improve even after a course of chemotherapy is begun, as well as to individuals whose disease worsens after having initially improved.

■ **treatment group**
group of patients assigned to receive a specified treatment.

■ **treatment ind**
program to provide experimental treatments to a class of patients lacking satisfactory alternative treatment.

■ **treatment interaction**
situation in which the effect exerted by a treatment is influenced by the level, or presence or absence, of some other factor or condition not related to treatment (e.g., one would say there is a treatment sex interaction if the test control treatment difference is in one direction for males and in the other direction, or is of a different order of magnitude, for females).

■ **treatment lag**
time required, or presumed to be required, for a treatment to exert its full effect.

■ **treatment protocol**
document that describes the treatment procedures used in a clinical trial.

■ **treatment side effect**
by product of treatment, either expected or unexpected, desired or undesired.

■ **treatment trial**
trial in which the test treatment consists of a procedure used for treatment of a specific disease or health condition. Therapeutic trial.

■ **trematodes**
flatworms known as flukes.

■ **tricarboxylic acid cycle (TC)**
metabolic pathway that incorporates acetyl COA, ultimately generating CO_2 and reducing power, also called the Krebs cycle and the citric acid cycle.

■ **trichome**
row of cells which have remained attached to one another following successive cell divisions. Trichomes are formed by many cyanobacteria and by species of *beggiatoa*.

■ **trickling filter method**
treatment method for small sewage plants in which a rotating arm of the filter sprays sewage onto a bed of rocks coated with a bio-film of organisms that aerobically degrades the wastes.

■ **triglyceride**
molecule consisting of three molecules of the same or different fatty acids bonded to glycerol.

■ **trimethoprim**
antimicrobial medication that interferes with folic acid synthesis.

■ **trimethoprim sulfamethoxazole**
combination of two antibiotics that is the preferred treatment for the prophylaxis and treatment of PCP. Active against a wide range of other organisms, possibly including *toxoplasma gondii*. Generally administered intravenously or (less often) orally for treatment of PCP, and orally for prophylaxis

■ **trimetrexate**
drug used for 'salvage' therapy of *pneumocystis carinii* pneumonia, when other treatments have failed. Trimetrexate is enormously toxic unless administered with leucovorin, which 'rescues' human cells from it's effects.

■ **triple blinded**
sometimes used in a jocular fashion to characterise a situation in which neither the patient, physician, nor statistician knows how the trial is designed or operated.

■ **triple blinded clinical trial**
double blinded clinical trial in which data analyses done for treatment monitoring are presented to the individual or group responsible for such monitoring in a way that con-

ceals the identity of the treatment groups.

- **t-RNA**
transfer RNA

- **trophic level**
describes the residence of nutrients in various organisms along a food chain ranging from the primary nutrient assimilating autotrophs to the predatory carnivorous animals.

- **trophozoite**
vegetative feeding form of some protozoa.

- **Trp operon**
operon that encodes the five enzymes of the pathway for tryptophan biosynthesis.

- **tubercle**
granuloma formed in tuberculosis.

- **tuberculosis (TB)**
bacterial infection caused by mycobacterium tuberculosis. TB bacteria are spread by airborne droplets expelled from the lungs when a person with active TB coughs, sneezes or speaks. Repeated exposure to these droplets can lead to infection in the air sacs of the lungs. The immune defences of healthy people usually prevent TB infection from spreading beyond a very small area of the lungs. If the body's immune system is impaired because of infection with HIV, aging, malnutrition or other factors, the TB bacterium may begin to spread more widely in the lungs or to other tissues.

- **tumble**
rolling motion of a motile cell that is caused by an abrupt change in the direction of rotation of flagella.

- **tumour necrosis factor**
macrophage produced cytokine that helps activate t cells. It is also thought to upregulate HIV replication, and may contribute to the pathogenesis of wasting.

- **tumor inducing (Ti) plasmid**
plasmid of *Agrobacterium tumefaciens* that enables the organism to cause tumors in plants. A derivative of the plasmid is used a vector by scientists to introduce DNA into plants. Also called the Ti plasmid.

■ **turbidity**
cloudiness, the turbidity of a bacterial suspension is proportional to the number of cells in that suspension.

■ **two tailed alternative hypothesis**
an alternative to the null hypothesis that specifies a range of permissible values that are symmetrically distributed about the null value.

■ **two tailed test (statistics)**
a statistical test of significance based on the null value of no difference versus the set of all alternative values (i.e., those that lie to the right and left of the null value).

■ **Tx**
common abbreviation for 'treatment'.

■ **tyndallisation**
repeated cycles of heating and incubation to kill spore forming bacteria.

■ **type I error (alpha error)**
deciding to reject the null hypothesis when the null hypothesis is in fact true. The investigator determines that there is something going on when in fact there is not.

■ **type II error (beta error)**
failing to reject the null hypothesis when the alternative hypothesis is in fact true. The investigator determines that there is nothing going on when in fact there is.

■ **ubiquitous**
present everywhere, common and prevalent

■ **ubiquity**
widespread prevalence.

■ **UHT**
abbreviation for ultra high temperature pasteurisation.

■ **ultraviolet light (UV)**
electromagnetic radiation with wavelengths between 175 and 350 nm, invisible.

■ **unblind**
to reveal the treatment assignment of an individual patient or group of patients to an individual or group of individuals associated with the trial (e.g., patients, study physicians, treatment effects monitoring committee) who have heretofore been denied this information.

■ **uncontrolled clinical trial**
clinical trial that does not involve a control treatment. Any study that does not have a control group made up of patients treated and followed over the same time period as those in a treated group.

■ **uniform treatment allocation**
scheme in which the assignment probability of any one treatment group is the same as for every other treatment group in a trial.

■ **uniporters**
transport systems that translocate a single molecule or ion.

■ **unsaturated**
refers to a fatty acid with one or more double bonds.

■ **upper limit of normal**
top of the normal range for a particular laboratory helps assure between lab comparability.

■ **upstream**
direction toward the 5' end of either an RNA molecule or the analogous (+) strand of DNA.

■ **uronic acid**
class of acidic compounds of the general formula HOOC $(CHOH)_n$ CHO that contain both carboxylic and aldehydic groups, are oxidation products of sugars, and occur in many polysaccharides; especially in the hemicelluloses.

■ **urticaria**
allergic skin reaction characterised by the formation of itchy red swellings.

■ **uterus**
hollow muscular organ located in the pelvic cavity of female mammals in which the fertilised egg implants and develops. Also called womb.

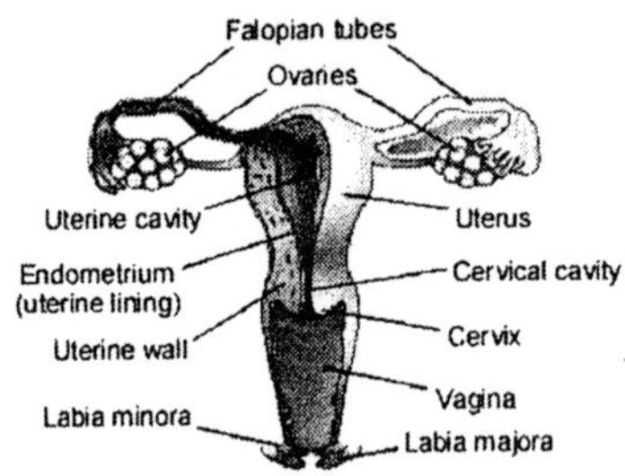

■ **V3 loop**
section of the gp120 protein on the surface of HIV. Appears to be important in stimulating neutralising antibodies.

■ **vaccination**
the act of administering a vaccine.

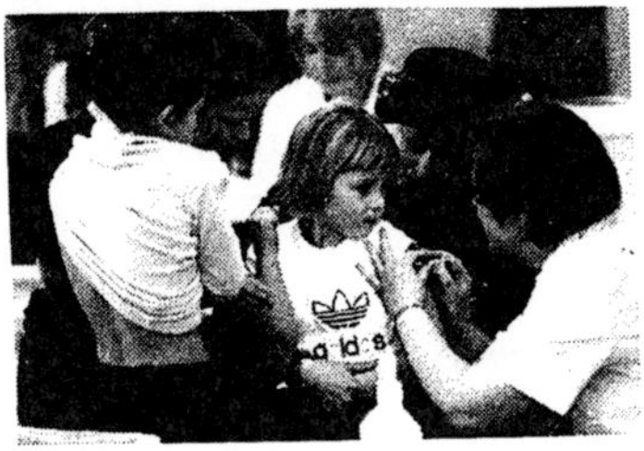

■ **vaccine**

preparation of living or dead micro-organisms or viruses or their components used to immunise a person or animal against a particular disease.

■ **vaccinia**

cowpox virus, formerly used in human smallpox vaccines. Employed as a vector in HIV vaccine research to transport HIV genes into the body.

■ **vadose zone**

unsaturated zone of soil above the groundwater, extending from the bottom of the capillary fringe all the way to the soil surface.

■ **vancomycin**

antimicrobial medication that interferes with peptidoglycan synthesis.

■ **variability (range)**

a measure of variability which describes the distribution as the difference between the largest and smallest values.

■ **variability (standard deviation (SD)**

measure of variability which describes the average distance of the observations from their mean. For example in a normal distribution, +1 SD from the mean includes 68% of the observations; +2 SD from the mean includes 95% of the observations; +3 SD from the mean includes 99.7% of the observations.

■ **variability, standard error of the mean (SEM)**

a measure of variability which describes the accuracy of the sample mean as an estimate of the population mean. SEM = SD /square root of the sample size.

■ **variable**

in this book, any trait, characteristic, test, measurement, or assessment that is recorded, or scheduled to be recorded, on patients enrolled, or to be enrolled, in a clinical trial.

■ **variable region**

the part of an antibody's structure that differs from one antibody to another.

■ **variable (continuous)**
continuous variables can assume all possible values along a continuum within a specified range, e.g., height, weight, blood pressure, cd4.

■ **variable (dependent)**
variable which has a value that is dependent upon the effect of one or more other independent variables. For example, diastolic blood pressure (dependent variable) can be dependent upon the effect of obesity (independent variable.)

■ **variable (discrete categorical)**
discrete variables have values that fall into a limited number of separate categories, e.g., gender (male/female), survival status (alive/dead), exposure status (exposed/nonexposed), blood type (A/B/AB/O.)

■ **variable (independent)**
variable which influences the value of the dependent variable. For example, obesity (independent variable) can influence the level of diastolic blood pressure (dependent variable).

■ **variable (quantile)**
measure of variability which divides the distribution into equal, ordered subgroups. For example, terciles are thirds, quartiles are quarters, and quintiles are fifths.

■ **variance**
degree to which a set of quantities vary a measure of the spread of scores in a distribution of scores, that is, a measure of dispersion. The larger the variance, the further the individual cases are from the mean. The smaller the variance, the closer the individual score are to the mean. Specifically, the population variance is the mean of the sum of the squared deviations from the mean score. The sample variance is computed by dividing the sum of squared deviations by the number in the sample minus 1. The standard deviation is the square root of the variance.

■ **variant**
variation of a particular strain of virus or infective agent; slightly different in form or function.

■ **varicella zoster virus (VZV)**
a virus in the herpes family that causes chickenpox during childhood and may reactivate later in life to cause herpes

zoster (shingles) in immunosuppressed individuals.

- **varix**
  painfully enlarge blood vessel, plural is varices
- **vector**
  anything capable of moving or transferring genetic material.
- **vegetative cell**
  typical, actively multiplying cell.
- **vehicle**
  inanimate carrier of an infectious agent from one host to another.
- **verification**
  process that is carried out to verify an item of information.
- **verify**
  to confirm or substantiate an item of information recorded in a data file or keyed for entry into the analysis database.
- **vertical evolution**
  acquisition of antimicrobial resistance through spontaneous mutation.
- **vertical transmission**
  transmission of HIV from mother to foetus.
- **vesicles**
  spherical structures, formed intracellularly, by some arbuscular mycorrhizal fungi.
- **viable**
  alive, able to reproduce.
- **viable but nonculturable**
  organisms that are alive but cannot be cultured on laboratory media.
- **viable count**
  measurement of the concentration of live cells in a microbial population.
- **vibrio (plural vibrios)**
  short, curved rod shaped bacterial cell.
- **villus (pl. Villi)**
  narrow protrusion from a membrane such as the intestinal lining.
- **viral burden/load**
  concentration of a virus in the body.
- **viral core**
  typically a virus contains an RNA (ribonucleic acid) or DNA (deoxyribonucleic acid) core of genetic material surrounded by a protein coat.
- **viral culture**
  laboratory method for growing viruses.

■ **viral envelope**
as related to HIV. It is spherical in shape with a diameter of 1/10,000 of a millimetre. The outer coat, or envelope, is composed of two layers of fat like molecules called lipids, taken from the membranes of human cells. Embedded in the envelope are numerous cellular proteins, as well as mushroom shaped HIV proteins that protrude from the surface. Each mushroom is thought to consist of a cap made of four glycoprotein molecules called gp120, and a stem consisting of four gp41 molecules embedded in the envelope. The virus uses these proteins to attach to and infect cells.

■ **viremia**
presence of virus in the blood.

■ **virion**
virus particle existing freely outside a host cell.

■ **viroid**
very exotic type of virus like particle that only infects plant cells and consists of a group of membrane less circular RNA's that neither code for nor contain any structural protein. They replicate without other viruses being present.

■ **viroid piece of RN**
that does not have a protein coat but does replicate within living cells.

■ **virology**
study of viruses and viral disease.

■ **virucide**
any agent that destroys or inactivates a virus.

■ **virulence**
degree of pathogenicity of a parasite.

■ **virus**
group of infectious agents characterised by their inability to reproduce outside of a living host cell. Viruses may subvert the host cells' normal functions, causing the cell to behave in a manner determined by the virus.

■ **visceral**
pertaining to the major internal organs.

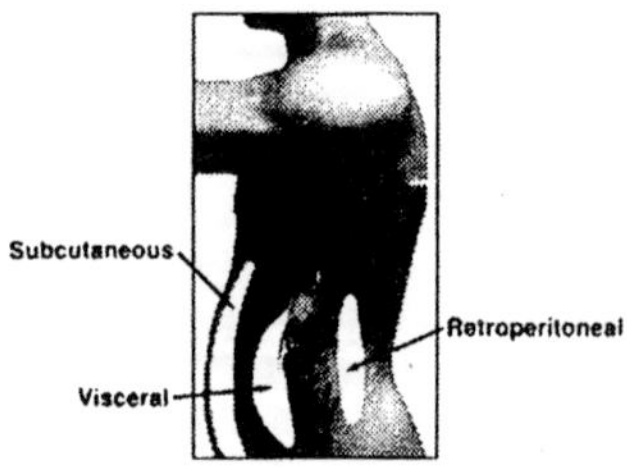

■ **visit driven data**
data such as laboratory mea-

surements or screening data that is collected on a fixed schedule.

■ **vitamin**
one of a group of organic compounds found in small quantities in natural foodstuffs that are necessary for the growth and reproduction of an organism; usually converted into coenzymes.

■ **vitreous humour**
gel like substance that fills the eyeball.

■ **volutin**
storage form of phosphate found inside certain bacterial cells. Because granules of volutin exhibit characteristic staining with the dye methylene blue, they are called metachromatic granules.

■ **wasting syndrome**
condition among HIV infected individuals characterised by involuntary weight loss of more than 10% of baseline body weight. Other symptoms may include chronic diarrhoea or chronic weakness and fever for more than 30 days, a CDC aids defining condition.

■ **water activity (AW)**
quantitative measure of the water available.

■ **water content**
water contained in a material expressed as the mass of water per unit mass of oven dry material.

■ **water moulds**
non photosynthetic members of the heterokons, similar to the fungi but not related genetically.

■ **water retention curve**
graph showing soil water content as a function of increasingly negative soil water potential.

■ **weathering**
all physical and chemical changes produced in rock by atmospheric agents.

■ **western blot**
laboratory test of blood for specific antibodies; more accurate than the elisa test, the western blot is used as a confirmatory test if an HIV elisa test is positive.

■ **whey**
liquid portion that remains after milk proteins coagulate during cheese making.

■ **white rot fungus**
fungus that attacks lignin, along with cellulose, and hemi cellu-

lose, leading to a marked lightening of the infected wood.

■ **woronin body**
spherical structure associated with the simple pore in the septa separating hyphal compartments of fungi in the phylum Ascomycota.

■ **xenobiotic**
compound foreign to biological systems. Often refers to human made compounds that are resistant or recalcitrant to biodegradation and decomposition.

■ **xerophile**
organism adapted to grow at low water potential, i.e., very dry habitats.

■ **yeast**
unicellular fungus.

■ **Yeast Artificial Chromosome(YAC)**
vector that can be used to clone segments of DNA up to a million nucleotides in length and used to introduce foreign DNA into the yeast *saccharomyces cerevisiae.*

■ **Z value**
increase in temperature required to reduce the decimal reduction time to one tenth of its initial value.

■ **Zerit**
brand name for stavudine.

■ **zithromax**
brand name for azithromycin

■ **zooplankton**
floating and swimming small animals and protozoa found in marine environments, usually in association with the phytoplankton.

■ **zoospore**
asexual spore formed by some fungi that usually can move in an aqueous environment via one or more flagella.

■ **zovirax**
brand name for acyclovir.

■ **zygospore**
thick walled resting spore resulting from fusion of two gametangia of fungi in the phylum zygomycota.

■ **zygote**
diploid cell formed by the sexual fusion of two haploid cells.

■ **zymogenous flora**
refers to micro-organisms, often transient or alien, that respond rapidly by enzyme production and growth when simple organic substrates become available. Also called copiotrophs.